Hemostasis and Coagulation

Guest Editor

HENRY M. RINDER, MD

CLINICS IN LABORATORY MEDICINE

www.labmed.theclinics.com

Consulting Editor
ALAN WELLS, MD, DMSc

June 2009 • Volume 29 • Number 2

SAUNDERS an imprint of ELSEVIER, Inc.

W.B. SAUNDERS COMPANY
A Division of Elsevier Inc.

1600 John F. Kennedy Boulevard ● Suite 1800 ● Philadelphia, Pennsylvania 19103-2899

http://www.theclinics.com

CLINICS IN LABORATORY MEDICINE Volume 29, Number 2

June 2009 ISSN 0272-2712, ISBN-13: 978-1-4377-1234-6, ISBN-10: 1-4377-1234-7

Editor: Katie Hartner
Developmental Editor: Donald Mumford

Reprints. For copies of 100 or more, of articles in this publication, please contact the Commercial Reprints Department, Elsevier Inc., 360 Park Avenue South, New York, New York 10010-1710. Tel. (212) 633-3813, Fax: (212) 462-1935, E-mail: reprints@elsevier.com.

Clinics in Laboratory Medicine (ISSN 0272-2712) is published quarterly by Elsevier Inc., 360 Park Avenue South, New York, NY 10010-1710. Months of issue are March, June, September, and December. Business and Editorial offices: 1600 John F. Kennedy Blvd., Suite 1800, Philadelphia, PA 19103-2899. Customer Service Office: 6277 Sea Harbor Drive, Orlando, FL 32887-4800. Periodicals postage paid at New York, NY and additional mailing offices. Subscription prices are $204.00 per year (US individuals), $321.00 per year (US institutions), $106.00 (US students), $234.00 per year (Canadian individuals), $405.00 per year (foreign institutions), $145.00 (foreign students). Foreign air speed delivery is included in all *Clinics* subscription prices. All prices are subject to change without notice. POSTMASTER: Send address changes to *Clinics in Laboratory Medicine*, Elsevier Periodicals Customer Service 11830 Westline Industrial Drive St. Louis, MO63146. **Customer Service: 1-800-654-2452 (US). From outside of the US, call 1-314-453-7041. Fax: 1-314-453-5170. E-mail: journalscustomerservice-usa@ elsevier.com (for print support) or journalsonlinesupport-usa@elsevier.com (for online support).**

Clinics in Laboratory Medicine is covered in *EMBASE/Exerpta Medica, MEDLINE/PubMed (Index Medicus), Cinahl, Current Contents/Clinical Medicine, BIOSIS* and *ISI/BIOMED.*

Printed and bound by CPI Group (UK) Ltd, Croydon, CR0 4YY
Transferred to Digital Print 2011

Contributors

GUEST EDITOR

HENRY M. RINDER, MD
Professor, Department of Laboratory Medicine, Yale University School of Medicine, New Haven, Connecticut

AUTHORS

ALICE CHEN, MD, PhD
Director of Molecular Laboratory; Associate Director of Blood Donor Center, Department of Pathology, St. Luke's Episcopal Hospital; and Adjunct Assistant Professor of Pathology, Baylor College of Medicine, Houston, Texas

KENDALL P. CROOKSTON, MD, PhD, FCAP
Department of Pathology, University of New Mexico, Albuquerque; TriCore Reference Laboratories; and United Blood Services of New Mexico, Albuquerque, New Mexico

CHARLES EBY, MD
Associate Professor, Department of Pathology and Immunology, Washington University School of Medicine, St. Louis, Missouri

YURI FEDORIW, MD
Assistant Professor, Departments of Pathology and Laboratory Medicine, University of North Carolina, Chapel Hill, North Carolina

BERNARD KHOR, MD, PhD
Director, Coagulation Laboratory; and Associate Professor, Harvard Medical School, Boston, Massachusetts

NANCY KRIZ, BS
Department of Laboratory Medicine, Yale-New Haven Hospital, Coagulation Laboratory Supervisor, New Haven, Connecticut

MARISA B. MARQUES, MD
Professor of Pathology, Division of Laboratory Medicine, Department of Pathology, University of Alabama at Birmingham, Birmingham, Alabama

PRASAD MATHEW, MD, FAAP
Department of Pediatrics and Ted R. Montoya Hemophilia Treatment Program, University of New Mexico, Albuquerque, New Mexico

VALERIE L. NG, PhD, MD
Professor Emeritus, Department of Laboratory Medicine, School of Medicine, University of California San Francisco; and Chairman, Department of Laboratory Medicine & Pathology, Alameda County Medical Center, Oakland, California

MARIE E. PEDDINGHAUS, MD
Department of Laboratory Medicine, Yale University School of Medicine, New Haven, Connecticut

PETER L. PERROTTA, MD
Associate Professor, Department of Pathology, West Virginia University Health Sciences Center; and Clinical Laboratories, West Virginia University Hospital, Morgantown, West Virginia

CHRISTINE S. RINDER, MD
Associate Professor, Yale University School of Medicine, New Haven, Connecticut

HENRY M. RINDER, MD
Professor, Department of Laboratory Medicine, Yale University School of Medicine, New Haven, Connecticut

ANNIKA M. SVENSSON, MD, PhD
Visiting Instructor, Department of Pathology, University of Utah, Salt Lake City; and ARUP Laboratories, Salt Lake City, Utah

JUN TERUYA, MD, DSc
Director, Center of Transfusion Medicine and Coagulation, Texas Children's Hospital; and Professor and Associate Chairman of Clinical Pathology, Baylor College of Medicine, Houston, Texas

CHRISTOPHER A. TORMEY, MD
Instructor in Laboratory Medicine, Department of Laboratory Medicine, Yale University School of Medicine, New Haven; and Pathology and Laboratory Medicine Service, VA Connecticut Healthcare System, West Haven, Connecticut

RICHARD TORRES, MD, MS
Associate Research Scientist, Department of Laboratory Medicine, Yale School of Medicine; and Department of Biomedical Engineering, Yale University, New Haven, Connecticut

KELLY T. TOWNSEND, BS, MT(ASCP) SH
Department of Pathology, University of New Mexico, Albuquerque; and TriCore Reference Laboratories, Albuquerque, New Mexico

ELIZABETH M. VAN COTT, MD
Chief Resident, Department of Pathology, Massachusetts General Hospital, Harvard Medical School, Boston, Massachusetts

BENJAMIN L. WAGENMAN, MD
Department of Pathology, University of New Mexico, Albuquerque; TriCore Reference Laboratories; and United Blood Services of New Mexico, Albuquerque, New Mexico

Contents

This article briefly details the physiologic and interdependent mechanisms of vascular hemostasis, with an eye toward how the laboratory can assist in diagnosing and maintaining the balance of procoagulant and anticoagulant functions. These functions include determining characteristics of the blood vessel wall, platelet components and receptor-ligand interactions critical for hemostasis, the regulation of thrombin generation and its effects, and the complex fibrinolytic pathways that complete the coagulation cascade.

Platelet-related bleeding is a pervasive and potentially life-threatening problem that can arise in both acute and chronic clinical settings. A growing number of laboratory assays have been developed to rapidly assess underlying platelet dysfunction in the bleeding patient. This article: (1) provides an overview of the current methods of platelet function testing, with a particular emphasis on recently developed "point-of-care" tests, (2) reviews evidencebased transfusion "triggers" and provides an update on new developments in platelet component therapy, and (3) outlines those initial studies that have demonstrated how point-of-care platelet function testing has helped lead to the development of targeted transfusion strategies for the acutely bleeding patient.

The heterogeneity of von Willebrand disease reflects the varied roles of von Willebrand factor in coagulation. Significant challenges remain in the detection, classification, and determination of bleeding risk in disorders related to von Willebrand factor. A clearer understanding of the specific disease mechanisms is essential to the development of improved methods for prognosis and management in this and other conditions with abnormalities of the von Willebrand factor system.

> The antiphospholipid syndrome (APS) is an autoimmune disorder presenting with tissue injury in various organs attributed to large or small vessel thrombosis or, in some instances, possible nonthrombotic inflammatory mechanisms, associated with in vitro evidence of antibodies to certain proteins, or proteinphospholipid complexes. Although the pathophysiology, diagnosis, and management of APS may seem clear and straightforward from a distance, closer inspection reveals a more complex, incomplete, and uncertain image. This article reviews the evolution of APS from the first description of lupus anticoagulant to the current criteria used to guide clinical research, critiques laboratory methods used to identify autoantibodies, comments on prognosis and management, and summarizes insights into the pathophysiology of this elusive disorder.

> Much has been learned about thrombotic thrombocytopenic purpura (TTP) and heparin-induced thrombocytopenia (HIT) and much remains a diagnostic and management challenge. While the pentad of thrombocytopenia, microangiopathic hemolytic anemia, fever, and renal and neurologic abnormalities characterize the clinical presentation of TTP, few patients present with all signs and symptoms. Worse yet, the pentad and its components are seen in other so-called thrombotic microangiopathies that demand different treatment approaches. HIT is another systemic disorder presenting with thrombocytopenia and/or thrombosis with potential devastating consequences whose diagnosis is difficult and management is still evolving. Highlights of the conditions and clinical and laboratory hints that allow physicians to diagnose TTP and HIT efficiently and offer patients the best available therapeutic interventions are presented.

> This discussion considers several important hypercoagulable states that predispose patients to venous, and in some instances, arterial thrombosis, focusing on activated protein C resistance/factor V Leiden, prothrombin G20210A, deficiencies of protein C, protein S or antithrombin, and antiphospholipid antibodies. The discussion includes the incidence of each hypercoagulable condition, the magnitude of the thrombotic risk it poses and synergistic interactions among the various hypercoagulable conditions. Salient advances in understanding the molecular pathogenesis of each condition are presented and discussed in the context of the interpretation and clinical utility of current laboratory testing and identifying potential targets of future testing. Finally, recommendations for laboratory testing are summarized.

The use of molecular diagnostic techniques in clinical and research hemostasis laboratories is increasing as genetic factors that affect the procoagulant and anticoagulant systems are identified. Many of these molecular alterations are associated with thrombotic tendencies, whereas others tip the hemostatic balance in favor of bleeding. In either scenario, molecular testing may serve as a primary diagnostic modality or may provide information that complements clot-based "functional" assays. The clinical application of DNA-based testing continues to expand since the discoveries of the factor V Leiden and prothrombin G20210A gene mutations. Indications for genetic testing continue to evolve as the underlying causes of hemostatic disorders are better understood. Further development of molecular assays depends on their proved utility in the clinical management and treatment of these complex multifactorial disorders.

Thromboelastography (TEG) as a method of assessing global hemostatic and fibrinolytic function has existed for more than 60 years. Improvements in TEG technology have led to increased reliability and thus increased usage. The TEG has been used primarily in the settings of liver transplant and cardiac surgery, with proven utility for monitoring hemostatic and fibrinolytic derangements. In recent years, indications for TEG testing have expanded to include managing extracorporeal membrane oxygenation (ECMO) therapy, assessing bleeding of unclear etiology, and assessing hypercoagulable states. In addition, TEG platelet mapping has been utilized to monitor antiplatelet therapy. Correlation between TEG platelet mapping and other platelet function tests such as the PFA-100 or platelet aggregation studies, however, has not been evaluated fully for clinical outcomes, and results may not be comparable. In general, the advantages of the TEG include evaluation of global hemostatic function using whole blood, a quick turn-around-time, the possibility of both point-of-care-testing and performance in central laboratories, the ability to detect hyperfibrinolysis, monitoring therapy with recombinant activated factor VII, and detection of low factor XIII activity. Potential applications include polycythemia and dysfibrinogenemia. Disadvantages of TEG include a relatively high coefficient of variation, poorly standardized methodologies, and limitations on specimen stability of native whole blood samples. In the pediatric setting, an additional advantage of the TEG is a relatively small sample volume, but a disadvantage is the difference in normal ranges between infants, especially newborns, and adults. In summary, TEG is an old concept with new applications that may provide a unique perspective on global hemostasis in various clinical settings.

THE CLINICS ARE NOW AVAILABLE ONLINE!

Access your subscription at:
www.theclinics.com

Preface

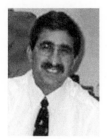

Henry M. Rinder, MD
Guest Editor

Physiologic hemostasis is maintained by a delicate balance of procoagulant and anti-coagulant influences in blood and blood vessels. This physiologic balance is most apparent clinically in small blood vessels, which must simultaneously maintain both liquid blood flow and the structural integrity of the vasculature. Bleeding in larger vessels can be managed operatively, but small-vessel bleeding requires local enhancement of clot formation, while simultaneously preserving organ perfusion. At the other end of the coagulation spectrum is the patient in whom prothrombotic factors predominate, leading to pathologic thrombosis; systemic anticoagulation then seeks to restore this hemostatic balance without unduly increasing bleeding risk. The laboratory plays a major role in guiding therapy that attempts to restore and maintain the optimum hemostatic balance. This brief overview of hemostasis physiology serves as a preface to the focused articles that follow. Readers will note that the articles have some sections in common; this purposefully reflects the redundancy and overlap of coagulation function and physiology. In addition, although this issue is primarily concerned with laboratory diagnosis, the function of the laboratory is inextricably tied to therapy for both bleeding and thrombosis. This aspect of laboratory medicine is not limited to the use of blood products, but is also linked to the critical needs of monitoring. Therefore, several sections of these articles discuss therapeutics, which the editor and authors consider to be well within the purview of laboratory medicine expertise.

Henry M. Rinder, MD
Department of Laboratory Medicine
Yale University School of Medicine
333 Cedar Street
PO Box 208035
New Haven, CT 05620-8035

E-mail address:
henry.rinder@yale.edu

Clin Lab Med 29 (2009) xi
doi:10.1016/j.cll.2009.06.003
0272-2712/09/$ – see front matter © 2009 Published by Elsevier Inc.

labmed.theclinics.com

Physiology of Hemostasis: With Relevance to Current and Future Laboratory Testing

Nancy Kriz, BS[a], Christine S. Rinder, MD[a,b], Henry M. Rinder, MD[a,c],*

KEYWORDS

- Hemostasis • Thrombosis • Hemorrhage • Thrombin
- Fibrinolysis • Blood platelets

Vascular damage triggers the initiation of clotting with the goal of producing a localized platelet-fibrin plug to prevent undue blood loss. This process is accompanied by rapid and sequential processes leading to clot containment, wound healing, clot dissolution, tissue regeneration, and remodeling. In healthy persons, all of these reactions occur continuously and in a balanced fashion such that bleeding is contained, yet blood vessels simultaneously remain patent to deliver adequate organ blood flow. When any of these hemostatic processes are disrupted because of inherited defects or acquired abnormalities, disordered hemostasis may result in either bleeding or thromboembolic complications.

Blood flow in the arterial and venous systems is, to a degree, disparate and imposes different needs on the coagulation system. In the pressurized arteries, relatively minor vascular damage can rapidly result in massive blood loss; the procoagulant response in arteries must rapidly arrest bleeding. Platelets are critical to this arterial response; they initially contain blood loss and then provide an active surface for soluble coagulation factors to localize and accelerate fibrin and—ultimately—clot formation. By contrast, in the venous circulation, the lesser flow rates produce slower bleeding, a feature that makes platelets somewhat less critical. Instead, the balance of venous hemostasis depends most on the rate of thrombin generation. These differences are

[a] Department of Laboratory Medicine, Yale-New Haven Hospital, Yale University School of Medicine, New Haven, CT, USA
[b] Department of Anesthesiology, Yale-New Haven Hospital, Yale University School of Medicine, New Haven, CT, USA
[c] Department of Internal Medicine (Hematology), Yale-New Haven Hospital, Yale University School of Medicine, New Haven, CT, USA
* Corresponding author. Department of Laboratory Medicine, Yale University School of Medicine, New Haven, CT 05620.
E-mail address: henry.rinder@yale.edu (H.M. Rinder).

Clin Lab Med 29 (2009) 159–174
doi:10.1016/j.cll.2009.06.004
labmed.theclinics.com
0272-2712/09/$ – see front matter © 2009 Elsevier Inc. All rights reserved.

further underscored therapeutically by the anticoagulant agents used in these distinct settings (ie, antiplatelet agents such as aspirin and clopidogrel) to prevent coronary and cerebral artery thrombus, compared with interventions that inhibit thrombin, including the heparins and warfarin, for treatment and prophylaxis of venous thromboembolic disease. Although weighted somewhat differently in the arterial and venous systems, the platelet and soluble coagulation systems work together to maintain overall hemostasis and wound healing.

This article briefly details the physiologic and interdependent mechanisms of vascular hemostasis, with an eye toward how the laboratory can assist in diagnosing and maintaining the balance of procoagulant and anticoagulant functions. These functions include determining characteristics of the blood vessel wall, platelet components and receptor-ligand interactions critical for hemostasis, and the complex fibrinolytic pathways that complete the coagulation cascade.

VASCULAR WALL PHYSIOLOGY
Anticoagulant Endothelial Cell Properties

Vascular endothelial cells (EC) exert a tonic anticoagulant activity, which helps to maintain blood fluidity. This activity is partially because of their passive barrier function separating blood from subendothelial collagen and tissue factor, both of which are highly procoagulant moieties. Healthy ECs actively regulate the hemostatic balance in their microenvironment via secreted products (**Table 1**). These products include prostacyclin and nitric oxide, both of which induce vascular smooth muscle relaxation and reduced shear when released in an abluminal direction. When secreted into the blood, they promote platelet cyclic adenosine monophosphate (cAMP) generation, thereby inhibiting platelet activation and aggregation.[1] ECs also secrete ADPase, which degrades platelet-released extracellular ADP, thereby limiting platelet recruitment into the growing platelet clot. Soluble coagulation factors are regulated by EC in a tonic and an inducible fashion. Tissue factor pathway inhibitor (TFPI) in its nascent circulating form blunts initiation of coagulation; early after coagulation activation, TFPI becomes primed for enhanced activity by exposure to small amounts of factor Xa.

Quiescent thrombomodulin and tissue plasminogen activator (t-PA) are localized at the EC extracellular matrix, ready to be activated by local formation of thrombin and fibrin, respectively, to carry out their anticoagulant and fibrinolytic functions. Thrombomodulin's activation by thrombin to subsequently down-regulate thrombin generation via its generation of activated protein C (APC) demonstrates the complex control of the coagulation pathway and even more so, the challenge to the clinical laboratory in

Table 1	
Endothelial cell coagulant properties	
Anticoagulant Properties of EC	**Procoagulant Properties of EC**
Vasodilatation	Vasoconstriction
Prostacyclin	E-selectin
Nitric oxide	P-selectin
ADPase	β1- integrins
Heparin sulfates	β2- integrins
Thrombomodulin	Platelet-EC adhesion molecule
Tissue factor pathway inhibitor	Factor VIII
Tissue plasminogen activator	Fibronectin

monitoring hemostasis. Tissue plasminogen activator (t-PA), produced by ECs, activates the plasminogen incorporated in the fibrin clot to form the serine protease, plasmin.[2] This reaction is kept specific for fibrin clot by the high affinity of plasminogen activator for fibrin. Fibrinolysis is regulated by the circulating plasminogen-activator inhibitor (PAI-1) that counteracts the action of t-PA and the plasmin inhibitors— alpha$_2$-antiplasmin and alpha$_2$-macroglobulin.[3] Thrombin activatable fibrinolysis inhibitor (TAFI) also tends to suppress fibrinolysis by removing carboxy-terminal lysine residues from fibrin to limit plasmin binding to fibrin clot.

Procoagulant Endothelial Cell Properties

When ECs are physically damaged or become activated to secrete their intracellular contents, their balance of coagulant properties shifts to favor a procoagulant state. This function is mediated by the ECs themselves and by the underlying subendothelial matrix that is exposed by vascular injury. Weibel-Palade bodies, granules located inside ECs, are secreted into the extracelluar fluid, releasing procoagulant von Willebrand factor (vWF) multimers and endothelin, which together with t-PA and angiopoietin, are targeted at fibrinolysis and wound remodeling, respectively. Activated ECs (eg, by toxins or secreted factors) express adhesive ligands on their surface, including the selectins (E-selectin and P-selectin), beta$_1$ and beta$_2$ integrins, and platelet-EC adhesion molecule-1 (**Table 1**). On the EC surface, integrins mediate adhesion and subsequent transendothelial migration of leukocytes into the tissues.

Exposed subendothelial matrix binds vWF multimers (**Fig. 1**) and contains other procoagulant, adhesive proteins, including thrombospondin, fibronectin, and collagen. These molecules function as ligands to capture platelets and as activators of adherent platelets. Collagen, in particular, is a platelet ligand and a strong platelet agonist; the latter capability causes platelets to undergo dense granule release and express conformationally active ligands, such as glycoprotein IIb/IIIa (GPIIb/IIIa). Another critical

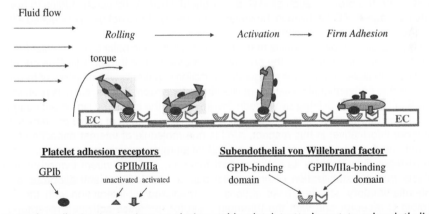

Fig. 1. The adhesive interactions producing stable platelet attachment to subendothelial vWF. The initial attachment between platelet GPIb and its binding domain on vWF is rapid but has a short half-life, and the result is a rolling movement from torque generated by flowing blood. The vWF-GPIb interaction produces transmembrane signaling and platelet activation. Platelets undergo shape change, and the GPIIb/IIIa surface receptor is transformed to an activated conformation capable of binding to its distinct domain on vWF. This secondary binding causes the platelet to firmly adhere to the exposed subendothelial vWF and is the basis of the growing platelet plug. EC, endothelial cell.

procoagulant mediator exposed by EC damage is tissue factor (TF), which is constitutively expressed by subendothelial smooth muscle cells and fibroblasts. TF also can be induced on cells (eg, monocytes), and this procoagulant induction may relate to the pathophysiology of antiphospholipid antibodies. (See the article by Eby on antiphospholipid syndrome, elsewhere in this issue.) As outlined in the section on soluble coagulation, TF is the major initiator of the soluble coagulation system that, with activated platelets, results in the formation of a definitive platelet-fibrin clot.

Testing of Vascular Dysfunction

Static laboratory testing of blood cannot reflect vascular function; in vivo assays that reflect the integrity of the vascular wall have been used in the past. The bleeding time is sensitive to abnormalities of connective tissue and the blood vessels and platelet numbers and function. The bleeding time has fallen out of favor, however, not only because of significant limitations with interobserver variability and poor predictive values but also because screening for platelet disorders has become possible with in vitro "bleeding time" tests such as the platelet function analyzer-100. (See the article by Tormey and colleagues on thrombocytopenia and platelet function, elsewhere in this issue.) The in vivo bleeding time can be prolonged by vascular fragility within the skin, but this finding does not differentiate etiologies (eg, between senile purpura and vitamin C deficiency). Multiple studies also have confirmed that the bleeding time has a poor predictive value for bleeding, especially in the operative setting. Because the physiology of the bleeding time test encompasses platelet and vascular function, it is clear that neither component of hemostasis is adequately evaluated by the bleeding time, at least for risk assessment, which is the main indication for testing. An alternative to the bleeding time—the tourniquet test for vessel fragility—involves the application of a tourniquet to provoke bleeding. This test is similarly limited as to specificity and does not discriminate between platelet dysfunction and a vascular bleeding disorder. Finally, any venous compression with a vasculopathy can cause a severe purpuric reaction and is generally contraindicated. Plasma levels of EC-secreted proteins such as vWF are frequently used in research studies to evaluate the degree of EC activation; however, these assays have not been correlated with diagnostics in the clinical laboratory arena.

It is possible that blood studies that offer a snapshot of the balance of vascular function may yield information on the clinical risk of bleeding or thrombosis. One current drawback in assessing soluble coagulation function in patients with a history of thrombosis is that conventional measures of vitamin K-dependent factors, such as protein C and S activity, are obviated by warfarin therapy. (See the article by Ng on anticoagulation monitoring, elsewhere in this issue.) Antigenic measures of active proteins may be more informative; in this respect, APC is one molecule of interest because of its ubiquitous function as a mediator of anti-inflammatory pathways and thrombin down-regulation. Besides its anticoagulant function, APC has direct cytoprotective effects through stabilization of endothelial barrier function and anti-apoptotic and anti-inflammatory activity. These actions are mediated by interaction with the EC protein C receptor and with the thrombin receptor, protease-activated receptor-1. Measurement of blood APC levels could provide an endpoint to assess thrombin-induced formation of functional thrombomodulin and determine the level of inhibition of factors VIIIa and Va in anticoagulated patients at risk of thrombosis.

Newly elucidated pathways of vessel/platelet-mediated hemostasis offer other mechanisms for testing vascular-ligand function. The recently described C1q–tumor necrosis factor receptor protein seems to physiologically block vWF-binding sites on vascular collagen, thereby preventing platelet interaction with collagen at arterial shear rates.[4] Activated clotting and bleeding times are not affected by infusion of the molecule, however. Whether C1q–tumor necrosis factor receptor protein blocks platelet-platelet aggregation is unknown, but nonhuman primate models support its antithrombotic function. If an acquired relative deficiency of this molecule occurs, this situation would presumably result in increased thrombotic risk, similar to deficiency of the vWF cleaving protease in the pathophysiology of thrombotic thrombocytopenic purpura. (See the article by Marques on TTP/HIT, elsewhere in this issue.) Whether measurement of this plasma protein will become an essential component of the laboratory evaluation of hypercoagulability is unclear currently.

PLATELET PHYSIOLOGY

Platelets contribute to vascular homeostasis in multiple ways. In the arterial circulation they are the first responders to breaks in vascular integrity, adhering to exposed vWF, recruiting passing platelets to form a platelet plug, and releasing vasoconstrictors to reduce blood loss. Factor XIII and platelet factor 4, both released from platelet granules during activation, protect the nascent clot from fibrinolysis. By contrast, in the venous circulation, the platelet's role is more ancillary, providing a surface replete with receptors for coagulation factors and a source of negatively charged phospholipids to optimize the kinetics of the soluble coagulation cascade. Adhesive ligands and growth factors, released from platelet granules, promote clot consolidation and wound healing, respectively.

Platelet-derived Demostasis

Platelets are anucleate cells between 2 and 4 μm in diameter with a volume between 6 and 11 fL. Platelets are derived from the megakaryocyte cytoplasm, with each megakaryocyte contributing approximately 1000 circulating platelets in its lifetime. Platelets are released in an ordered fashion from the megakaryocyte; megakaryocytes have an active cytoskeleton and invaginations that form proplatelets and then release them into the circulating blood after a maturation time of approximately 4 days. When platelets are released into the circulation, they survive between 7 and 10 days. Platelets leave the circulation presumably through a combination of senescence and consumption as part of the daily maintenance of vascular structural integrity. For the latter, in normal healthy individuals few platelets are needed; approximately 7100 platelets/μL are used daily for "housekeeping hemostasis" when vascular structures are not challenged by recent surgery or trauma and when there is no systemically enhanced platelet consumption (eg, sepsis). The normal platelet count range is between 150,000 and 450,000/μL; based on a survival time of 7 to 10 days, between 15,000 and 45,000/μL of platelets exit the circulation each day. Most daily platelet turnover is a result of senescence and not consumption for maintenance of hemostasis.

When platelet function was described by the in vivo bleeding time early in the twentieth century, a platelet count in the normal range and a bleeding time less than 8 minutes indicated normal platelet function. The bleeding time requires a critical threshold for a functional platelet mass and is prolonged when platelets are less than 100,000/μL, however, regardless of whether those platelets function normally. Clinically, this means that the in vivo bleeding time reflects platelet function for counts of more than 100,000/μL but cannot be used to assess platelet function or connective tissue disease when thrombocytopenia is present. Ample studies have shown that the bleeding time is an operator-dependent, highly variable in vivo assay that can leave scars. Consequently, most laboratories have switched to "in vitro bleeding time" tests; for example, the platelet function analyzer-100, which uses anticoagulated whole blood to examine "closure time." The platelet count limitation is also true for the newer in vitro "bleeding times," but not to the same extent. The platelet function analyzer-100 may be better able to distinguish between thrombocytopenia and abnormal platelet function when platelet counts are between 50,000/μL and 100,000/μL. Platelet counts lower than that value definitely prolong the closure times such that the additional presence of platelet function cannot be discerned.

Shear-induced Adhesion

Platelet–vessel wall interaction has been well characterized at the high flow velocities of the arterial circulation. The interaction between the vasculature and flowing blood, as shown on the left side of **Fig. 1**, creates parallel planes of blood moving at different velocities; the blood closest to the vessel wall moves slower than blood closer to the center of the vessel. These different velocities create shear stress that is greatest at the vessel wall and is least at the center of the vessel. Shear rate changes inversely with the vessel diameter, with levels estimated to vary between 500/s in larger arteries and 5000/s in the smallest arterioles. Shear rates at the surface of atherosclerotic plaques with modest (50%) stenosis reach 3000 to 10,000/s, with even greater shear at more clinically significant stenoses. The high-velocity aspect of arterial blood flow actually opposes the tendencies to clot by (1) limiting the time available for procoagulant reactions to occur and (2) disrupting cells and proteins that are not tightly adherent to the vessel wall. Shear stress of more than 100,000/s can directly activate platelets independent of any platelet agonist; once the vessel wall is damaged and bleeding occurs, platelets can rapidly and decisively respond to the loss of endothelial integrity while they simultaneously resist the tendency to be swept downstream.[5]

One of the forces that enhances platelet readiness for wall adhesion in the arterial circulation is radial dispersion, which is the tendency of larger cells (erythrocytes and leukocytes) to stream in the center of the vessel, where shear is lowest. This process effectively pushes the smaller platelets toward the vessel wall and optimally positions them to respond to hemostatic challenges. This size-dependent flow also may explain the seemingly paradoxic ability of red blood cell transfusions to slow or even eliminate bleeding in patients with severe uremia. This effect also underscores the importance of platelets in arterial hemostasis; reductions in platelet number or function may be associated with severe arterial hemorrhage after surgery or trauma. By contrast, the lesser shear forces experienced in the venous circulation permit more random cell movement and greater time for coagulation reactions to occur. The minimum requirements for platelet number and function in venous hemostasis are correspondingly less stringent.

In the setting of high-velocity blood flow at an arterial bleeding site, platelets must activate and adhere to the injured vessel nearly instantaneously. Two molecules present in the subendothelium are critical for this process: vWF and collagen. Control of bleeding in vessels under the highest shear stresses absolutely depends on the presence and function of vWF. (See the article by Torres on vWD, elsewhere in this issue.) vWF is a large molecule synthesized as multimeric strings in ECs and megakaryocytes, and multimeric vWF is constitutively secreted into blood and stored in Weibel-Palade bodies of ECs. The ultralarge vWF multimers are the most active at binding platelets, particularly when unfolded by shear stress after tethering to the vessel surface. The multimeric forms of vWF, which are immobilized by adherence to exposed subendothelial collagen, bind to the glycoprotein Ib (GPIb)/IX-V complex on the platelet surface when normally cryptic loci on vWF are exposed by high shear stress (**Fig. 1**). This binding is rapid but low-affinity, and those bonds frequently rupture as a result of the high shear stress present at those locations. The transmembrane signaling produced by the GPIb-V-IX-vWF interaction produces loss of the normal platelet discoid shape (shape change) and conformational change in another platelet receptor, GPIIb/IIIa. With the velocity of the platelet slowed because of transient binding, this latter receptor can bind to a different locus on vWF, a bond of sufficiently high affinity to arrest the platelet.

Ligands

One important regulator of this process of platelet binding and activation through vWF is the circulating vWF-cleaving protease present in plasma: a disintegrin and metallo-proteinase with a thrombospondin type 1 motif, member 13 (ADAMTS-13). In small diameter arteries in which the shear stress is highest, platelets must be able to bind transiently to vWF via GPIb-V-IX then securely via GPIIb/IIIa at a different vWF site to withstand the local shear. For this function, the high multimeric forms of vWF are the most effective, providing multiple binding sites for platelets as they are uncoiled by the shear that makes adhesion so problematic. ADAMTS-13 modulates the hemostatic activity of vWF by cleaving the ultra-large multimers into smaller fragments that have reduced overall affinity for platelet binding. Paradoxically, the cleavage sites for this regulatory enzyme on vWF are normally cryptic but become exposed by the same uncoiling that provides platelets with their locus for binding via GPIb-V-IX. ADAMTS-13 is, in turn, regulated by thrombin. Besides directly activating platelets, thrombin causes proteolysis of ADAMTS-13, thereby promoting large vWF multimer persistence and enhanced platelet recruitment into areas of vessel injury. These regulators, together with local factors such as shear, the platelet count, and the levels of vWF, maintain vascular integrity in the arterial circulation. Under ideal conditions, vWF size is maintained in a range such that sufficient large multimers are available for arterial hemostasis, yet platelet plugs are restrained from growing to a degree that produces arterial occlusion.

Pathologic loss of the ADAMTS-13 cleaving protease activity can allow ultra-large vWF multimers to persist in the circulation, multimers that support unchecked platelet adhesion that is not predicated on any vascular insult, producing widespread microvascular thrombosis. At more moderate shear rates, GPIb-V-IX-vWF adhesion is supplemented by platelet binding to subendothelial collagen, an adhesive moiety that is capable of arresting the platelet by binding to GPIa/IIa (**Box 1**). Subendothelial vWF and collagen act cooperatively to initiate platelet adhesion, with the former predominating at higher shear. Collagen is unique in that it can anchor platelets at one locus by binding to platelet GPIa/IIa and can activate platelets at a second locus by binding to platelet GPVI, and both platelet receptors are critical for physiologic platelet function. The congenital absence of any of the platelet adhesion receptors—GPIIb/IIIa, GPIb/IX-V, GPVI, or GPIa/IIa—results in a significant hemostatic defect, correctable only by platelet transfusion.[6] This finding is further reinforced by the α chain of GPIb normally serving as a cofactor for thrombin activation of platelets through the GPV receptor and the protease activated receptor. Similarly to defects in platelet receptors, decreases in the vWF ligand, especially the larger multimeric forms, can lead to bleeding.

Once a layer of platelets adheres to the site of injury, vWF bound to GPIb/IX-V on the luminal side of the adherent platelets serves to recruit additional platelets from the flowing blood into the growing platelet plug. Platelet recruitment is further enhanced by platelet activation and release of serotonin and ADP, which serve to activate and adhere platelets from the circulation to the growing platelet clot. Platelet activation is actually a series of interdependent processes[7] with five major effects: (1) local release of ligands essential to stabilizing the platelet-platelet matrix, (2) continued recruitment of additional platelets, (3) vasoconstriction of smaller arteries to slow

---

Box 1
Platelet coagulant properties

Receptor-ligand interactions promoting adhesion

GPIb/IX/V-vWF

GPIIb/IIIa-fibrinogen and GPIIb/IIIa-vWF

GPIa/IIa-collagen

P selectin-P selectin glycoprotein ligand-1

Receptor-ligand interactions mediating activation

GPV-thrombin

GPVI-collagen

Secreted alpha-granule proteins

Ligands (fibrinogen, fibronectin, thrombospondin, vitronectin, vWF)

Enzymes (α2-antiplasmin, factors V, VIII, and XI)

Antiheparin (platelet factor 4)

Secreted dense-granule agonists

ADP, serotonin

Secreted cytosolic components

Factor XIII, Thrombin-activatable fibrinolysis inhibitor

Membrane components

Thromboxane A2 formation, phosphatidylserine expression

---

bleeding, (4) localization and acceleration of platelet-associated fibrin formation, and (5) protection of the clot from fibrinolysis.

Activation

The basis of the platelet plug is a platelet-ligand-platelet matrix with fibrinogen, fibronectin, and vWF serving as bridging ligands. Both fibrinogen and vWF are endocytosed from plasma and stored in alpha granules inside the resting platelet. Both molecules are released with activation, and both can bind to a GPIIb/IIIa receptor on each of two platelets, thereby linking them. Platelet GPIIb/IIIa undergoes a calcium-dependent conformational change that allows it to bind to a locus containing the amino acid sequence arginine-glycine-aspartate (RGD) on any fibrinogen, fibronectin, or vWF molecule. Each fibrinogen molecule has two RGD sites on its polar ends, and the larger vWF multimers have several RGD sites, all capable of binding to conformationally altered GPIIb/IIIa and creating the platelet-ligand-platelet matrix integral to a platelet plug. GPIIb/IIIa is the most abundant glycoprotein on the platelet surface, with approximately 50,000 copies on the resting platelet and additional GPIIb/IIIa receptors within the platelet cytosol that are mobilized to the surface after activation.

Platelets are also recruited into the platelet plug by local agonists (collagen, epinephrine, and thrombin) and by platelet release of agonists into the local microenvironment. Collagen (as noted previously) and thrombin interact with their specific platelet receptors to activate platelets strongly. Although circulating epinephrine by itself is not a powerful platelet agonist, stimulation of the alpha-adrenergic receptor on platelets primes them for synergistic activation by low thrombin doses and relatively weak agonists such as ADP. One activating compound released directly from the platelet is thromboxane A_2 (TxA_2), which is formed in the platelet cytosol after cyclo-oxygenase-1 (COX-1)–mediated cleavage of arachidonic acid and then released into the clot milieu. TxA_2 is a platelet agonist and a vasoconstrictor, and it is rapidly degraded to its readily measurable inert byproduct, thromboxane B_2. Platelet COX-1 activity is irreversibly inhibited by aspirin, thereby blocking TxA_2 formation for the lifetime of that platelet. Aspirin irreversibly and covalently binds to a specific serine residue on COX-1 and causes steric hindrance of the active site, a tyrosine molecule across from the serine residue. Nonsteroidal anti-inflammatory drugs (NSAIDs) do not covalently bind through acetylation at serine. Instead, they reversibly and competitively bind at the active, catalytic tyrosine site. Unlike aspirin, the antiplatelet effects of NSAIDs depend on the continual presence of plasma levels of the NSAID.

COX-2 is an induced isoform within leukocytes that mediates inflammation and pain. Because mature platelets do not possess COX-2 activity, one rationale for development of the highly selective COX-2 inhibitors for inflammatory diseases was the avoidance of bleeding caused by platelet dysfunction by not affecting platelet COX-1 activity. It seems that vascular ECs require COX-2 activity to synthesize the antithrombogenic compound, prostacyclin (**Table 1**). Selective COX-2 inhibition can produce down-regulation of EC prostacyclin coupled with preserved platelet prothrombotic function, a combination that may tip the hemostatic balance in favor of clot formation. Large-scale clinical trials have shown that some highly selective COX-2 inhibitors increase the likelihood of hypertension and vascular arterial events, including myocardial infarction and stroke.[8]

Other platelet agonists are liberated into the extracellular fluid after fusion of the dense and alpha granules with the platelet canalicular membrane allows extrusion of granule contents. The dense granules contain serotonin that, similar to TxA_2, is a platelet agonist and a vasoconstrictor. Another dense granule constituent, ADP, acts purely as a platelet agonist through the G protein-linked $P2Y_{12}$ receptor and has no vasoactive properties (**Box 1**). This $P2Y_{12}$ receptor is the site of action of the metabolite of the antiplatelet agent, clopidogrel, which inhibits ADP-induced activation. The importance of TxA_2- and serotonin-induced vasoconstriction is not entirely clear; however, vasoconstriction, by decreasing the vessel diameter, may increase shear stress and facilitate recruitment of platelets to the injured site. Shear force seems to be capable of independently activating platelets and, by virtue of its ability to uncoil vWF, promote platelet adhesion. The importance of dense granule release to the maintenance of hemostasis is underscored by the severe bleeding seen in congenital dense granule deficiencies (eg, Hermansky-Pudlak syndrome). Another membrane change that occurs with platelet activation is the coordinated internalization of surface phosphatidylcholine and externalization of phosphatidylserine (ie, membrane flip-flop). Phosphatidylserine at the platelet surface provides the negatively charged phospholipid cofactor necessary for ideal kinetics of the soluble coagulation cascade. Platelet activation serves to amplify platelet adhesion and optimizes the platelet surface for interaction with soluble coagulation factors, which allows for explosive generation of thrombin requisite for a fibrin clot.[9]

SOLUBLE COAGULATION
Coagulation Models

The "Cascade" model of soluble coagulation as first described more than 40 years ago features two starting points that converge to a common pathway leading to thrombin and fibrin generation. This model allowed great strides to be made in identifying the proteolytic reactions that culminate in fibrin clot and dovetailed well with the prothrombin time/partial thromboplastin time (PT/aPTT) assays guiding warfarin and heparin dosing, respectively. Although workable for some clinical scenarios, bleeding in a disease such as hemophilia contradicts the model's prediction that when one of these pathways is dysfunctional, activity of the other should be sufficient to maintain adequate clot formation. (See the article by Crookston and colleagues on hemophilia and factor deficiency elsewhere in this issue.) The total absence of any bleeding diathesis in factor XII-deficient patients with aPTT times that are immeasurably prolonged further undermines this model as an apt conceptual framework for in vivo clotting.

More recent models have made significant strides in clarifying the dynamics of in vivo coagulation (**Fig. 2**). The balance of coagulation is characterized by continuous, low-grade factor activation and coordinated assembly of enzyme complexes, which are promptly down-regulated by circulating inhibitor proteins. These enzyme complexes consist of serine proteases, their co-factors, and zymogen substrates. In the absence of overt blood vessel disruption, enzyme complex formation and the resultant thrombin generation are minute and relatively slow. Circulating endogenous anticoagulants are sufficient to inactivate these procoagulant complexes and prevent

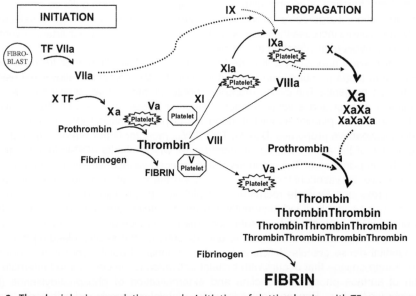

Fig. 2. The physiologic coagulation cascade. Initiation of clotting begins with TF exposure on a cell (eg, fibroblasts), which then combines with small amounts of circulating VIIa to form the extrinsic Xase complex and generate Xa. Xa forms the prothrombinase complex with Va and prothrombin, generating small amounts of thrombin, which begin to cleave fibrinogen into weak fibrin monomers in the initiation phase of coagulation. Feedback activation of factors by thrombin, especially when performed on the activated platelet surface, is responsible for propagation of the coagulant response. Thrombin generates XIa, which in turn activates IX; the TF-VIIa complex (before its shutdown by TFPI) also generates IXa. Thrombin-activated VIIIa then combines with IXa to from the intrinsic Xase complex, generating large amounts of Xa on the platelet surface, which in combination with Va, massively amplifies thrombin production. The large amounts of thrombin generate enough fibrin monomers for a stable fibrin clot.

inappropriate clot formation.[10] Once a procoagulant stimulus occurs that generates significant amounts of activated factors, however, formation of these enzyme complexes is rapidly amplified, in part by its assembly on a favorable membrane (phospholipid) surface, leading to intense thrombin—and subsequent fibrin—formation. Activation of soluble coagulation can be divided into two phases: (1) the initiation phase, successful completion of which gives rise to (2) the propagation phase (**Fig. 2**).

Clot Initiation

Coagulation in vivo follows exposure of the blood to a source of TF, typically on the surface of a fibroblast brought into contact with blood via a break in the vessel wall. The intrinsic or contact pathway of coagulation plays no role in the earliest events in clotting. The initiation phase (left side of **Fig. 2**) begins as the exposed TF binds to factor VIIa, picomolar amounts of which are present in the circulation at all times. This VIIa-TF complex catalyzes the conversion of small amounts of factor X to Xa, which generates nanomolar amounts of thrombin. The seemingly trivial amount of thrombin formed during this initiation phase sparks the inception of the propagation phase (right side of **Fig. 2**), successful completion of which culminates in explosive thrombin generation and, ultimately, fibrin deposition. More than 96% of the total thrombin that is generated during clotting occurs during the propagation phase.

Clot Propagation

Thrombin generated during the initiation phase is a potent platelet activator, supplying the developing clot with an activated platelet surface membrane and abundant platelet-released factor V, which is promptly activated to Va by thrombin. Factor VIII, conveniently brought to the bleeding site by its carrier, vWF, is also activated by thrombin, a step that causes its release by vWF. VIIIa then complexes with the picomolar amounts of factor IXa generated by the TF-VIIa complex during the initiation phase to create the VIIIa-IXa complex. The formation of this complex on the platelet surface heralds the switch of the primary path of Xa generation from the TF-VIIa complex (the extrinsic Xase) to the intrinsic Xase (the VIIIa-IXa complex). This switch is of significant kinetic advantage, with the intrinsic Xase complex exhibiting 50-fold higher efficiency than the extrinsic Xase. The bleeding diathesis associated with hemophilia is testament to the physiologic importance of the exuberant thrombin generation engendered by the switch from extrinsic to intrinsic Xase. The aPTT, which measures the initiation phase of clotting begun by an artificial in vitro stimulant, is prolonged by severe deficiencies in either VIII or IX, but it is the ability to ramp up thrombin generation during the propagation phase, a function not evaluated by the aPTT, that causes the bleeding in hemophilia.

The activated platelet expresses receptors for VIIIa, and IXa, and binding of these active proteases in complex with membrane phosphatidylserine enhances the binding of the enzyme's substrate, factor X, thereby producing the markedly greater kinetic efficiency of the intrinsic Xase complex as compared with the extrinsic Xase complex. Assembly of the prothrombinase complex similarly depends on the activated platelet surface for optimum activity. Like the Xase complex, the membrane-bound prothrombinase complex activates prothrombin with a rate enhancement 300,000-fold higher than free Xa acting on prothrombin in solution. Platelet-bound Xa is the rate-limiting enzyme in prothrombin cleavage for the initiation and propagation phases of clotting; its substrate, prothrombin, binds to GPIIb/IIIa on both activated and unactivated platelets. The net kinetic advantage conferred by platelet binding is such that assembly of the entire reaction on the platelet membrane is a 13 million-fold increase in catalytic efficiency over that of the same proteases free in solution.

What role do other "intrinsic pathway" factors play in coagulation? Evidence is growing that factor XI further amplifies the propagation phase of coagulation. Levels of factor Xa are particularly rate-limiting once the switch is made to the intrinsic Xase where its generation is dependent on the IXa-VIIIa enzyme complex. Although small amounts of IXa are generated by the TF-VIIa complex, IXa generation in this manner is limited by TFPI. To generate Xa in amounts sufficient to fuel the propagation phase, a kinetically superior source of IXa is required. Factor XI is another zymogen activated by small amounts of initiation phase-generated thrombin, but this activation is restricted to the activated platelet surface. Platelet-bound XIa activates IX on the platelet surface, thereby favoring assembly of the intrinsic Xase complex in a location where its kinetics are optimized. Binding to the platelet surface protects XIa from its inhibitor, protease nexin 2. XIa generation on the activated platelet is instrumental for providing IXa in amounts sufficient to maintain peak Xa generation via the efficient intrinsic Xase complex. There is also evidence for parallel feedback activation of XI by the contact system, a finding that demands re-evaluation of the role of the contact system in physiologic blood coagulation. Some evidence indicates that the balanced pro- and anticoagulant function of the contact system allows for a "null" phenotype with deficiency of factor XII, high-molecular-weight kininogen, or prekallikrein.[11]

Limiting Soluble Coagulation

Endogenous anticoagulants can either inactivate formed thrombin or prevent thrombin generation. (See the article by Van Cott and colleagues on hypercoagulability, elsewhere in this issue.) The most important anticoagulant of the former type is antithrombin (AT). AT is physiologically present at more than twice the concentration ($3.2 \, \mu mol/L^{-1}$) of the highest local thrombin concentration ($1.4 \, \mu mol/L^{-1}$) that can be reached during clotting, and AT activity against thrombin is potentiated 1000-fold by endogenous EC-associated heparin sulfate proteoglycans. Platelet surface membranes and platelet-released platelet factor 4 protect thrombin from inactivation at the site of the clot. Any thrombin that escapes into the circulation is immediately (< 1 min) inhibited by plasma AT, however, and in the microenvironment of healthy ECs, which bind approximately 60,000 molecules of AT per cell, free thrombin is neutralized almost instantaneously. The thrombin that is generated early is particularly dependent on protection by the activated platelet membrane for sufficient time to transition from initiation to the propagation phase.

Among endogenous anticoagulants that target thrombin generation, the earliest in the coagulation process is TFPI, which inactivates factor Xa and the TF-VIIa complex. TFPI is constitutively released by ECs into the microvasculature. Under normal conditions, TFPI is largely localized to the endothelial surface by binding to EC-associated glycosaminoglycans but can be displaced by heparin. Nascent TFPI has direct activity only against Xa, but after exposure to Xa, TFPI acquires activity against the TF-VIIa complex. During the initiation phase, platelet-bound Xa is protected from inactivation by TFPI and AT. Preservation of the small amounts of Xa that are generated during this early stage of coagulation is critical to formation of the nanomolar amounts of thrombin needed to begin the propagation phase of clotting.

Activated protein C (APC) has anticoagulant, anti-inflammatory, and profibrinolytic properties that make it an important regulator of thrombosis and inflammation. Like TFPI, protein C becomes activated only after coagulation is underway. Formed thrombin binds to thrombomodulin, a proteoglycan associated with endothelial and monocyte cell surfaces. Thrombomodulin-bound thrombin loses its ability to activate platelets and activates protein C. On the EC surface, nascent protein C binds to EC protein C receptor, which posits it for activation by the adjacent thrombomodulin-bound thrombin. Once activated, in a reaction that is enhanced by EC protein C receptor and protein S, APC inactivates factors VIIIa and Va, components of the Xase and prothrombinase complexes, respectively, thereby limiting procoagulant self-amplification. The factor V Leiden mutation confers APC resistance and a hypercoagulable phenotype. (See the article by Perrotta on molecular diagnostics elsewhere in this issue.) As with other coagulation factors, the activated platelet membrane protects VIIIa and Va from APC inactivation. In addition to its effects on thrombin generation, APC neutralizes plasminogen activator inhibitor-1 (PAI-1) to enhance clot remodeling. APC has anti-inflammatory properties as well; recombinant APC reduces tumor necrosis factor-α production after endotoxin challenge, and protein C-deficient mice (heterozygotes) exhibit higher levels of proinflammatory cytokines with systemic endotoxemia.

The liver is the major site of synthesis of all coagulation factors. In liver disease, however, factor VIII levels are not generally diminished because VIII is also produced by ECs and the reticuloendothelial system. (See the article by Ng on liver disease elsewhere in this issue.) The subset of coagulation factors that depend on vitamin K for synthesis includes prothrombin (II), VII, IX, and X, and the anticoagulants, proteins C and S. Posttranslational modification (through a vitamin K–dependent carboxylase) of the amino-terminal domain of these proteins adds 10 to 12 γ-carboxyglutamate residues, which are critical for calcium binding and determining the functional three-dimensional structure of the proteins and their proper binding orientation to membrane surfaces. Warfarin blocks vitamin K epoxide reductase and decreases generation of vitamin K (from vitamin K epoxide) in the vitamin K cycle.

Laboratory Testing of Coagulation

The cascade model of clotting that divides early events into two parallel pathways — one an extrinsic and the other an intrinsic pathway — is no longer viewed as an accurate representation of physiologic events contributing to in vivo coagulation. For purposes of laboratory testing, however, this model is useful for interpreting the two assays most commonly used to evaluate coagulation, the PT and PTT. The PTT measurement is based on in vitro contact activation (eg, plasma stimulation with a negatively charged compound such as kaolin). It is worth noting that most of the commonly used laboratory tests of soluble coagulation measure the kinetics of the initiation phase only. (See the article by Ng on PT/PTT assay considerations elsewhere in this issue.) The PT and PTT have as their endpoints the first appearance of fibrin gel, which occurs with less than 5% of the total reaction complete, and only minimal levels of prothrombin have been activated. The PT/PTT are sensitive for detecting congenital abnormalities associated with severe factor deficits (eg, hemophilia) and for guiding heparin/warfarin therapy. It is important to note that "normal" factor levels change with aging, from the pediatric to adult period[12] and with progression to elderly status.[13] Neither factor levels nor current clotting tests yield information relevant to thrombin generation during the propagation phase, which determines whether a persistent clot forms or whether the endogenous anticoagulants and fibrinolytic regulators constrain it from excess growth.[14]

CLOT VIABILITY AND MATURATION

Evidence is growing that initial formation of a thrombus does not ensure sustained hemostasis. Events initiated during thrombus generation that are critical to its stability operate after the clot is formed, whether fibrin-rich in the venous or platelet-rich in the arterial circulation.

Fibrin Clot Architecture

The architecture of a fibrin clot is surprisingly variable, and although genetic factors unquestionably play a role in determining clot structure, two dominant factors are the local thrombin and fibrinogen concentrations, whose reaction yields the fibrin strands.[15] A thrombin-rich microenvironment typically results in thinner, more tightly cross-linked fibers, which makes the overall fibrin clot virtually impermeable to lytic enzymes, as opposed to thrombin-poor locations, in which the fibrin strands are thicker and the structure more porous, which makes the clot vulnerable to thrombolysis. Similarly, high fibrinogen concentrations are associated with large thrombi whose tight, rigid meshwork makes them less deformable and more lysis-resistant. Low fibrinogen concentrations, by contrast, produce a less compact clot that is highly lysis-prone.

Fibrin Cross-linking by Factor XIIIa

Factor XIII also plays a critical role in stabilizing the nascent clot. XIII circulates in the plasma and is stored within platelets. Fully 50% of total fibrin-stabilizing activity in blood resides in the platelet and is released by activation. In plasma, XIII is a tetrameric molecule consisting of 2 A-subunits, which contain the active site of the enzyme, and 2 B-subunits, which increase the zymogen's plasma half-life but must be dissociated for full enzyme activity. Platelet factor XIII, by contrast, is a dimer that contains only the 2 A-subunits. Both forms of the zymogen require thrombin cleavage and fibrin as a cofactor, but plasma XIII activation proceeds at a considerably slower rate than its platelet counterpart because of the need for dissociation of the B-subunits. Thrombin-activated XIIIa binds to fibrin and cross-links the fibrin units, which renders them less permeable and more resistant to lysis. XIIIa cross-links the major plasmin inhibitor, α2-antiplasmin, directly to fibrin, positing it for neutralization of any invading plasmin.

FIBRINOLYSIS

The fibrinolytic system operates to prevent fibrin from occluding healthy vessels. During clot formation, Xa and thrombin stimulate healthy ECs to release t-PA and urokinase-type plasminogen activator, both capable of cleaving plasminogen into plasmin. The vast excess of plasminogen present in the plasma dictates that under normal circumstances, the concentration of these enzymes is rate-limiting for plasmin formation. The kinetic efficiency of t-PA is improved by at least an order of magnitude by the presence of fibrin, thus helping keep t-PA most active in the microenvironment of the clot. By contrast, urokinase-type plasminogen activator seems to require binding to activated platelets for its ability to liberate plasmin.

Acting to contain fibrinolysis are the plasma mediators that either inactivate formed plasmin (eg, α2-antiplasmin and possibly α2-macroglobulin) or block plasmin formation, foremost of which is plasminogen activator inhibitor-1 (PAI-1). PAI-1 is present in several-fold molar excess in the plasma and is released by activated platelets, thereby protecting clots from premature lysis. PAI-1 plasma levels can be highly variable in part because of its circadian pattern of secretion but also because of polymorphisms of the PAI-1 gene. The 4G promoter region polymorphism of PAI-1 is associated with higher PAI-1 levels and a higher risk of thromboembolic disease. Another mediator that limits fibrinolysis in the vicinity of the clot is TAFI. TAFI is synthesized in an inactive form by the liver and circulates in the plasma, possibly in a complex with plasminogen. TAFI cleaves specific fibrin lysine residues that would otherwise promote binding of fibrinolytic enzymes (eg, plasmin). TAFI requires either plasmin or thrombin for activation; however, thrombin activation of TAFI requires extraordinarily large amounts of free thrombin. By contrast, EC-associated thrombomodulin potentiates thrombin-induced TAFI activation 1250-fold, making this an essential cofactor and one that is predominantly available only at the blood-vessel interface. In addition to the EC surface, macrophages are also critical to fibrinolysis. Macrophages degrade fibrin clot through lysosomal proteolysis by a plasmin-independent mechanism. The macrophage binds to fibrin(ogen) through its surface integrin receptor, CD11b/CD18; this binding is followed by internalization of the complex into the lysosome, where fibrin(ogen) is degraded.

Tissue repair and regeneration are the physiologic endpoints of clotting, eventually leading to dissolution of the fibrin-based clot. Besides t-PA and urokinase, the intrinsic pathway activators kallikrein, XIIa, and XIa generate active plasmin from plasminogen. Plasminogen binding to cell surface receptors promotes its own activation to plasmin by placing it in proximity to t-PA and fibrin clot and protects plasmin from inactivation by circulating (not clot-bound) α2-antiplasmin. Plasmin eventually dissolves the fibrin matrix to produce soluble fibrin peptides and D-dimer and activates metalloproteinases that further degrade damaged tissue. Fibroblasts and leukocytes migrate into the wound, the latter mediated by selectin binding; these inflammatory cells act in concert with growth factors secreted by leukocytes and activated platelets (eg, transforming growth factor-β) to enhance vascular repair and tissue regeneration.

FUTURE STUDIES: INTERINDIVIDUAL VARIABILITY AND THE EXTREMES OF "NORMAL"

The understanding of hemostasis physiology has been advanced by kinetic models in research laboratories using the interplay of cells and soluble coagulation factors. In such models, thrombin is clearly an important, if not central, coordinator of hemostatic function and is a target for measurement to assess hemostatic function and risk. The PT/aPTT do not begin to measure the full physiology of the hemostatic response, however, and the platelet contribution to clotting is absent in such tests. It remains to be seen whether newer measurements such as endogenous thrombin potential or the refinement of older methods such as thromboelastography can better quantitate global hemostatic function. (See the article by Teruya on global hemostasis testing elsewhere in this issue.)

Translation of hemostasis research methods into clinical laboratory assays is an ongoing process. The approach to hemostasis testing and interpretation may need to undergo a sea of change, however. The concept of the normal range for hemostasis factors may not be adequate for predicting outcomes. Measuring an individual's capacity to generate activated mediators (or their byproducts) and their kinetics has shown an extreme range of biologic variability. For example, total amounts and peak rates of thrombin formation and platelet amplification of thrombin generation demonstrate a remarkable breadth of "normal." Our ability to derive the most useful information from sophisticated coagulation testing may demand more than a simple normal range, similar to our clinical understanding of individualizing risk factors as predictors of a patient's response to hemostatic challenge. For the latter, one apparent success for the laboratory is the evolving use of D-dimer threshold values for predicting the risk of recurrent venous thromboembolism.[16] An individualized approach to anticoagulation in this instance, rather than fixed anticoagulation duration based on population means, may improve the balance of thrombotic versus bleeding outcomes.

REFERENCES

1. Jackson SP. The growing complexity of platelet aggregation. Blood 2007;109: 5087–95.

2. Oliver JJ, Webb DJ, Newby DE. Stimulated tissue plasminogen activator release as a marker of endothelial function in humans. Arterioscler Thromb Vasc Biol 2005;25:2470–9.
3. Lijnen HR. Pleiotropic functions of plasminogen activator inhibitor-1. J Thromb Haemost 2005;3:35–45.
4. Lasser G, Guchhait P, Ellsworth JL, et al. C1qTNF-related protein (CTRP-1): a vascular wall protein that inhibits collagen-induced platelet aggregation by blocking vWF binding to collagen. Blood 2006;107:423–30.
5. Ruggeri ZM, Mendolicchio GL. Adhesion mechanisms in platelet function. Circ Res 2007;100:1673–85.
6. Nurden AT, Nurden P. Inherited disorders of platelets: an update. Curr Opin Hematol 2006;13:157–62.
7. Yin W, Czuchlewski D, Peerschke EI. Development of proteomic signatures of platelet activation using surface-enhanced laser desorption/ionization technology in a clinical setting. Am J Clin Pathol 2008;129:862–9.
8. Antman EM, DeMets D, Loscalzo J. Cyclooxygenase inhibition and cardiovascular risk. Circulation 2005;112:759–70.
9. Lane DA, Phillippou H, Huntington JA. Directing thrombin. Blood 2005;106: 2605–12.
10. Brummel-Ziedins K, Vossen CY, Rosendaal FR, et al. The plasma hemostatic proteome: thrombin generation in healthy individuals. J Thromb Haemost 2005;3: 1472–81.
11. Blat Y, Sieffert D. A renaissance for the contact system in blood coagulation? Thromb Haemost 2008;99:457–60.
12. Monagle P, Barnes C, Ignjatovic V, et al. Developmental haemostasis: impact for clinical haemostasis laboratories. Thromb Haemost 2006;95:362–72.
13. Yamamoto K, Takeshita K, Kojima T, et al. Aging and plasminogen activator inhibitor-1 (PAI-1) regulation: implication in the pathogenesis of thrombotic disorders in the elderly. Cardiovasc Res 2005;66:276–85.
14. Hemker HC, Dieri RA, Beguin S. Thrombin generation assays: accruing clinical relevance. Curr Opin Hematol 2004;11:170–5.
15. Scott EM, Ariens R, Grant PJ. Genetic and environmental determinants of fibrin structure and function: relevance to clinical disease. Arterioscler Thromb Vasc Biol 2004;24:1558–66.
16. Legnani C, Palareti G, Cosmi B, et al. Different cut-off values of quantitative d-dimer methods to predict the risk of venous thromboembolism recurrence: a post-hoc analysis of the PROLONG study. Haematologica 2008;93:900–7.

Platelet-Related Bleeding: An Update on Diagnostic Modalities and Therapeutic Options

Marie E. Peddinghaus, MD[a], Christopher A. Tormey, MD[a,b],*

KEYWORDS

- Platelet-related bleeding • Platelet function testing
- Platelet transfusion therapy

Platelets (PLTs) play a fundamental role in hemostasis and represent the first line of defense in the prevention and cessation of hemorrhagic episodes.[1] As such, quantitative and qualitative PLT disorders can be problematic in that they can predispose patients to spontaneous bleeding episodes, or manifest as severe complications during trauma or invasive procedures. Although PLT-related bleeding was previously encountered primarily in thrombocytopenic patients with oncologic disorders and/or rare congenital PLT defects, the routine use of anti-PLT agents like aspirin has caused a surge in the reported cases of PLT-related bleeding.[2–4]

For many years, the only laboratory means for acutely determining PLT bleeding risks were basic tests to quantitate the numbers of circulating PLTs. As such, much of the approach to transfusion therapy has previously centered on "trigger" PLT counts. In addition, some crude "in vivo" assays, such as the template bleeding time, have been used to gain insight into functional PLT defects and other bleeding disorders such as von Willebrand disease. Over time, a number of studies have revealed that the template bleeding time is a poor screening test for disorders of hemostasis and, as such, this assay has been largely abandoned for this purpose.[5,6] Traditional light transmission aggregometry is also a tool that is routinely used to assess PLT function, however this assay is not easily applied in the acute setting.

Based on a growing need for assays that could quickly and easily identify PLT inhibition in an individual, a number of commercial point-of-care (POC) tests of PLT function have been recently developed.[7] These assays, in combination with traditional PLT

---

[a] Department of Laboratory Medicine, Yale University School of Medicine, 333 Cedar Street, PO Box 208035, New Haven, CT 06520, USA
[b] Pathology and Laboratory Medicine Service, VA Connecticut Healthcare System, West Haven, CT 06516, USA
* Corresponding author. Department of Laboratory Medicine, Yale University School of Medicine, 333 Cedar Street, PO Box 208035, New Haven, CT 06520.
E-mail address: christopher.tormey@yale.edu (C.A. Tormey).

Clin Lab Med 29 (2009) 175–191
doi:10.1016/j.cll.2009.03.004
0272-2712/09/$ – see front matter. Published by Elsevier Inc.

labmed.theclinics.com

counts, provide a much wider assessment of the totality of PLT coagulation status. Although the primary end point of many of these POC assays is to determine if anti-PLT regimens are efficacious in inhibiting PLT activity in patients at risk for cardiovascular diseases, the insight gained from these tests can also help to guide an appropriate response for presumed PLT-related bleeding.

Thus, the goals of this article are to review issues relevant to PLT-related bleeding. We briefly summarize the most common causes of bleeding associated with PLT disorders. We also detail the recent advancements made in PLT function testing with a particular emphasis on new POC modalities and their applications in various clinical settings. Further, we update the reader on developments in PLT transfusion therapy, including newly licensed components and potential future directions. Finally, we outline those initial studies that have shown that POC PLT function assays are useful in assessing hemorrhage risk and composing "targeted" transfusion strategies in patients with PLT-related bleeding.

PLATELET-RELATED BLEEDING: ETIOLOGIES IN BRIEF

PLT-related bleeding can be tied to one of two primary causes: thrombocytopenia and/or PLT dysfunction. **Table 1** summarizes the most common etiologies underlying each of these disorders. For patients with significant thrombocytopenia (ie, PLT counts ≤50,000/μL), this problem is most often attributable to a hypoproliferative bone marrow. Various chemotherapeutic and hematopoietic progenitor cell transplantation regimens result in the delivery of marrow toxic drugs, suppressing PLT counts, and raising the risk for hemorrhage.[8] Another frequently encountered cause of thrombocytopenia is PLT destruction. In many cases, pathogenic antibodies can arise after the administration of drugs like heparin.[9] Antibiotics and autoimmune disorders are other common causes of antibody-mediated PLT destruction.[10,11] Recently, dilutional thrombocytopenia associated with the infusion of massive quantities of crystalloids, colloids, red blood cells (RBCs), and plasma has been recognized as another important cause of morbidity and mortality in bleeding patients.[12] In these scenarios, replacement of one to two whole blood volumes consisting of individual blood components and ongoing consumption serve to reduce baseline PLT counts by greater than 50%, thereby increasing the risk for bleeding complications.

Dysfunction that is attributable to anti-PLT agents is arguably the most common cause for PLT-related bleeding in patients with normal PLT counts. Because of an aging US population and the great number of individuals with coronary artery and peripheral vascular disease, more and more physicians are placing patients on routine anti-PLT therapy.[13] While reducing the risks associated with myocardial infarction and stroke, this trend has led to an increase in the number of patients presenting with PLT-related bleeding. Gastrointestinal bleeds, in particular, are a well-known side effect of anti-PLT therapy.[2–4] Although much less frequent than bleeding related to anti-PLT agents, uremia in hospitalized individuals is also gaining in recognition as an important cause of PLT dysfunction and PLT-related bleeding.[14] Via mechanisms that are not well-understood, uremia inhibits the adhesion and aggregability of endogenous and even transfused PLTs.[14] In addition to these acquired PLT function disorders, clinicians must also contend occasionally with the rare inherited PLT disorders such as Glanzmann thrombasthenia and Bernard-Soulier syndrome.[15]

THROMBOCYTOPENIA ASSESSMENT: ADVANCES IN LABORATORY DIAGNOSTICS

Significant advances have been made in the ability to quickly and accurately quantitate PLT counts.[16] Using automated flow cytometric techniques, modern hematology

Table 1
Common causes of PLT-related bleeding

PLT Problem	Etiology	Common Causes
Thrombocytopenia	Hypoproliferation	Chemotherapy
		Metastatic illness
		Hematopoietic disease
		Hepatic failure/decreased thrombopoietin
	Consumption	Acute bleeding
		Fever, sepsis
	Destruction	Hypersplenism
		Microangiopathic anemia
		Anti-PLT antibodies (autoimmune)
		Drug-induced antibodies
	Dilution	Massive transfusion
		Fluid or volume overload
Dysfunction	Acquired abnormalities	Anti-PLT medications (eg, aspirin, clopidogrel)
		Uremia
		Surgical bypass circuits
	Congenital abnormalities	Bernard-Soulier disease
		Glanzmann thrombasthenia
		Storage pool disorders

Abbreviation: PLT, platelet.

analyzers can rapidly process large numbers of patient specimens and report counts ranging from 1×10^3 PLTs/μL up to greater than 1×10^6 PLTs/μL with great precision.[16,17] However, despite these advances, data generated from assessment of PLT counts on standard laboratory analyzers reveals virtually no information regarding the causes for thrombocytopenia. The advent of modified PLT quantitation, in the form of reticulated PLT counting, now provides clinicians with the ability to distinguish thrombocytopenia attributable to lack of production from thrombocytopenia caused by PLT consumption or destruction.

Reticulated Platelet Count

In this assay, peripheral blood PLTs are stained with thiazole orange or other nucleic acid-binding dyes and interrogated by flow cytometry to detect intracellular RNA.[18] High levels of RNA should be detected only in those PLTs that have been recently released from the bone marrow. Thus, reticulated PLTs refer to those circulating PLTs with high RNA content, analogous to newly produced RBC reticulocytes. In general, patients demonstrating high percentages of reticulated PLTs (>20% to 50% of total PLTs) are representative of groups with destructive thrombocytopenia and a hyperproliferative marrow.[19,20] On the other hand, thrombocytopenia accompanied by a lesser percentage of reticulated PLTs generally indicate a hypoproliferative marrow.[19,20] A substantial advantage of the assay is that it provides insight into marrow regenerative capacity without the need for invasive testing of the marrow.[21] Automated cell counters now produce reticulated PLT values as a routine function, sometimes termed the "immature" platelet fraction or percentage.

The reticulated PLT count has been used in many settings including assessment of reconstitution of bone marrow following hematopoietic progenitor cell transplantation,[22] gauging the efficacy of anti-PLT therapy in patients with coronary artery disease,[23,24] provision of insight into the risk for vaso-occlusive crises in patients with sickle cell disease, and even in the basic evaluation of inflammatory diseases such as ulcerative colitis.[25]

PLATELET FUNCTION ASSESSMENT: NEW TESTING MODALITIES

Whether a patient has too few PLTs, or PLTs that are unable to properly function, PLT-related bleeding ultimately arises because of an inability to form a strong and sustainable PLT plug at the site of a vascular lesion or injury.[1] Unfortunately, only those disorders leading to a decrease in PLT count can be readily identified by standard laboratory hematology analyzers. Thus, patients with underlying PLT defects that do not result in thrombocytopenia may appear to have normal hemostatic pathways. It is in these patients that tests of PLT function have the most utility.

In the past, in vitro laboratory assessment of PLT function could be carried out only through traditional aggregometry studies, often referred to as light transmission aggregometry, turbidimetric aggregometry, or optical aggregometry.[26] Typically in these studies, PLT-rich plasma (PRP) preparations are exposed to varying doses of the PLT agonists collagen, epinephrine, ristocetin, adenosine diphosphate (ADP), and arachidonic acid. Aggregation is measured optically as a function of light passage before and after the addition of the agonists. Although some advancements have recently been made to improve the speed of specimen analysis (eg, whole blood rather than PRP analysis),[27] and to broaden the scope of testing (eg, dense granule ATP release via lumiaggregation),[28] traditional aggregometry remains labor intensive, yields results that are difficult to interpret, and is not readily performed in the acute care setting. Although this form of PLT function analysis clearly has an important place in the evaluation of patients with complex acquired or congenital PLT bleeding disorders, a new generation of POC instruments has been introduced to hasten turnaround time and simplify data interpretation. In addition, specimens analyzed by these instruments and platforms require little processing and thus more properly fit the mold of a POC test. **Table 2** provides a brief description of each of these POC platforms; details regarding the various systems are provided in the sections that follow.

Single Platelet Counting

Single PLT counting (SPC) does not refer to a particular instrument, but rather is a technique that allows one to determine the percentage contribution of "single" PLTs to an aggregated clot.[29] Because SPC essentially measures aggregation via cell counting, it is classified as impedance aggregometry.[30,31] With this technique, a baseline PLT count is measured via standard cell counting in fresh whole blood. Next, an agonist(s) is added to the whole blood, shear is induced by shaking or agitation of the mixture, and a repeat PLT count is performed on the post-agonist specimen. The addition of the agonist(s) and the application of shear (either via manual shaking or stir bar) cause the formation of large PLT aggregates. These aggregates are too large to be counted as single PLTs by standard laboratory analyzers and only small numbers of "single" PLTs are counted. Any PLTs uninvolved in aggregate formation are presumed to be dysfunctional and/or inhibited. The percentage of platelet aggregation is calculated by the following formula:

$$\% \text{ Aggregation} = [(\text{Baseline PLT count} - \text{Post-agonist PLT count}) \div \text{Baseline PLT count}] \times 100$$

In general, aggregation of more than 70% of PLTs in response to potent agonists (eg, collagen or ADP) is consistent with "normal" global PLT function.

Table 2
POC platelet function instruments and platforms

Technique	Commercial Instrument/ Platform	Agonists/Reagents	Function Measured	Current Applications[a]
Single platelet counting	ICHOR/Plateletworks	ADP, collagen, arachidonic acid (commercial kit)	Aggregation	Cardiac surgery, anti-PLT therapy monitoring
Optical aggregometry	VerifyNow	ADP, arachidonic acid, thrombin receptor peptide	Aggregation	Anti-PLT therapy monitoring
Optical aggregometry and adhesion	PFA-100 analyzer	ADP, collagen, epinephrine	Adhesion, aggregation	Cardiac surgery, acquired PLT dysfunction (non-iatrogenic), vWD screening, anti-PLT therapy monitoring
Plate-based aggregometry and adhesion	Impact cone and plate(let) analyzer	Extracellular matrix, shear	Adhesion, aggregation	Anti-PLT therapy monitoring
Thromboelastography	TEG 5000 hemostasis analyzer	Kaolin (ADP, arachidonic acid for PLT mapping)	Clot strength and stability (PLT function)	Cardiac and hepatobiliary surgery (anti-PLT therapy monitoring)

Abbreviations: ADP, adenosine diphosphate; PFA, platelet function analyzer; PLT, platelet; POC, point-of-care; TEG, thromboelastography; vWD, von Willebrand disease.
[a] Current applications refers to clinical settings where the given platforms have been thoroughly investigated and used in published trials and/or case series.

SPC has been applied in several clinical settings, but has been most extensively evaluated in determining the extent of PLT dysfunction during interventional cardiology procedures and cardiothoracic surgery involving bypass.[32,33] Although SPC can be readily applied by laboratory staff with access to PLT agonist reagents and standard cell counters, a commercial kit and analyzer are currently marketed (ICHOR/Plateletworks, Helena Laboratories, Beaumont, Texas). This commercial kit offers individually aliquotted doses of the PLT agonists ADP, collagen, and arachidonic acid. After baseline PLT counts, specimens of citrated whole blood are added to each agonist tube for post-agonist counting. The ICHOR/Plateletworks platform, like other SPC assays, has been primarily used in the setting of cardiac surgery and to gauge responses to anti-PLT therapy.[34,35]

SPC offers several advantages for POC PLT function testing including rapid turnaround time, easy reporting of data, and an ability to use preexisting hematology laboratory technology (ie, a cell counter) rather than specialized instruments to perform functional testing. In addition, unlike some other platforms, SPC is less likely to be adversely affected by mild-moderate thrombocytopenia and anemia. However, SPC does have some drawbacks. It can be somewhat laborious in that it involves manual manipulation, including pipetting of reagents (or whole blood) and application of shear. These steps can be time consuming and each introduces the possibility for laboratory accidents and errors. Further, the assay may not reflect true physiologic PLT function as the shear induced by stirring or shaking does not equate to that encountered in vivo. In addition, SPC provides insight only into aggregation; thus, it is not a useful tool in the evaluation of patients with disorders of PLT adhesion including von Willebrand disease and Bernard-Soulier syndrome. Data interpretation could also be somewhat difficult, particularly if patients demonstrate giant PLTs or other cellular fragments which interfere with the counting process.

Optical Aggregometry

Optical aggregometers in the POC setting are very similar, in principle, to those used for traditional light aggregometry. Both instruments are designed to measure light transmittance through a PLT milieu before and after the addition of PLT agonists. Unlike traditional aggregometers, however, POC instruments have been designed to be used with fresh whole blood to minimize specimen preparation and processing and to maximize turnaround time.

The most widely used commercial POC optical aggregometer is the VerifyNow platform (Accumetrics, San Diego, California). In addition to using the agonists arachidonic acid (for aspirin-related dysfunction), ADP (for P2Y12 inhibitors), and thrombin-receptor activating peptide (TRAP, for PLT GPIIb-IIIa inhibitors), this platform also uses fibrinogen-coated particles to enhance aggregation.[30,31] Once PLTs are activated by one of these three agonists, they bind the fibrinogen-coated particles resulting in aggregate formation and an increase in light transmission.[36] In this platform, results are reported as reaction or aggregation units, with levels of inhibition corresponding to satisfactory or unsatisfactory dosing of anti-PLT agents (eg, <550 aspirin resistance units correlates with evidence for adequate aspirin inhibition).[36] Trials and studies reported using the VerifyNow systems have centered primarily on the efficacy of anti-PLT therapy in patients with acute coronary events.[37–39] The results of these studies indicate that routine monitoring of patients on anti-PLT therapy can detect those who are subtherapeutic and who may then benefit from enhanced anti-PLT regimens. As yet, few studies have correlated VerifyNow results with the need for transfusion intervention in patients with acute bleeding episodes caused by anti-PLT therapy.

VerifyNow is advantageous because it is a whole blood POC analyzer with little need for specimen processing or pipetting. In this sense, it is the truest representation of a POC device among the various PLT function assays.[31] In addition, the variety of agonists allows clinicians to gauge the inhibitory effects of several different anti-PLT agents, providing greater specificity with regard to detection of abnormal results. Like SPC, however, VerifyNow provides little information regarding PLT adhesion and is not an ideal screen for some PLT bleeding disorders or von Willebrand disease. In addition, aggregation results in this platform can be affected by underlying RBC and PLT counts, which may limit the application of this modality in the acute care setting.[31] Finally, VerifyNow requires the purchase of specialized equipment and reagents which could be costly for some small hospital-based laboratories.

Adhesion and Aggregation—Optical and Plate-Based Platforms

The broadest assessment of functional PLT activity is performed by assays that reflect both PLT aggregation and adhesion functions. Currently, two commercial POC platforms (the platelet function analyzer, or PFA-100, and the cone and plate[let] analyzer) provide insight into these two functions. The methodology used to reflect adhesion and aggregation are quite different in these instruments, and each platform is discussed separately in the following paragraphs.

The PFA-100 (Dade Behring Inc, Deerfield, Illinois) is a whole blood–based POC instrument in which patient specimens are pipetted into cartridges containing combinations of collagen/epinephrine and collagen/ADP for activation.[40–42] The activated PLTs are then streamed toward an aperture to induce shear and, upon contact, PLT adhesion takes place. Subsequently, aggregation between PLTs at the primary aperture site and those streaming toward the aperture should ensue. Over time, PLT adhesion and aggregation yield a solid plug, sealing the aperture.[42] The time frame between PLT activation/streaming and aperture closing is measured and this "closure time" directly correlates with PLT adhesion and aggregation functionality. In general, closure times of less than 170 to 180 seconds (for collagen/epinephrine reagents) and less than 110 to 120 seconds (for collagen/ADP reagents) are consistent with normal PLT function.[42]

The PFA-100 is arguably the most widely studied and used PLT function POC instrument in the world.[42] PFA-100 usage has been reported in a variety of clinical settings including, but not limited to, assessment of bleeding risk and transfusion therapy in cardiac surgery,[43,44] evaluation of the extent of PLT dysfunction in uremia,[45,46] screening and follow-up for patients with von Willebrand disease,[47,48] and evaluating the extent of PLT inhibition in patients taking anti-PLT agents such as aspirin and clopidogrel.[49–51] An excellent and extensive review of the myriad studies involving the PFA-100 was recently composed by Favaloro.[42]

The PFA-100 is highly advantageous in that it is an automated, whole blood–based system that reflects both adhesion and aggregation. As such, it is a useful screening tool for PLT function disorders and von Willebrand disease. In addition, the PLT flow aspects of PFA-100 analysis induce significant automated shear within the instrument leading to a more physiologically valid representation of PLT function.[31] The PFA-100 does have some drawbacks. Despite the automation of the system, there is a need for manual pipetting of whole blood into the reagent cartridges. Adhesion and aggregation are also dependent upon underlying PLT and RBCs, such that anemia (eg, hematocrit <30%) and/or thrombocytopenia (eg, PLT counts <100,000/μL) may result in prolongation of closure time even in patients with normal PLT function.[42,52,53] Additionally, the relationship between blood group O and decreased von Willebrand antigen levels also appears to correlate with prolonged closure times in healthy adults, a factor that should be considered in individuals with abnormal PFA-100 results.[54] Finally, as with the other POC tests, there is little specificity associated with prolongation of a closure time. Although this factor is generally advantageous for hemostasis screening, it adds a layer of complexity for the clinician interested solely in the evaluation of PLT-related bleeding disorders.

The cone and plate(let) platform (Impact Cone and Plate(let) Analyzer, DiaMed AG Corporation, Canton, Ohio) also assesses both adhesion and aggregation properties of PLTs but does so via an entirely unique format. In this system, whole blood aliquots are added to a plate coated with a thrombogenic extracellular matrix substrate and then are subsequently exposed to substantial shear (approximately 2000 s^{-1}) via a rotating Teflon cone.[55–57] The interaction between the thrombogenic plate surface and the shear serves to activate the PLTs, resulting in their adhesion and aggregation on the plate surface. After the activation process is completed, the plates are stained (typically with a May-Grünwald stain) and microscopically analyzed to determine the percentage of plate surface covered by PLT aggregates.[56,57] The percentage of surface covered correlates with PLT function.

Like other POC PLT function devices, most clinical studies of the cone and plate(let) platform have been performed to determine the efficacy anti-PLT regimens. Several studies have shown that this assay is useful to detect the degree of inhibition of PLTs in patients with acute coronary syndromes and predict needs for alternative intervention.[56,58–60] The cone and plate(let) platform is similar to the PFA-100 in that it provides insight into both the adhesive and aggregation properties of PLTs. As such, it is a better screen for patients with generalized hemostatic defects ranging from PLT dysfunction to von Willebrand disease. By inducing shear, cone and plate(let) testing best approximates the physiologic environment of the circulating PLT.[31] Despite these advantages, cone and plate(let) testing does share many of the same limitations of other POC analyzers including lack of specificity in diagnosing PLT disorders and the need for pipetting of whole blood onto the plate for analysis.[31]

Thromboelastography

Thromboelastography (TEG) exploits the viscoelastic properties of clotting whole blood to provide information about the integrity of the coagulation cascade (see Chapter by Teruya in this issue of Clinics).[61] TEG involves the mixture of whole blood and the prothrombotic reagent kaolin within an instrument cuvette.[61] As the liquid whole blood begins to solidify, a sensitive detector pin placed within the cuvette generates an electronic signal reflecting the strength and speed of clot formation, which is summarized on a graphical plot.[61] As such, TEG plots reflect the entirety of the process of clot formation by providing insight into both PLT function and coagulation factor activity. Recent modifications of the TEG platform have been made to specifically enhance its utility in assessing PLT dysfunction. A PLT mapping assay (TEG 5000 PlateletMapping Assay, Haemonetics, Braintree, Massachusetts) uses the PLT agonists ADP and arachidonic acid to reflect PLT contribution to clot formation.[31,61] As such, modified TEG can be better applied as a specific tool in the assessment of PLT dysfunction.

Standard, or unmodified, TEG has been used for many years in cardiac and hepatobiliary surgery. In this setting, it has shown to be efficacious in predicting the risk for bleeding and eliminating or diminishing unnecessary transfusions.[62–66] Uniquely for POC coagulation analyzers, TEG is also being explored as a means to predict the risk for development of thrombosis.[61] The specific application of TEG PLT mapping has thus far been most extensively evaluated to gauge an individual's response to anti-PLT agents like aspirin and clopidogrel.[61,67–69] Further studies are needed to define the role of PLT mapping in the diagnosis and management of acute bleeding.

TEG has many advantages over other coagulation analyzers in that it provides an assessment of the entirety of the coagulation system. Although this previously may have been considered a drawback in the evaluation of PLT-specific bleeding disorders, PLT mapping modifications may help to overcome this particular obstacle. In addition, like other POC instruments, whole blood is directly analyzed on TEG instruments, although pipetting of specimens is required. Limitations of TEG include a relatively slow turnaround time and a complicated data output tracing, both of which may restrict its use in the POC setting. The advent of a rapid TEG platform and automated interpretation of tracings could alleviate some of these concerns.[61] In addition, there are some reports of variability with validation and standardization of the instrument.[61] Unlike other POC platforms, the instrument is very sensitive to environmental disturbances and vibrations, a factor that can markedly influence results or invalidate test runs. As such, consideration must be given to anchoring the machine in an appropriate area of the laboratory and organizing the environment to avoid vibrational disturbances.

PLATELET TRANSFUSION THERAPY: UPDATE ON COMPONENTS

Once a patient has been diagnosed with either thrombocytopenia or a PLT dysfunction disorder, an important step in management is determining if PLT transfusion therapy is warranted. Commonly used PLT transfusion "trigger" guidelines, based primarily on PLT counts, are presented in **Table 3**.[70–72] Unfortunately, many of the currently accepted PLT count guidelines result from standard practice rather than evidence compiled from clinical studies. The results of ongoing trials will be very helpful in determining appropriate "transfusion triggers" for the prevention and treatment of PLT-related bleeding.[73]

Random-Donor Platelets

In addition to understanding when a PLT transfusion is warranted, it is equally important to appreciate the most appropriate transfusion product for a patient. Perhaps the most reliable distinction between PLT products is their collection method. One method to produce a PLT unit is via centrifugation of a whole blood donation. The whole blood unit is first placed into a soft spin to separate the PRP.[71] The PRP is then subjected to a harder spin to form the PLT pellet and PLT-poor plasma. Once the PLTs are separated, they are resuspended in approximately 50 mL of plasma to form a PLT concentrate.[71] Because transfusion of individual PLT concentrates would be inefficient for most adults, hospital-based blood banks typically combine 4 to 6 individual PLT units together to yield a "pool" of random-donor platelets.

Although pooling of PLT concentrates on-site at hospitals and blood banks has been the standard of practice for many years, a platform recently licensed by the Food and Drug Administration (FDA) allows for the pooling of up to six random PLT units before storage.[74,75] These prestorage-pooled PLT products are superior, in many ways, to PLTs pooled after storage. Most importantly, prestorage-pooled units are of sufficient volume to allow sampling for bacterial contamination by culture methods.[75] Septic transfusion reactions due to bacterial contamination of PLTs remain a significant problem for transfusion services.[76] In addition, prestorage-pooled products are convenient in that they do not require hospital-based blood banks to pool, test, or manipulate PLT units. This leads to a PLT product that can be more rapidly issued from the blood bank.[74]

Table 3
Platelet transfusion triggers

Indication for PLT Transfusion	Appropriate PLT Count Threshold Trigger	PLT Dose
Prophylactic transfusion to prevent spontaneous hemorrhage	≤10,000/μL	1 random-donor pool -or- 1 apheresis PLT
Minor invasive procedures[a]	≤ 20,000/μL -or- On anti-PLT therapy	1 random-donor pool -or- 1 apheresis PLT
Major invasive procedures[b]	≤ 50,000/μL -or- On anti-PLT therapy	1 random-donor pool -or- 1 apheresis PLT
Significant hemorrhage: WHO Grades 2–3[c]	≤ 50,000/μL -or- On anti-PLT therapy	1 random-donor pool -or- 1 apheresis PLT
Significant hemorrhage: WHO Grade 4[c]	≤ 100,000/μL -or- On anti-PLT therapy	1 to 2 random-donor pool -or- 1 to 2 apheresis PLT

Abbreviations: PLT, platelet; WHO, World Health Organization.
[a] Examples of minor invasive procedures include lumbar puncture. Bone marrow biopsies can be safely performed at counts <20,000/μL.[71,72]
[b] Examples of major invasive procedures include hepatic biopsy, paracentesis, thoracentesis, tooth extraction, central line or catheter insertion, and most major surgeries (non-neurological).[71,72,106] For major neurological surgeries, a PLT count threshold of >100,000/μL may be appropriate.
[c] Grade 2 hemorrhage on the WHO scale refers to clinically significant bleeding that does not require red blood cell transfusion; grade 3 hemorrhage refers to large blood loss requiring red cell transfusion; and grade 4 hemorrhage, in this setting, refers to an intracerebral or retinal bleed.

Apheresis (Single-Donor) Platelets

Although whole blood–derived PLTs were once the most frequent PLT product transfused in the United States, donations from apheresis volunteers are becoming vastly more prevalent. It is estimated that more than 80% of all transfused PLTs in the United States are derived from apheresis collection.[77] Much of the appeal of single-donor PLTs arises from the fact that two or three PLT doses from one donor can be collected as a result of advancements in apheresis technology. This is far superior to the individual PLT concentrate typically obtained from one whole-blood donation.

Apheresis PLTs offer other theoretical advantages. By definition, a single-donor PLT should cause fewer donor exposures overall, yielding a reduction in transfusion-transmitted diseases and leukocyte-induced HLA alloimmunization.[71] However, there is little evidence to suggest that apheresis PLTs are superior to pooled concentrates. The advent of modern nucleic acid testing has reduced infectious risks, whereas routine leukocyte filtration has significantly diminished the potential for alloimmunization. Currently, apheresis and random-donor PLTs are considered medically equivalent in almost all cases. If, however, an HLA-compatible donor is specifically donating for an HLA alloimmunized patient, then PLT collection via apheresis is clearly the product of choice.

Cryopreserved and Lyophilized Platelets

The short shelf life (about 5 days) of PLT components often results in problematic shortages for hospital-based transfusion services and blood banks. As such, several other pathways for PLT transfusion have been explored. The cryopreservation of PLTs is one such option. Traditionally, attempts at cold storage have been limited because PLTs exposed to cold temperatures are rapidly cleared upon infusion.[78] As such, cold PLT storage is not performed in the United States and cold-stored products are not licensed by the FDA; however, evidence that glycosylation of cold-stored PLTs may prevent their rapid clearance after infusion has renewed interest in pursuing cryopreserved PLT units.[78,79] At present, there are indications that glycosylation may not be entirely adequate to overcome the cold-storage lesion; recent data suggest that glycosylation does not adequately protect PLTs stored in the cold for greater than 48 hours.[80] As such, refinement of the glycosylation process and a greater number of studies involving long-term cold PLT storage are necessary before this product is available for clinical use in the United States.

An alternative to cold PLT storage is the provision of a freeze-dried, lyophilized PLT product. Several studies have shown that the lyophilization process, wherein PLTs are dehydrated and then rehydrated for use, can yield viable PLTs to participate in primary and secondary hemostasis.[81,82] In fact, efforts to produce a commercial lyophilized PLT product (Stasix, Entegrion Inc, Research Triangle Park, North Carolina) are currently under way.[83] In addition to helping to overcome PLT shortages, this type of product might also be useful as a tool in immune-mediated PLT refractoriness. It is conceivable that patients with a history of PLT alloimmunization could "bank" lyophilized PLTs when their counts are elevated and have them stored for subsequent use during future chemotherapy or other PLT-toxic therapies.

FUTURE GOALS AND DIRECTIONS: TARGETED PLATELET THERAPY IN HEMOSTASIS MANAGEMENT

In this article, we have summarized some of the latest technologies and platforms that can be used for PLT diagnostics. Included among these are assays designed to reflect PLT dysfunction in patients with otherwise normal PLT counts. We have also reviewed recent developments and advances in PLT transfusion therapy. It is evident that the increased ability of clinicians to detect PLT dysfunction can have an impact on guiding PLT transfusion therapy.[84–86] As such, it is our belief that the continued use of POC PLT function assays will lead to better and more accurate transfusion therapy by targeting patients with hemostatic abnormalities directly attributable to PLT inhibition.

Indeed, several small trials and studies have been published that have documented success in this approach to the bleeding patient. The largest number of studies correlating PLT function testing and PLT transfusion have been performed in the settings of cardiac and hepatobiliary surgery. Specifically, studies evaluating the use of TEG, cone and plate(let) testing, PFA-100, and SPC have demonstrated that routine use of PLT function tests can better identify patients at risk of postoperative bleeding.[43,49,65,66,87–94] Earlier identification of patients at risk for PLT-related bleeding has led to more aggressive transfusion management for these patients. In addition, for bleeding patients without evidence of PLT dysfunction, POC tests have been shown to reduce unnecessary transfusions in these groups. If no PLT dysfunction is evident, clinicians are prompted to investigate other causes of hemorrhage. This is yet another benefit of PLT function testing in the bleeding patient.

The reported uses of PLT function testing to guide transfusion therapy are more limited than in other clinical settings. Some of the conditions in which POC PLT function tests have been used to guide transfusion therapy and predict bleeding risks include massive trauma, traumatic brain injury, Bernard-Soulier syndrome, and patients with poor increases in PLT count post-transfusion.[95–101] To date, these studies have shown limited benefit of such testing. More clinical trials are necessary to clearly define the role of PLT function testing for bleeding encountered outside of the operating room.

In addition to potential uses in acute bleeding, others have championed the use of PLT function testing as a means to gauge the need for prophylactic PLT transfusion in critical care settings.[73,86] For instance, the question of when to transfuse the non-bleeding, thrombocytopenic neonate is complex with few clear guidelines.[72,102] In this setting, there is little evidence to suggest that prophylactic transfusion is of benefit, and some studies even suggest that unnecessary PLT transfusion actually leads to increased neonatal morbidity and mortality.[102,103] As such, some authors have advocated for the use of PLT function testing to determine the need for PLT transfusion in neonatal intensive care units.[104,105] One obvious limitation of such an approach is that many POC assays do not provide reliable results at very low PLT counts. However, as technology improves and new advances are made, it is likely that such an approach to prophylactic PLT transfusion will expand to other patient care arenas.

REFERENCES

1. Nachman RL, Rafii S. Platelets, petechiae, and preservation of the vascular wall. N Engl J Med 2008;359(12):1261–70.
2. Aronow HD, Steinhubl SR, Brennan DM, et al. Bleeding risk associated with 1 year of dual antiplatelet therapy after percutaneous coronary intervention: insights from the Clopidogrel for the Reduction of Events During Observation (CREDO) trial. Am Heart J 2009;157(2):369–74.
3. O'Riordan JM, Margey RJ, Blake G, et al. Antiplatelet agents in the perioperative period. Arch Surg 2009;144(1):69–76 [discussion: 76].
4. Tan VP, Yan BP, Kiernan TJ, et al. Risk and management of upper gastrointestinal bleeding associated with prolonged dual-antiplatelet therapy after percutaneous coronary intervention. Cardiovasc Revasc Med 2009;10(1):36–44.
5. Peterson P, Hayes TE, Arkin CF, et al. The preoperative bleeding time test lacks clinical benefit: College of American Pathologists' and American Society of Clinical Pathologists' position article. Arch Surg 1998;133(2):134–9.
6. Cariappa R, Wilhite TR, Parvin CA, et al. Comparison of PFA-100 and bleeding time testing in pediatric patients with suspected hemorrhagic problems. J Pediatr Hematol Oncol 2003;25(6):474–9.
7. Dempfle CE, Borggrefe M. Point of care coagulation tests in critically ill patients. Semin Thromb Hemost 2008;34(5):445–50.
8. Narimatsu H, Emi N, Kohno A, et al. High incidence of secondary failure of platelet recovery after autologous and syngeneic peripheral blood stem cell transplantation in acute promyelocytic leukemia. Bone Marrow Transplant 2007;40(8):773–8.
9. Selleng K, Selleng S, Greinacher A. Heparin-induced thrombocytopenia in intensive care patients. Semin Thromb Hemost 2008;34(5):425–38.
10. Kenney B, Stack G. Drug-induced thrombocytopenia. Arch Pathol Lab Med 2009;133(2):309–14.
11. Gernsheimer T. Epidemiology and pathophysiology of immune thrombocytopenic purpura. Eur J Haematol Suppl 2008;80:3–8.
12. Levy JH. Massive transfusion coagulopathy. Semin Hematol 2006;43(1 Suppl 1): S59–63.

13. De Luca G, Marino P. Antithrombotic therapies in primary angioplasty: rationale, results and future directions. Drugs 2008;68(16):2325–44.
14. Escolar G, Diaz-Ricart M, Cases A. Uremic platelet dysfunction: past and present. Curr Hematol Rep 2005;4(5):359–67.
15. Peyvandi F, Cattaneo M, Inbal A, et al. Rare bleeding disorders. Haemophilia 2008;14(Suppl 3):202–10.
16. Briggs C, Harrison P, Machin SJ. Continuing developments with the automated platelet count. Int J Lab Hematol 2007;29(2):77–91.
17. Lehto T, Hedberg P. Performance evaluation of Abbott CELL-DYN Ruby for routine use. Int J Lab Hematol 2008;30(5):400–7.
18. Ault KA, Rinder HM, Mitchell J, et al. The significance of platelets with increased RNA content (reticulated platelets). A measure of the rate of thrombopoiesis. Am J Clin Pathol 1992;98(6):637–46.
19. Salvagno GL, Montagnana M, Degan M, et al. Evaluation of platelet turnover by flow cytometry. Platelets 2006;17(3):170–7.
20. Rinder HM, Munz UJ, Ault KA, et al. Reticulated platelets in the evaluation of thrombopoietic disorders. Arch Pathol Lab Med 1993;117(6):606–10.
21. Monteagudo M, Amengual MJ, Munoz L, et al. Reticulated platelets as a screening test to identify thrombocytopenia aetiology. QJM 2008;101(7):549–55.
22. Michur H, Maslanka K, Szczepinski A, et al. Reticulated platelets as a marker of platelet recovery after allogeneic stem cell transplantation. Int J Lab Hematol 2008;30(6):519–25.
23. Guthikonda S, Alviar CL, Vaduganathan M, et al. Role of reticulated platelets and platelet size heterogeneity on platelet activity after dual antiplatelet therapy with aspirin and clopidogrel in patients with stable coronary artery disease. J Am Coll Cardiol 2008;52(9):743–9.
24. Cesari F, Marcucci R, Caporale R, et al. Relationship between high platelet turn-over and platelet function in high-risk patients with coronary artery disease on dual antiplatelet therapy. Thromb Haemost 2008;99(5):930–5.
25. Kayahan H, Akarsu M, Ozcan MA, et al. Reticulated platelet levels in patients with ulcerative colitis. Int J Colorectal Dis 2007;22(12):1429–35.
26. Shah U, Ma AD. Tests of platelet function. Curr Opin Hematol 2007;14(5):432–7.
27. Mengistu AM, Mayer J, Boldt J, et al. Whole-blood aggregometry: are there any limits with regard to platelet counts? Acta Anaesthesiol Scand 2009; 53(1):72–6.
28. Podczasy JJ, Lee J, Vucenik I. Evaluation of whole-blood lumiaggregation. Clin Appl Thromb Hemost 1997;3:190–5.
29. Falcon C, Arnout J, Vermylen J. Platelet aggregation in whole blood—studies with a platelet counting technique—methodological aspects and some applications. Thromb Haemost 1989;61(3):423–8.
30. Michelson AD, Frelinger AL 3rd, Furman MI. Current options in platelet function testing. Am J Cardiol 2006;98(10A):4N–10N.
31. Michelson AD. Methods for the measurement of platelet function. Am J Cardiol 2009;103(3 Suppl):20A–6A.
32. Siotia A, Buckland R, Judge HM, et al. Utility of a whole blood single platelet counting assay to monitor the effects of tirofiban in patients with acute coronary syndromes scheduled for coronary intervention. Thromb Haemost 2006;95(6): 997–1002.
33. Akowuah E, Shrivastava V, Jamnadas B, et al. Comparison of two strategies for the management of antiplatelet therapy during urgent surgery. Ann Thorac Surg 2005;80(1):149–52.

34. Campbell J, Ridgway H, Carville D. Plateletworks: a novel point of care platelet function screen. Mol Diagn Ther 2008;12(4):253–8.
35. Mobley JE, Bresee SJ, Wortham DC, et al. Frequency of nonresponse antiplatelet activity of clopidogrel during pretreatment for cardiac catheterization. Am J Cardiol 2004;93(4):456–8.
36. VerifyNow Instructions For Use (Accumetrics SD, CA) [package insert]. 2008.
37. Marcucci R, Gori AM, Paniccia R, et al. Cardiovascular death and nonfatal myocardial infarction in acute coronary syndrome patients receiving coronary stenting are predicted by residual platelet reactivity to ADP detected by a point-of-care assay: a 12-month follow-up. Circulation 2009;119(2):237–42.
38. Saw J, Madsen EH, Chan S, et al. The ELAPSE (Evaluation of Long-Term Clopidogrel Antiplatelet and Systemic Anti-Inflammatory Effects) study. J Am Coll Cardiol 2008;52(23):1826–33.
39. van Werkum JW, Harmsze AM, Elsenberg EH, et al. The use of the VerifyNow system to monitor antiplatelet therapy: a review of the current evidence. Platelets 2008;19(7):479–88.
40. Jilma B. Platelet function analyzer (PFA-100): a tool to quantify congenital or acquired platelet dysfunction. J Lab Clin Med 2001;138(3):152–63.
41. Kundu SK, Heilmann EJ, Sio R, et al. Description of an in vitro platelet function analyzer—PFA-100. Semin Thromb Hemost 1995;21(Suppl 2):106–12.
42. Favaloro EJ. Clinical utility of the PFA-100. Semin Thromb Hemost 2008;34(8): 709–33.
43. Wahba A, Sander S, Birnbaum DE. Are in-vitro platelet function tests useful in predicting blood loss following open heart surgery? Thorac Cardiovasc Surg 1998;46(4):228–31.
44. Lasne D, Fiemeyer A, Chatellier G, et al. A study of platelet functions with a new analyzer using high shear stress (PFA 100) in patients undergoing coronary artery bypass graft. Thromb Haemost 2000;84(5):794–9.
45. Escolar G, Cases A, Vinas M, et al. Evaluation of acquired platelet dysfunctions in uremic and cirrhotic patients using the platelet function analyzer (PFA-100): influence of hematocrit elevation. Haematologica 1999;84(7):614–9.
46. Ho SJ, Gemmell R, Brighton TA. Platelet function testing in uraemic patients. Hematology 2008;13(1):49–58.
47. Dean JA, Blanchette VS, Carcao MD, et al. von Willebrand disease in a pediatric-based population—comparison of type 1 diagnostic criteria and use of the PFA-100 and a von Willebrand factor/collagen-binding assay. Thromb Haemost 2000;84(3):401–9.
48. van Vliet HH, Kappers-Klunne MC, Leebeek FW, et al. PFA-100 monitoring of von Willebrand factor (VWF) responses to desmopressin (DDAVP) and factor VIII/VWF concentrate substitution in von Willebrand disease type 1 and 2. Thromb Haemost 2008;100(3):462–8.
49. Bevilacqua S, Alkodami AA, Volpi E, et al. Risk stratification after coronary artery bypass surgery by a point-of-care test of platelet function. Ann Thorac Surg 2009;87(2):496–502.
50. Mueller T, Dieplinger B, Poelz W, et al. Utility of the PFA-100 instrument and the novel multiplate analyzer for the assessment of aspirin and clopidogrel effects on platelet function in patients with cardiovascular disease. Clin Appl Thromb Hemost 2008; in press.
51. Crescente M, Di Castelnuovo A, Iacoviello L, et al. Response variability to aspirin as assessed by the platelet function analyzer (PFA)-100. A systematic review. Thromb Haemost 2008;99(1):14–26.

52. Ortel TL, James AH, Thames EH, et al. Assessment of primary hemostasis by PFA-100 analysis in a tertiary care center. Thromb Haemost 2000;84(1):93–7.
53. Eugster M, Reinhart WH. The influence of the haematocrit on primary haemostasis in vitro. Thromb Haemost 2005;94(6):1213–8.
54. Haubelt H, Anders C, Vogt A, et al. Variables influencing Platelet Function Analyzer-100 closure times in healthy individuals. Br J Haematol 2005;130(5): 759–67.
55. Savion N, Varon D. Impact—the cone and plate(let) analyzer: testing platelet function and anti-platelet drug response. Pathophysiol Haemost Thromb 2006; 35(1-2):83–8.
56. Spectre G, Brill A, Gural A, et al. A new point-of-care method for monitoring anti-platelet therapy: application of the cone and plate(let) analyzer. Platelets 2005; 16(5):293–9.
57. Varon D, Dardik R, Shenkman B, et al. A new method for quantitative analysis of whole blood platelet interaction with extracellular matrix under flow conditions. Thromb Res 1997;85(4):283–94.
58. Shenkman B, Matetzky S, Fefer P, et al. Variable responsiveness to clopidogrel and aspirin among patients with acute coronary syndrome as assessed by platelet function tests. Thromb Res 2008;122(3):336–45.
59. Lev EI, Osende JI, Richard MF, et al. Administration of abciximab to patients receiving tirofiban or eptifibatide: effect on platelet function. J Am Coll Cardiol 2001;37(3):847–55.
60. Shenkman B, Schneiderman J, Tamarin I, et al. Testing the effect of GPIIb-IIIa antagonist in patients undergoing carotid stenting: correlation between standard aggregometry, flow cytometry and the cone and plate(let) analyzer (CPA) methods. Thromb Res 2001;102(4):311–7.
61. Hobson AR, Agarwala RA, Swallow RA, et al. Thrombelastography: current clinical applications and its potential role in interventional cardiology. Platelets 2006; 17(8):509–18.
62. Luddington RJ. Thrombelastography/thromboelastometry. Clin Lab Haematol 2005;27(2):81–90.
63. Ewe K. Bleeding after liver biopsy does not correlate with indices of peripheral coagulation. Dig Dis Sci 1981;26(5):388–93.
64. Dorman BH, Spinale FG, Bailey MK, et al. Identification of patients at risk for excessive blood loss during coronary artery bypass surgery: thromboelastography versus coagulation screen. Anesth Analg 1993;76(4):694–700.
65. Shore-Lesserson L, Manspeizer HE, DePerio M, et al. Thromboelastography-guided transfusion algorithm reduces transfusions in complex cardiac surgery. Anesth Analg 1999;88(2):312–9.
66. Kang Y. Transfusion based on clinical coagulation monitoring does reduce hemorrhage during liver transplantation. Liver Transpl Surg 1997;3(6):655–9.
67. Lev EI, Ramchandani M, Garg R, et al. Response to aspirin and clopidogrel in patients scheduled to undergo cardiovascular surgery. J Thromb Thrombolysis 2007;24(1):15–21.
68. Tantry US, Bliden KP, Gurbel PA. Overestimation of platelet aspirin resistance detection by thrombelastograph platelet mapping and validation by conventional aggregometry using arachidonic acid stimulation. J Am Coll Cardiol 2005;46(9):1705–9.
69. Swallow RA, Agarwala RA, Dawkins KD, et al. Thromboelastography: potential bedside tool to assess the effects of antiplatelet therapy? Platelets 2006;17(6): 385–92.

70. Slichter SJ. Evidence-based platelet transfusion guidelines. Hematology Am Soc Hematol Educ Program 2007;2007:172–8.
71. Slichter SJ. Platelet transfusion therapy. Hematol Oncol Clin North Am 2007; 21(4):697–729, vii.
72. Rebulla P. Platelet transfusion trigger in difficult patients. Transfus Clin Biol 2001; 8(3):249–54.
73. Blajchman MA, Slichter SJ, Heddle NM, et al. New strategies for the optimal use of platelet transfusions. Hematology Am Soc Hematol Educ Program 2008;2008: 198–204.
74. Vassallo RR, Murphy S. A critical comparison of platelet preparation methods. Curr Opin Hematol 2006;13(5):323–30.
75. Heddle NM, Barty RL, Sigouin CS, et al. In vitro evaluation of prestorage pooled leukoreduced whole blood-derived platelets stored for up to 7 days. Transfusion 2005;45(6):904–10.
76. Dodd RY. Bacterial contamination and transfusion safety: experience in the United States. Transfus Clin Biol 2003;10(1):6–9.
77. The 2007 National Blood Collection and Utilization Survey Report. 2007. Available at: http://www.hhs.gov/ophs/bloodsafety/2007nbcus_survey.pdf. Accessed February 22, 2009.
78. Jhang JS, Spitalnik SL. Glycosylation and cold platelet storage. Curr Hematol Rep 2005;4(6):483–7.
79. Hoffmeister KM, Josefsson EC, Isaac NA, et al. Glycosylation restores survival of chilled blood platelets. Science 2003;301(5639):1531–4.
80. Wandall HH, Hoffmeister KM, Sorensen AL, et al. Galactosylation does not prevent the rapid clearance of long-term, 4 degrees C-stored platelets. Blood 2008;111(6):3249–56.
81. Read MS, Reddick RL, Bode AP, et al. Preservation of hemostatic and structural properties of rehydrated lyophilized platelets: potential for long-term storage of dried platelets for transfusion. Proc Natl Acad Sci U S A 1995;92(2):397–401.
82. Fischer TH, Bode AP, Parker BR, et al. Primary and secondary hemostatic functionalities of rehydrated, lyophilized platelets. Transfusion 2006;46(11):1943–50.
83. Bode AP, Fischer TH. Lyophilized platelets: fifty years in the making. Artif Cells Blood Substit Immobil Biotechnol 2007;35(1):125–33.
84. Dickinson KJ, Troxler M, Homer-Vanniasinkam S. The surgical application of point-of-care haemostasis and platelet function testing. Br J Surg 2008;95(11):1317–30.
85. Despotis GJ, Goodnough LT. Management approaches to platelet-related microvascular bleeding in cardiothoracic surgery. Ann Thorac Surg 2000;70 (2 Suppl):S20–32.
86. Sweeney JD. The blood bank physician as a hemostasis consultant. Transfus Apher Sci 2008;39(2):145–50.
87. Gerrah R, Brill A, Tshori S, et al. Using cone and plate(let) analyzer to predict bleeding in cardiac surgery. Asian Cardiovasc Thorac Ann 2006;14(4):310–5.
88. Cammerer U, Dietrich W, Rampf T, et al. The predictive value of modified computerized thromboelastography and platelet function analysis for postoperative blood loss in routine cardiac surgery. Anesth Analg 2003;96(1):51–7, table of contents.
89. Avidan MS, Alcock EL, Da Fonseca J, et al. Comparison of structured use of routine laboratory tests or near-patient assessment with clinical judgement in the management of bleeding after cardiac surgery. Br J Anaesth 2004;92(2): 178–86.

90. Shaffer KE, Pearman DT, Galen RS, et al. A rapid platelet function assay used to regulate platelet transfusion prophylaxis following cardiopulmonary bypass surgery. J Extra Corpor Technol 2004;36(2):145–8.

91. Rahe-Meyer N, Winterhalter M, Boden A, et al. Platelet concentrates transfusion in cardiac surgery and platelet function assessment by multiple electrode aggregometry. Acta Anaesthesiol Scand 2009;53(2):168–75.

92. Gerrah R, Snir E, Brill A, et al. Platelet function changes as monitored by cone and plate(let) analyzer during beating heart surgery. Heart Surg Forum 2004; 7(3):E191–5.

93. Coakley M, Reddy K, Mackie I, et al. Transfusion triggers in orthotopic liver transplantation: a comparison of the thromboelastometry analyzer, the thromboelastogram, and conventional coagulation tests. J Cardiothorac Vasc Anesth 2006;20(4):548–53.

94. Ranucci M, Nano G, Pazzaglia A, et al. Platelet mapping and desmopressin reversal of platelet inhibition during emergency carotid endarterectomy. J Cardiothorac Vasc Anesth 2007;21(6):851–4.

95. Panzer S, Eichelberger B, Koren D, et al. Monitoring survival and function of transfused platelets in Bernard-Soulier syndrome by flow cytometry and a cone and plate(let) analyzer (Impact-R). Transfusion 2007;47(1):103–6.

96. Carr ME Jr. Monitoring of hemostasis in combat trauma patients. Mil Med 2004; 169(12 Suppl):11–5, 14.

97. Salama ME, Raman S, Drew MJ, et al. Platelet function testing to assess effectiveness of platelet transfusion therapy. Transfus Apher Sci 2004;30(2):93–100.

98. Hardy JF, de Moerloose P, Samama CM. Massive transfusion and coagulopathy: pathophysiology and implications for clinical management. Can J Anaesth 2006; 53(6 Suppl):S40–58.

99. Nekludov M, Bellander BM, Blomback M, et al. Platelet dysfunction in patients with severe traumatic brain injury. J Neurotrauma 2007;24(11):1699–706.

100. Kaufmann CR, Dwyer KM, Crews JD, et al. Usefulness of thrombelastography in assessment of trauma patient coagulation. J Trauma 1997;42(4):716–20 [discussion: 720–2].

101. Geeraedts LM Jr, Kaasjager HA, van Vugt AB, et al. Exsanguination in trauma: a review of diagnostics and treatment options. Injury 2009;40(1):11–20.

102. Roberts I, Stanworth S, Murray NA. Thrombocytopenia in the neonate. Blood Rev 2008;22(4):173–86.

103. Baer VL, Lambert DK, Henry E, et al. Do platelet transfusions in the NICU adversely affect survival? Analysis of 1600 thrombocytopenic neonates in a multihospital healthcare system. J Perinatol 2007;27(12):790–6.

104. Christensen RD, Paul DA, Sola-Visner MC, et al. Improving platelet transfusion practices in the neonatal intensive care unit. Transfusion 2008;48(11):2281–4.

105. Christensen RD. Advances and controversies in neonatal ICU platelet transfusion practice. Adv Pediatr 2008;55:255–69.

106. McVay PA, Toy PT. Lack of increased bleeding after paracentesis and thoracentesis in patients with mild coagulation abnormalities. Transfusion 1991;31(2): 164–71.

Laboratory Testing for von Willebrand Disease: Toward a Mechanism-Based Classification

Richard Torres, MD, MS[a,b,*], Yuri Fedoriw, MD[c]

KEYWORDS

- von Willebrand factor • von Willebrand disease
- Laboratory testing • Methods • Mechanisms • Classification

Nearly 85 years since von Willebrand disease (vWD) was first described, aspects of the definition and classification of the disorder remain a work in progress. The disease is widely regarded as being the most commonly inherited coagulation disorder, with a global prevalence of up to one person per 10,000. Physicians have long identified a wide variability in the severity and natural history of vWD.[1] Currently, aspects of the framework for vWD categorization are being reorganized in light of the observed clinical heterogeneity, driven by an increasing understanding of the genetic basis for the molecular mechanisms that underlie the disease. Part of the importance of improving diagnostic precision lies in our limited ability to accurately predict the risk of bleeding of individuals affected by the disorder. This fact is particularly true for patients with borderline values of von Willebrand factor antigen (vWF:Ag) levels, most of whom fall within the current category of Type 1 vWD. Subcategories have long been recognized, but physicians and surgeons continue to struggle with the uncertainties of bleeding risk in a whole host of patients, which may lead to delayed procedures and inadequate or unnecessary therapy. With a broader perspective on vWF, we may consider that a more complete understanding of the pathophysiology of vWD and the further development of laboratory assessment of vWF function are

[a] Department of Laboratory Medicine, Yale School of Medicine, 333 Cedar Street, P.O. Box 208035, New Haven, CT 06520-8035, USA
[b] Department of Biomedical Engineering, Yale University School of Engineering and Applied Science, 55 Prospect Street, New Haven, CT 06511, USA
[c] Department of Pathology and Laboratory Medicine, CB# 7525, 101 Manning Drive, University of North Carolina, Chapel Hill, NC 27599-7525, USA
* Corresponding author. Department of Laboratory Medicine, Yale School of Medicine, P.O. Box 208035, New Haven, CT 06520-8035.
E-mail address: richard.torres@yale.edu (R. Torres).

Clin Lab Med 29 (2009) 193–228
doi:10.1016/j.cll.2009.06.005
0272-2712/09/$ – see front matter © 2009 Elsevier Inc. All rights reserved.

important in the management of patients with common clinical conditions, many of which result in vWF abnormalities and abnormal coagulation.

Our difficulties predicting the risk of bleeding stem largely from limitations of modern laboratory techniques. Although invaluable in the diagnosis of vWD, typical vWD laboratory tests have problems with standardization, reproducibility, and temporal variability. These difficulties, coupled with the diversity of abnormalities that are inherent to the disease, have contributed to a vast literature with sometimes conflicting results and created significant confusion. The research use of molecular testing has been able to address some of the issues of ambiguity in diagnosis and is helping to elucidate genetic abnormalities at the root of vWD. Molecular diagnosis is shedding light into subclasses of the disease that had been anticipated and, as in other areas of medicine, may be close to becoming the definition of specific disease types. However, gene properties and the sheer number of genetic abnormalities associated with vWD have impaired our ability to develop a simple and practical molecular classification. Through the painstaking process of genotypic/phenotypic correlation and the further characterization of bleeding risk, we can begin to fine-tune our diagnostic approach to maximize the clinical utility and begin to develop a more complete view of the mechanistic and genetic basis for abnormalities in vWF.

PHYSIOLOGY OF VON WILLEBRAND FACTOR
von Willebrand Factor Form and Function

A mechanistic description of the pathology of vWD requires knowledge of the role of vWF in coagulation and the structural basis for its function. This role can be described from a conceptual point of view as a form of mechanochemical transducer converting vascular damage into activation of coagulation. In simple terms, the process begins with damage to endothelial cells exposing underlying collagen (**Fig. 1**). Because vWF exists in circulation as a multimer of vWF dimers, it has the flexibility to form extended string-like forms when subjected to high shear rates (approximately > 2000/s).[2,3] The vWF becomes anchored to the subendothelial collagen, and this large multimer is twisted and stretched by shear stresses from the overlying flowing blood. In the laminar flow profile of blood, red blood cells tend to be more concentrated in the central portion of vessels, pushing platelets toward the margins. This allows extended vWF to reach out and grab flowing platelets, taking hold of platelet membrane glycoprotein Ibα (GPIbα) molecules through the vWF-A1 domain. The GPIbα interaction has a relatively high rate of turnover, which allows the platelet to essentially roll from vWF molecule to vWF molecule.[4] The tethered platelet can become stabilized by stronger binding to vWF and coming into direct contact with the subendothelial collagen through activated receptors α2β1 integrin and glycoprotein GPVI.[5] The binding process then results in a conformational change on the important glycoprotein GPIIb/IIIa (also known as integrin αIIbβ3), allowing further binding to vWF and fibrinogen.[6] The resulting chain reaction of continued platelet and coagulation factor cascade activation culminates in thrombin production, fibrinogen splitting, and the formation of a platelet/fibrin clot. vWF also participates in these other steps by serving as the carrier protein of the essential coagulation protein factor VIII. Through its binding of factor VIII, vWF acts as a "fight ready" clotting factor reserve that can be made available quickly at a site of injury. Although there is a buffering aspect to this factor VIII binding, the vWF role as a factor VIII carrier is predominantly passive.

From Gene to Protein

The gene structure of vWF is relevant in terms of molecular characterization of the disease and explaining the difficulties associated with developing genetic testing for

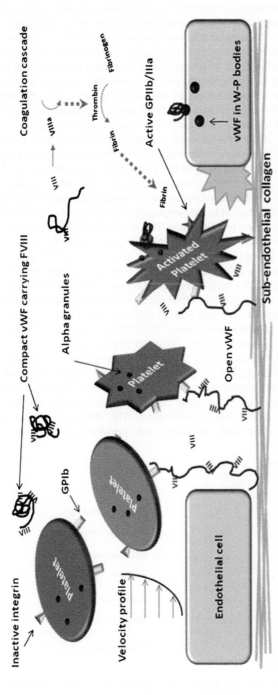

Fig. 1. Overview of vWF function. Circulating inactive platelets are loosely trapped by collagen-bound vWF that has stretched in response to the shear stresses at endothelial cell injury sites. The platelets roll atop vWF molecules and undergo shape-change and activation, which allows the platelets to bind collagen directly through integrins. The factor VIII carried on vWF can then interact with the coagulation cascade to promote the generation of thrombin and eventually fibrin strands. The newly formed fibrin can then crosslink platelets through the activated GPIIb/IIIa receptor, forming the basis for a platelet-fibrin clot.

screening and diagnosis. Located on chromosome 12p13, the vWF gene is large—spanning 178 kb and consisting of 52 separately expressed regions. The vWF gene product (2813 amino acids) is composed of a 22 amino acid signal prepeptide and a 741 amino acid propeptide (vWFpp) located at the N-terminus of the mature 2050 amino acid vWF subunit. Frequent and nonrandomly distributed cysteine residues provide anchors for dimerization later in processing. The pro-vWF, composed of the vWFpp and mature vWF subunit, is arranged into structural domains with sequence and functional homology to well-characterized protein motifs. They are labeled linearly as D1-D2-D′-D3-A1-A2-A3-D4-B1-B2-B3-C1-C2-CK (**Fig. 2**). The multifaceted functions of the mature vWF can be attributed to these structural domains, and mutations within these conserved regions often explain the observed phenotypes.

vWF is synthesized in endothelial cells and megakaryocytes in a process that includes extensive postsynthesis modification.[7,8] After directed transport to the endoplasmic reticulum, there is uncoupling of the prepeptide signal sequence and initial glycosylation. The propeptide chaperones dimerization of the vWF subunits through disulfide bonds within the C-terminal CK-domain.[9] The glycosylation and dimerization precede the subsequent transport to the Golgi apparatus and linkage of the dimers via disulfide bonds near the amino terminal ends. This process yields a distribution of vWF multimers, primarily composed of the largest molecules, including some with more than 40 dimers and a molecular weight of more than 20 MDa.[10,11] vWF is further sulfated and glycosylated within the Golgi. The propeptide is removed during the dimerization process within the trans-Golgi compartment, remains loosely associated to the assembled vWF, and along with other microenvironmental factors (such as pH) is responsible for storage of vWF into platelet alpha granules and the Golgi-derived Weibel-Palade bodies of endothelial cells.[12] The vWFpp, permanently dissociated from mature vWF after secretion, is also released into circulation in a 1:1 ratio with each vWF monomer. A relatively short half-life (2 hours) contributes to a circulating concentration one-tenth that of multimerized vWF (1 μg/mL versus 10 μg/mL).[13,14]

Constitutive and secretagogue-dependent vWF release pathways have been extensively studied, but the precise signaling cascade mediating the distribution and trafficking of vWF is incompletely understood. The Weibel-Palade bodies are regulated storage vesicles and, as such, are convincingly implicated in the

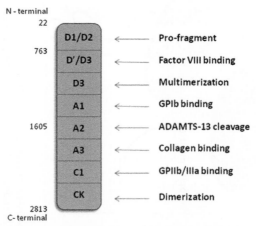

Fig. 2. The domains of vWF protein. Motifs correspond to specific vWF functions. The pre-vWF fragment is not shown (1–22), but the current standard amino acid naming convention begins at the first portion of the prepeptide.

secretagogue-dependent release. Recent evidence also points to steady state, delayed, basal secretion through Weibel-Palade bodies to be the primary means of vWF release into the circulation.[15] Megakaryocytes are not believed to contribute significantly to this steady-state vWF level and platelet vWF in alpha granules is mainly of low multimer number.[16] A significant reserve is present in endothelial cells and the secretagogue-mediated granule exocytosis releases multimers that are larger and more biologically active than those released via the constitutive pathway.

Population-based reference ranges for plasma vWF are broad, and individual subjects show considerable variability on repeat testing because of the complex genetic and environmental factors regulating expression of vWF.[17] Within the normal population without a bleeding diathesis and wild type vWF gene, blood type is the single most important qualifier of baseline vWF. vWF release, however, contributes only part of the "steady state" vWF level and multimer distribution.

von Willebrand Factor Multimers, Degradation, and ADAMTS-13

The largest mature vWF multimeric structures have the capability to extend to 2 μm, making it the largest human plasma protein, but it is further modified as it enters the circulation. Initially secreted as ultra-large multimers reaching 80 monomers large, the metalloproteinase ADAMTS-13 cleaves these molecules at a specific amino-acid junction (Y^{1605}-M^{1606}) in the A2 portion of any of the exposed units. It produces a distribution of multimers down to dimer form with a molecular weight of 556 kD. ADAMTS-13 has received a great deal of attention lately with the recognition that antibody-mediated inhibition of this protein is the cause of nonfamilial thrombotic thrombocytopenia purpura (TTP). Diagnostic tests to assess its activity and its inhibitors have evolved. In normal patients, the higher functionality of larger multimers likely relates to an increased ability to extend under shear stresses and longer reach available for platelet trapping. Degraded products are removed from circulation via as-yet-unclear mechanisms, but it seems to be related to the expression of H antigens on the multimers and is independent of multimer size.[18] Intermediate degradation products correspond to dim bands that appear between bright bands in intermediate- or high-resolution gel electrophoresis (see the section on multimer analysis; **Fig. 3**). The net distribution of multimers achieves a "steady state" when the balance of synthesis, secretion, degradation, and removal is reached. The relative kinetic rates of these steps define the total concentration and relative distribution of vWF multimers in peripheral blood. Normally, the distribution is such that most vWF dimers exist in intermediate multimer form. Alterations in any of these steps lead to the range of multimer abnormalities detected on gel electrophoresis.

Response to Desmopressin

Endothelial cells are the specific source of rapid increases in vWF in response to the therapeutic agent desmopressin (DDAVP). DDAVP is a vasopressin analog that stimulates secretion of vWF, vWFpp, and factor VIII, apparently through a V2-receptor and cAMP mediated activation of endothelial cells.[19] It is often used as a diagnostic/therapy-evaluation tool. A standard challenge protocol involves a baseline measure of vWF:Ag and vWF:ristocetin cofactor (RCof) and/or vWF:collagen binding (CB) levels, with a measure of the same tests 1 hour after infusion of 0.3 μg/kg body weight of DDAVP. A 4-hour measure is sometimes also obtained for clearer determination of half-life. Therapeutically, similar levels are used. Most (but not all) type 1 patients respond with normalization of levels of all tests at 1 hour. Few type 2 and no type 3 patients normalize. Some type 1 patients respond with supranormal levels of antigen and activity. Other type 1 patients have partial responses; at the Yale-New Haven

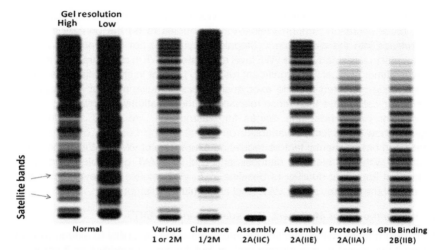

Fig. 3. Schematic representation of representative vWF multimer gels. Low-resolution gels show a distribution of multimers and are able to resolve broad patterns of small, intermediate, and large multimers. Higher resolution gels are needed to visualize satellite bands representing degradation products and flank main multimers. Various patterns are characterized predominantly by the main features of total intensity, distribution of sizes, and abnormalities of the satellite bands corresponding to different molecular mechanisms as discussed in the text.

Hospital laboratory, we consider 1-hour post-DDAVP levels that remain less than 75 IU/dL as a suboptimal response. Levels that remain less than 50 IU/dL we deem as abnormal responses, which may correspond to type 2 and type 3 patients. The weakly responsive type 1 patients also may require factor replacement therapy to prevent more serious bleeding complications with even minor trauma. These findings usually indicate characteristic molecular abnormalities (see later discussion). Although the DDAVP challenge is generally considered to be safe, there is significant cost and it is not without risks; hence, attempts at developing alternative methods for identification of nonresponders, such as the vWF propeptide to vWF antigen ratio and spectroscopic multimer measurements, which are discussed in the laboratory testing section.

VON WILLEBRAND'S DISEASE CLASSIFICATION: CONCEPT EVOLUTION

Excessive bleeding with minor trauma is one of the principal presenting symptoms of von Willebrand disease of all types. The severity and initial presentation, however, are highly variable, reflecting the broad pathophysiologic heterogeneity. Inherited forms with strong penetrance and forms with severe symptoms are more easily recognized. Even von Willebrand himself, aside from describing clinical and genetic characteristics that make vWD distinct from hemophilia A, noted the variability in clinical behavior within the broader disease category. As with any diagnostic evaluation, the goal in investigating a chief complaint of excessive bleeding is disease classification as a means to better predict the natural history of—corresponding to the need for and potential effect of— therapeutic intervention. An early formal attempt at classification in vWD was published in 1987 by Ruggeri and Zimmerman.[20] It used the traditional three-category system: initially designated by roman numerals and limited to just type I (partial quantitative deficiency and type II) qualitative deficiencies, with the subsequent addition of a type III (absence of vWF protein). The classification originated from the compilation of published reports of vWD variants as characterized mainly by patterns on agarose gel electrophoresis. This initial effort was a great step forward in disease classification but had significant drawbacks, primarily that new variants were quickly identified that did not fit well within categories and that the complexity was such that it became unwieldy for practicing physicians. These problems were compounded by the difficulties associated with gel electrophoresis, which made it (and to a large degree still do) impractical as a routine diagnostic test. It illustrates the early recognition that the three subtype classification system is a gross simplification of the variety of disease mechanisms.

With the further development of ristocetin-based functional tests for vWD and to address the limitations of the 1987 effort, a new classification was published in 1994 by Sadler[21] that simplified the categorization into the three main types and four type 2 subcategories: 2A, 2B, 2N, and 2M, all of which are still in use. Type 1 and type 2 vWD and the subtypes were determined on the basis of total vWF antigenic level (vWF:Ag) and ratios of vWF:Ag to vWF:RCof and low-resolution gel electrophoresis patterns. The conceptual framework is that the principal clinically important distinctions to be made are overall risk of bleeding and responsiveness to DDAVP. Most cases of vWD are mild forms that tend to have mild to moderately decreased antigen levels, proportionally decreased RCof activity levels, a normal distribution of multimers, and good response to therapeutic administration of DDAVP. These "type 1" cases should be distinguished from the more severe type 2A cases that generally have disproportionately low activity levels corresponding to lack of more functionally active large multimers. Types 2B, 2N, and 2M represent special cases with the specific mechanisms of increased binding to GPIb on platelets, impaired factor VIII binding mimicking hemophilia, and impaired binding to GPIb, respectively. Severe cases of vWD fall into the "type 3" category, which manifest as nearly complete absence of vWF. Outside this simplified framework lies pseudo-vWD, which represents a defect in the GPIb molecule on the platelets rather than on the vWF protein, and acquired vWD, which results from antibody formation directed toward the multimeric protein and other mechanisms related to increased clearance. The originally designated Vincenza type of vWD, characterized by increased clearance of multimers, has been variably classified as type 1 and type 2M.

This simplified scheme has survived for 15 years with minor adjustments described in a 2006 update from the Working Party on vWD Classification of the International Society on Thrombosis and Haemostasis, which maintained the categories as defined in 1994 but broadened the definition of type 1 to include small abnormalities in multimer patterns and eliminated the restriction to mutations in the vWF gene.[22] In practical terms, this allows for the clinical designation of type 1 vWD in patients with a history of excessive bleeding and low vWF for whatever combination of reasons. Limitations remain. An important aspect is the heterogeneity in mechanism, bleeding risk, and DDAVP responsiveness of cases labeled as type 1, type 2A, and type 2M. Another is the demarcation between individuals with low but hemostatic levels of vWF and individuals with true type 1 vWD. As molecular information gets correlated with the various subtypes described, additional clues are acquired that can help us further stratify risk and responsiveness. What is certainly becoming clear is that multiple factors contribute to overall bleeding risk in vWD.

LABORATORY TESTING METHODS

Identifying methods to accurately and reproducibly monitor vWF activity and stratify bleeding risk has been a primary goal of clinical laboratory testing and research for decades. Reproducing the complexity and in vivo requirements of vWF-mediated coagulation in the laboratory has been a stumbling block for accurate diagnosis and classification, however. Many of the testing assays and platforms depend on nonphysiologic intermediaries that can somewhat effectively recapitulate portions of the in vivo microenvironment. Although the current phenotypic working classification is not tied to specific testing platforms, a discrete panel of readily available assays usually can discriminate between the broad subtypes of vWD. These classic assays, including vWF antigen (vWF:Ag), vWF activity (vWF:RCof), and factor VIII, also enjoy the added benefit of uniform sample requirement (citrated platelet poor-plasma) and can be ordered retrospectively on samples previously drawn for standard coagulation prolife testing (PT/INR,PTT). Additional testing is often required for further clinically relevant subclassification, particularly for type 2 disease. This discrimination usually can be achieved with multimer gel electrophoresis. Low-resolution gels are most often used, but higher resolution gels can reveal more subtle abnormalities that are recognized to have clinical implications. Unfortunately, gel methods are laborious and difficult to perform reproducibly, which makes them impractical for many laboratories. They remain in many ways the gold standard for vWD evaluation.

Two tests have become more frequent in the initial evaluation and monitoring of vWD, both designed to improve on vWF:RCof as a functional screen for the characterization of type 2 defects. One is the collagen binding assay (vWF:CB) and the other is the platelet functional analyzer (PFA-100) clotting time. The vWF:CB has demonstrated increased sensitivity to large multimers and has proven itself at least as a useful adjunct to the traditional tests. The PFA-100 has shown utility as a substitute to the unwieldy bleeding time. (See the article by Tormey and colleagues, elsewhere in this issue.) As we gain clinical experience with the use of these tests, we will be better able to define their role. Like traditional tests, however, they have fundamental limitations.

The ever-increasing list of available tests for vWF assessment can help classify and stratify risk but also can contribute to the confusion that surrounds typing systems, particularly because they may have unpredictable results in some of the less common variants of this very heterogeneous disorder and because they do not incorporate the genetic mutation information that is accumulating. Still, with an understanding of the basic principles underlying the various tests, it becomes possible to interpret results in light of this growing body of genotypic and mechanistic knowledge.

von Willebrand Factor Antigen

Several methods are in general use for the determination of total vWF antigen concentration. The two principal techniques that have supplanted the traditional Laurell immunoelectrophoresis are a bead aggregation immunoturbidometric assay (Dade Behring and Stago) and enzyme linked immunosorbent assay (ELISA)-based systems using a variety of commercially available antibodies (Abs). The turbidity assay measures the increase in bead-affected turbidity that results from the antibody mediated clumping of Ab coated beads when cross-linked by vWF. Immunosorbent assays are most often sandwich-based methods that have wells coated with vWF antibody; plasma levels are detected with either enzyme-linked colorimetric or fluorescence-linked anti-vWF antibodies. The levels are calibrated with pooled standards derived from more than 200 donors designated as 100 IU/dL by the World Health Organization (WHO) International Standards and correspond to a normal percentage of 100%. All the methods demonstrate relatively good intra-assay and interassay reproducibility on quality assurance surveys, certainly better than activity measures, but variable sensitivity to clinical interference, such as with rheumatoid factor, in bead-based tests has been described.[23]

Specific aspects to consider when interpreting vWF:Ag values are discussed in the section on diagnostic issues and include blood type variability, reactive increases, and disease threshold values. It is worth noting that the WHO standard itself has had problems of drift over successive evaluations resulting in a revaluation of the international unit standard in 2001.[24] In general, however, bleeding risk correlates with antigen level and so values should be somewhat interpreted as a marker of bleeding propensity regardless of cause.

von Willebrand Factor: Ristocetin Cofactor Activity

Ristocetin is an actinomycete-derived antibiotic initially used in the treatment of staphylococcal infections in the early 1950s, which unexpectedly induced several hematologic complications, including thrombosis. It induces platelet aggregation via vWF-GPIbα interaction that depends somewhat on the larger, more biologically active vWF multimers. The ability of ristocetin to induce platelet-vWF-dependent platelet aggregation in vitro has been exploited in the laboratory setting. The vWF:RCof assay is based on the capacity of plasma vWF to agglutinate formalin fixed reagent platelets in the presence of ristocetin. This differs from the platelet aggregation ristocetin test, which uses the patient's native unfixed platelets and is much more susceptible to inadvertent activation and spurious results. Similar to the platelet aggregometry ristocetin test, however, comparison of serially diluted patient plasma aggregometry profiles to normal/reagent plasma aggregometry profiles using the fixed platelets provides a quantitative estimate of vWF activity, most frequently expressed as a percent of normal, calibrated to international units per deciliter. As such, calibration curves are critically important, and because of the intrinsic variability of the agglutination, accuracy depends on the number of repeats on a given sample. As expected, inter- and intra-assay variability is high, and the WHO international standard has seen excessive variations on successive measurements, resulting in revaluation.[24]

When interpreted in the context of vWF:Ag and factor VIII level, however, vWF activity testing provides a reasonable stratification of most patients within the traditional phenotypic classification of vWD. In patients with type 1 disease (accounting for most cases), there is a proportional decrease in vWF:RCof and factor VIII level with respect to vWF:Ag. This relationship can be numerically expressed as a ratio of vWF:RCof/vWF:Ag, with values more than 0.7 (close to 1.0) highlighting the quantitative deficiencies (type 1) and ratios less than 0.7 suggesting qualitative defects (type 2). These findings are particularly relevant in classic type 1 disease. Unfortunately, when antigen or activity levels fall into the 20 IU/dL range or below, the ratios become less reliable indicators of multimer size distribution. Multimer analysis (or potentially the collagen binding assay) is nearly always needed for confirmation. It has also been proposed that ratios between 0.5 and 0.7 may be seen in both types, especially with some of the less sensitive cofactor activity assays, and that specificity for type 2 occurs only below 0.5. Regardless, activity measurements also can be measured after DDAVP administration to monitor efficacy and help in the classification of some rarer variants. It should be noted that this assay does not account for plasma antigenic concentration of vWF, and decreased activity is noted in qualitative and quantitative vWF deficient states. Additional testing on a separate platform is necessary for a complete initial evaluation, including vWF:Ag and factor VIII in cases with a decreased cofactor activity.

Relatively recently, an assay was introduced comprised of a fully automated latex agglutination-based system that is commercially available.[25-27] The HemosIL VWF

Activity assay (Instrumentation Laboratory, Lexington, Massachusetts) uses latex particles conjugated to monoclonal antibodies directed against the vWF GPIbα binding site. The activity of vWF to bind the latex beads is proportional to the turbidity of solution measured by standard spectrophotometric means. Direct comparison of this assay with vWF:RCof shows excellent concordance; however, additional testing either by classic ristocetin aggregometry or other functional testing may be warranted for confirmation of abnormal results. As with the analogous antigen assay, some falsely elevated levels may be seen in the presence of autoantibodies to rheumatoid factor, and absolute values tend to be higher than with the conventional agglutination assay.

A recombinant GPIbα-based ELISA assay also has been introduced. A variant uses a sandwich antibody conformation, with one Ab recognizing a bound conformation of recombinant GPIbα for capture and a polyclonal Ab for detection.[28] The assay is run under conditions of artificial ristocetin stimulation and levels depend on antigen concentration, but the activity-to-antigen ratio using this ELISA-based assay seems to have excellent sensitivity for deficiencies of high molecular weight multimers and reportedly lower coefficients of variation than agglutination based assays. As more clinical experience is acquired, its overall utility will become clearer.

Multimer Analysis (Gel Electrophoresis)

With all its limitations, the gold standard in determining vWF multimer distributions remains gel electrophoresis. Unfortunately, the difficulties associated with this type of testing severely limit its use. The technical challenges lie in creating reproducible vWF multimer patterns, which makes calibrated quantitative determinations virtually impossible. A standard method for multimer analysis involves preparation of 1% to 1.2% (low resolution) or 1.5% to 2% (intermediate resolution) SDS-agarose gels with electrophoresis for approximately 16 hours, followed by anti-vWF antibody-coated nitrocellulose filter electroblotting, washing, and radiolabeled or enzyme-linked second antibody-based detection of bands.[29,30] Several variations exist, including techniques that speed up and improve reproducibility of gels, but in general the test is laborious and time-consuming and suffers from numerous sources of variability, including gel thickness, homogeneity, heat and evaporation, current fluctuation, blotting efficiencies, and detection exposure. As a result, typically only reference laboratories offer the test on a routine basis, usually with turnaround times of a week or more, and they report only qualitative interpretations.

Multimer analysis by gel electrophoresis provides valuable diagnostic information. At its simplest, low resolution, gel electrophoresis can identify gross abnormalities in the distribution of multimers, as would be expected in most types 2A, 2B, and 3 of vWD. These figures can be contrasted with the more normal distribution expected in types 1 and 2M. As illustrated in **Fig. 3**, intermediate- and high-resolution gels have the added capability of identifying abnormalities that arise from specific mechanisms that directly relate to bleeding risk. Many of these result in abnormalities in the so-called "satellite bands," which represent the asymmetric degradation products of ADAMTS-13 activity. Normally, low-resolution gels can identify the smallest 556 kD homodimer and show multimer separation up to approximately 10 to 15 dimers. Higher resolution gels can resolve the satellite bands from at least the 2- to 6-mers, which may be decreased, increased, or of abnormal size/mobility as a result of the specific mechanistic defect in vWF synthesis or metabolism. The use of this technique for identification of subtle abnormalities that correspond to polymorphisms or frank vWD mutations seems to be on the rise and may be increasingly helpful in the future for stratification of risk and therapy as more of these defects are correlated with clinical and genetic information. (See the section on mechanistic classification.)

Collagen Binding Assay

The assessment of the ability of vWF to bind collagen as a functional assay was first reported more than 20 years ago. The current favored procedure involves a standard sandwich ELISA with collagen coated wells for capture and polyclonal anti-vWF for labeling and detection. Controversy over the relative sensitivity of the various forms of this assay has affected support of its use. The conflict stems mainly from the observation that type III collagen, as first used, seems to bind relatively indiscriminately to multimers of all sizes, whereas a combination of types I and III collagen in an approximate proportion of 19:1 seems to be much more selective for only the largest multimers.[31] It is this latter mixture that is deemed as having the best ability to sensitively and specifically identify abnormalities in the distribution of multimers. Unfortunately, the commercial collagen-binding assays available remain restricted to type III collagen, which, in purified form, seems to still have discriminatory advantage over the RCof assays in detecting relative decreases in large multimers, only not sufficient to warrant replacement of gel multimer evaluation. Home-brewed assays using the collagen combination are likely to be superior when properly validated. A remaining area of contention is the behavior of this assay in patients with type 2M, which is reportedly either low or borderline in most cases. This may reflect ambiguities in type 2M diagnosis itself.

Monitoring the response of vWF:CB to DDAVP administration also has been proposed for determination of the appropriateness of therapy and the potential need for factor replacement.[32] Additional data would be helpful in confirming the clinical utility of this approach. What does seem rather clear is that laboratories vary in their ability to distinguish between types 1 and 2 of vWD and that the RCof/Ag ratio and even gel electrophoresis (especially low resolution) may not be sufficiently sensitive or specific.[31] It is likely that there could be improvement with the incorporation of a well-validated collagen binding assay as part of the repertoire of vWF testing tools.

Platelet Functional Analyzer-100 in von Willebrand Disease

The PFA-100 was introduced in 1995 by Dade-Behring as a simple, more practical and rapid substitute method for the cumbersome bleeding time traditionally used as a screening test in the evaluation of platelet function.[33] In principle, the PFA-100 closure time is a measure of overall ex vivo platelet-based coagulant function. A PFA-100 cassette contains a membrane coated with the platelet activators collagen and epinephrine or collagen and ADP that stimulate platelet activation. On this membrane is a small orifice (150 µm) through which citrated whole blood is aspirated, creating a high shear stress that more closely simulates in vivo conditions for vWF-related platelet tethering and clot formation. The amount of time from flow start to occlusion is a measure of overall platelet function (clotting time). Time is measured in seconds, and normal ranges are generally recommended to be determined at a given laboratory. This latter property is especially important because there are no whole blood control samples available for calibration. For the Yale-New Haven Hospital laboratories, the normal ranges are 80 to 180 seconds for collagen and epinephrine and 60 to 110 seconds for collagen and ADP, which fall within the distribution of normal ranges reported in other laboratories.[34] Values more than 300 seconds are reported as "nonclosures." As is typical of platelet function assays, low platelet counts and aspirin use affect results, and care must be taken in specimen preprocessing so as to avoid inadvertent premature platelet activation. The PFA-100, however, is far more robust than traditional aggregometry because samples need not be drawn immediately next to the analyzer and sample preparation is minimal.

The platelet activation measured in response to agonists depends on vWF binding to GPIbα. Like other platelet function tests, PFA-100 closure time depends on adequate amounts of functional vWF. In principle, the PFA-100 closure time has been shown to be sensitive as a screening and diagnostic tool in vWD. Under real testing conditions, however, the sensitivity drops somewhat and is estimated to be 85% to 90%.[34] A criticism of the use of PFA-100 in screening, particularly as it pertains to type 1 diagnoses, is that closure time correlates rather closely with vWF:Ag levels and that the antigen levels tend to be more reliable. The closure time also has been correlated to age, blood type, and a variety of other clinical states, but it is unclear how much of this correlation is related directly to vWF levels. The specificity depends greatly on the clinical indication for the test (pretest probability), although this becomes less important for screening or monitoring therapy.

Studies also indicate that the PFA-100 closure time is most sensitive to high molecular weight multimers, likely reflecting the relative importance of these large multimers in vivo. This feature is shared by the other vWF functional tests, namely vWF:RCof and vWF:CB assays. Of these, the latter is the more sensitive to high molecular weight multimers. The PFA-100 is simpler to perform and less labor intensive with a comparable sensitivity, however. Unfortunately, in our laboratory's experience, sample platelet/preprocessing sensitivity reduces reproducibility and causes occasional unsatisfactory specimens. The lack of reliable and readily available standardized control material limits confidence in results. By comparison, our long experience with RCof activity counterbalances it's shortcomings of the PFA-100. It would be considered highly unusual for a patient with type 2 or type 3 vWD to have a PFA-100 closure time within the normal range, although there are a few reported instances for some type 2 patients. Currently, clinicians at our institution use both functional tests on a regular basis.

From a monitoring point of view, the PFA-100 has some characteristics that make it clinically useful, likely related to its high molecular weight multimers bias. Post-DDAVP testing shows correlation between what is loosely considered therapeutic by antigen methods and the correction of closure time. This is particularly true in type 1 patients who often respond to DDAVP infusions. In a recent article by van Vliet and colleagues,[35] discrepancies were found between correction of values in type 2 post-factor VIII/vWF concentrate patients using RCof and CB assays versus PFA-100 results. The speculation is that this reflects a higher sensitivity of the PFA-100 to high molecular weight multimers, allowing this method to detect potentially clinically important deviations from the normal multimer size distribution. Although the sensitivity of the specific vWF:CB assay used in this study is not clear, testing of all parameters post-DDAVP is likely to yield clinically useful information. Additional studies confirming the clinical relevance are needed.

Platelet Aggregation (Low- and High-dose Ristocetin)

As in the ristocetin-induced activity plasma-based assay, ristocetin can be used to induce the patient's own platelets to aggregate. The additional challenge in this test is that platelets are exquisitely sensitive to inadvertent activation and do not withstand storage and transport well. The test must be performed with the patient near the instrument so that the sample can be tested immediately. The procedure itself is relatively straightforward and involves mixing patient platelet-rich plasma with ristocetin and monitoring turbidity. As platelets agglutinate, turbidity increases and a characteristic curve with high-dose ristocetin results in decreased light transmittance over the course of minutes. When there is a defect in GPIbα and vWF-mediated platelet agglutination, transmittance is preserved to some degree. The RCof assay using a standardized formalin-fixed platelet reagent serves this purpose better. The PFA-100 also can test overall GPIbα/vWF-mediated platelet function using a far more convenient procedure. Where the RIPA is most useful is in the evaluation of agglutination in the presence of low doses of ristocetin ($\leq$ 0.5 mg/mL versus 1.0 and 1.5 mg/mL). A normal response is lack of agglutination using this reduced stimulation. Patients with vWF abnormalities that result in increased GPIbα binding aggregate platelets with low-dose ristocetin, which allows detection of type 2B disease. An important limitation that applies equally to all endogenous platelet assessment tests is that the test does not work properly in patients with thrombocytopenia. Because type 2B patients are susceptible to low platelet counts, they may need to wait for the thrombocytopenia to subside before the confirmatory RIPA test can be done.

Another potentially important application of the RIPA test described involves the distinction between whether the abnormality for hyperresponsive vWF-GPIbα binding lies in the vWF or the GPIb on the platelets, corresponding to type 2B vWD and platelet type vWD (PT-vWD), respectively.[36,37] In this method, patient platelets and plasma are separated and tested together or in cross-mixture with control platelets or plasma. Patients with a platelet GPIbα defect show a normal negative response when their plasma is tested with control platelets and a persistently elevated response when their platelets are tested with normal plasma. The addition of high vWF concentrates such as cryoprecipitate also has been used, with the theory that overwhelming with normal vWF can overcome the low-dose ristocetin aggregation in type 2B. These tests are labor intensive and prone to artifact from the additional platelet manipulation and the ambiguities of platelet aggregation, but they may assist in pinpointing this diagnosis in patients with vWD.

von Willebrand Factor Propeptide

Measures of the vWF propeptide (ie, the D1-D2 portion of the immature vWF protein), have been demonstrated as having potential clinical use in the prediction of DDAVP responsiveness.[38–40] Specifically, high ratios of pro-vWF to vWF:Ag are associated with reduced circulating survival of mature vWF, one of the general mechanisms postulated to be responsible for type 1 vWD. The theory is that the propeptide degradation and removal is independent of the mature vWF degradation and removal, so increased removal of antigen increases the relative propeptide amount. This interpretation is supported by the differing half-lives: 2 to 3 hours for vWFpp and 8 to 12 hours for mature vWF (probably longer in non–blood type O patients) and the relative constancy of vWFpp half-lives in patients with reduced vWF plasma survival. Patients with increased ratios are also associated with a series of particular vWF gene mutations affecting assembly. They are often classified initially as type 1 patients, but they may be best categorized as type 2A (IIE).

The vWF propeptide level measurement is based on selective immunologic detection in a standard ELISA. A limitation lies in that the anti-vWFpp antibody (known as Mango) is only available as a research use only reagent kit from GTI Diagnostics. Its general use in the routine subclassification of vWD remains to be fully demonstrated.

Flow Cytometry for von Willebrand Disease

Detection of platelet aggregation and detection of vWF binding to platelets with fluorescently labeled antibodies by flow cytometry has been proposed as an alternate or complementary method for vWD diagnosis and monitoring.[41–43] There are some theoretical differences between results obtained by these methods and the corresponding functional and quantitative values obtained in the RCof/CB assays and the antigen levels. The platelet aggregation involves the use of patient platelet-rich plasma incubated with ristocetin, followed by particle size detection. More activation is reflected in the higher distribution of particle sizes, with more of the larger particles corresponding to activated platelet aggregates. In this regard, it is more analogous to the PFA-100 in that the patient's own components are used, with the difference that the less discriminate platelet activator ristocetin is used. As would be expected, the quantitation of vWF seems to correlate well to the antigen detection by traditional methods. Putative advantages of flow methods are high sensitivity, small volumes, and speed of results. Although cost, standardization, and labor intensity may be argued to be comparable in theory, in practical terms, a clear advantage has not been demonstrated. This is particularly true in light of the rather extensive specimen preprocessing dilutions, count adjustments, and incubations used. The ability of these flow tests to detect abnormalities in multimer distribution has not been shown, which raises questions about the relative use of the methods as proposed. Results thus far merit further exploration, however.

Factor VIII and Factor VIII-vWFB

The measurement of coagulation factor VIII is routinely used in the evaluation of patients for vWD. Apart from being helpful in the identification of the relatively common hemophilia A, levels of factor VIII are usually low or low-normal in the different types of vWD and are low in the variant that results in low factor VIII binding (type 2N). The method of choice is based on the degree of correction of PTT in factor VIII–deficient plasma, which is standardized against international standards and reported as a percentage of normal or IU/dL. Antigen-based chromogenic assays are also available and produce satisfactory results.

In the specific vWD subtype 2N, its differentiation from hemophilia A can be made by using antibodies that detect the bound conformation of factor VIII with vWD. This factor VIII-vWF binding test demonstrates a disproportionately low level of binding to factor VIII, relative to the vWF antigen concentration in the vWD variant, whereas it is proportional to the vWF concentration in hemophilia.

Other Approaches: Correlation Spectroscopy

Alternative methods for the detection of vWF antigen concentration and multimer distribution are being pursued. One such method being studied by Torres and Levene[44] involves the use of correlation spectroscopy. The principle is based on the relative differences in Brownian motion translational mobility of multimers of different sizes. Fluctuation analysis, including autocorrelation and photon counting, of fluorescently tagged antibody bound molecules in small volumes of their native plasma allows determination of differences in the concentration and distribution of vWF multimers between patients and controls and potentially reveals conformational changes and binding defects. It has the advantages of minimal preparation, rapid analysis, small volumes, and low expense. The preliminary data show potential for the eventual routine evaluation of vWF multimers in a variety of patients for diagnosis and monitoring of coagulation abnormalities, although further studies are needed and are currently in progress.

General Test Considerations

Freeze-thaw cycles cause variable degradation of multimers, resulting in uninterpretable results because of artifactually low antigen levels and RCof activity. Similarly, slow thawing methods can inadvertently cause cryoprecipitation with variable decreases in observed values. The recommendation for storage is that collection be followed by a quick spin for preparation of platelet-poor plasma, which should then be frozen separately in smaller aliquots. Samples should be thawed at 37°C for several minutes and used quickly thereafter, particularly for tests that are sensitive to high molecular weight multimers. Although low-resolution multimer analysis seems to remain relatively unaffected for gross abnormalities on refrozen and rethawed specimens, degradation can be detected within a few hours using sensitive techniques, even in the absence of high molarity urea or low ionic buffer (unpublished observations).

DIAGNOSTIC ISSUES
Blood Type, Race, Antigen Levels, and Type 1 Disease

A significant challenge in identifying people affected with vWD is the relationship between ABO blood type and vWF levels. Correlations have been established in large blood donor studies and subsequently confirmed by others. **Table 1** shows data from four such analyses. The first often-quoted study is based on 1117 blood donors in Wisconsin.[45] The second study is a pedigree analysis of families containing members with idiopathic thrombosis.[46] The third study evaluated the blood group and vWF antigen level association with a history of thrombosis in patients presenting to a hemostasis clinic.[47] The last evaluated the genetic polymorphism/mutation Y1584C in normal blood donors in the United Kingdom.[48]

Several points are worth noting. First, it is evident that there is significant variation in normal levels as determined at different institutions. The use of different methods (and slightly different units) does not account for the variation observed given that method correlation studies and other published measured ranges have validated the relative consistency of the various techniques. The revaluation of the WHO IS calibration standard in 2001 may have had an influence on measures because it represents a 6% increase in reported antigen levels.[24] Regardless, although surveys from various countries have shown acceptable interassay and interinstitution variation, this comparison demonstrates that a significant need remains for individual institutions to establish their own reference ranges based on their specific populations.

A consistent finding, however, is that a strong correlation exists between blood type and vWF:Ag levels: significantly lower vWF antigen levels are associated with type O blood, somewhere on the order of 25% to 30% lower than non–type O individuals. For vWD, it is relevant that normal blood type O donors have ranges that overlap

Table 1
Correlation of ABO blood type with vWF:Ag levels in four different studies

	Study 1 (Gill 1987) IEP	Study 2 (Souto 2000) ELISA	Study 3 (Scheleef 2004) Particle Immunoassay		Study 4 (Davies 2007) Particle Immunoassay	
	Blood Donors (1117)	Familial Idiopathic Thrombophilia (328)	Controls (236)	Thrombosis (355)	Wild-Type Donors (5000)	Y1584C Donors (100)
	vWF:Ag (2 SD) (U/dL)	vWF:Ag (% Normal)	vWF:Ag (IU/dL)	vWF:Ag (IU/dL)	vWF:Ag (IU/dL)	vWF:Ag (IU/dL)
Type O	75 (36–157)	77 ± 27	103 ± 25	123 ± 42	95 ± 29	58 ± 14
Type A	106 (48–234)	114 ± 40	117*	161*	124 ± 37	98 ± 34
Type B	117 (57–241)	103 ± 30	140 ± 30*	165 ± 30*	131 ± 37	108 ± 38
Type AB	123 (64–238)	137 ± 34	135 ± 20*	180 ± 25*	137 ± 43	119 ± 20

Method and corresponding units are described. Standard deviations are given where available. Values with asterisk (*) are estimates from graphical representation of data.

significantly with antigen levels considered to be in the VWD range. Not shown here is that this correlation is heavily influenced by race. Non-white individuals have significantly higher vWF:Ag levels, so much so that even type O non-white persons have levels that approximate average normal levels and non–type O non-whites have the highest baseline vWF:Ag.[49] These observations have prompted the suggestion that blood type- and even race-specific normal ranges be used.

As to the reason for the blood type and vWF:Ag correlation, recent evidence points to increased clearance in blood type O individuals as a potential mechanism of the observed trend.[50] There is some indication that H-type carbohydrate antigenic determinants on vWF play a role in this clearance.[51] This might explain the variation in blood type A, which has been shown to be influenced by the H antigen expression differences seen in blood types A_1O versus A_2O versus AA. A key consideration is that bleeding symptoms correlate better with overall vWF antigen levels than with levels relative to blood type-specific ranges. That is, blood type O individuals are generally at higher risk for excessive bleeding and, according to the third study mentioned earlier, are less likely to become hypercoagulable. It is also relevant that normal blood type and race-specific ranges would be challenging and costly to define for a given institution, with large patient number requirements. As a result, the recommendation is that blood typing not be used for the clinical purpose of evaluating coagulopathy and that vWF:Ag levels be considered an imperfect but direct measure of bleeding risk after site-specific validation of overall normal ranges. Importantly, the distribution sensitive activity assays seem to show a similar association by blood type,[52] so ratios are not affected, which further obviates the need for blood type-specific reference ranges.

Study 4 from **Table 1** shows that baseline vWF levels across blood types are also reduced with the presence of the Y1584C polymorphism but that donors with blood type O have the bulk of the disease-range antigen levels. Still, it seems that the primary determinant of bleeding risk in these patients remains the vWF antigen level, making this type of polymorphism determination unnecessary for clinical purposes.

Another relevant point for accurate assessment of risk is that vWF levels also vary in response to conditions such as pregnancy, inflammatory illness, hyperthyroidism, and exercise. In an interesting (if odd) demonstration of the sensitivity of vWF levels, subjects had levels increase three- to fourfold in response to an induced syncopal episode.[53] Practically, values of vWF:Ag less than 50 IU/dL or 50% of normal pool, in the proper clinical setting, are suggestive. If vWF:RCof levels are also less than 50% with low antigen levels, suspicion should be higher. Antigen or activity levels less than 30 IU/dL (some advocate 20 IU/dL) increase specificity a great deal with relation to a true diagnosis of vWD, identifiable mutations, and more severe bleeding symptoms. In the end (see later discussion), studies still suggest that bleeding scores are better predictors of future bleeding episodes than vWF levels in isolation, particularly histories of postoperative bleeding. The PFA-100 closure times, when properly used, also could be useful in excluding a bleeding propensity. Repeat testing at a later date reduces the chance of misclassifying in light of confounding effects such as an acute phase reaction or illness.

A conceptual framework for interpreting vWF:Ag levels and mutations can be formed from this and similar studies (**Fig. 4**). It seems evident that overall vWF associated bleeding risk is the result of the complex compound effect of blood type–related natural vWF:Ag levels plus the combination of any mutations that may affect the synthesis, release, conformation, binding, degradation, or clearance of vWF. There are likely other unidentified mechanisms. Certainly, other coagulation components also modulate this risk. In short, we can reinforce the view that we need more data

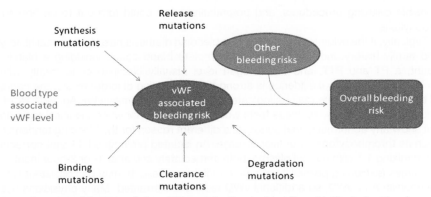

Fig. 4. Conceptual framework for vWF contribution to bleeding risk illustrates the dependence on multiple factors.

and better tools. In any case, the antigen and activity levels that are derived from the multimer distribution remain critically important parameters, even if the specific contribution to overall bleeding risk in individual cases cannot be defined fully.

Bleeding Score and Diagnostic Approach

Although bleeding history is a natural part of assessing bleeding risk, it was only relatively recently that standardization in bleeding history for vWD assessment evolved. In 2006, a questionnaire published by the European Union multicenter group studying the Molecular and Clinical Markers for Diagnosis and Management of Type I Von Willebrand Disease (MCMDM-1 VWD) showed excellent discrimination between individuals at increased risk of bleeding with vWF abnormalities and unaffected individuals.[54] It is derived from a more extensive bleeding score system that has the significant drawback of requiring approximately 40 minutes for completion. The newer abbreviated questionnaire is available at http://www.euvwd.group.shef.ac.uk/bleed_score.htm. This quicker, simplified approach includes questions on frequency and severity of excessive bleeding as the result of tooth extraction, surgery, oral cavity conditions, minor wounds, nosebleeds, menorrhagia, gastrointestinal problems, postpartum, hematomas in muscles, and hemarthroses and bleeding into the central nervous system. Points are added based on positive bleeding episodes ranging from no bleeding postsurgical or traumatic bleeding (−1) to need for blood transfusion or desmopressin therapy (+4). Total points range from −3 to 45, but a threshold of points (bleeding score 4) correlates with risk of vWD as determined by complete testing using vWD diagnostic guidelines that use traditional tests. The sensitivity using this threshold for identifying cases with abnormal vWF testing is reportedly near 100% and specificity is approximately 87%.[55] By all measures, it serves well as an initial screen.

In using the bleeding score system, however, it should be noted that the validation was performed on patients who were almost exclusively over 15 years of age. Younger patients may present with a more limited personal history. In these cases, the family history may be more important and the physician faces more of a judgment call in terms of additional testing. In borderline cases, there is a risk of falsely labeling a patient with vWD, which leads to unnecessary cost and worry, possible delaying procedures, and potentiating what could turn out to be harmful prophylaxis.

Typically, if the evidence points to a true bleeding diathesis based on clinical history and family history, indicated tests are: complete blood count, including a platelet count, a PT and PTT, and a fibrinogen level (usually obtained concurrently with PTT). When the clinical evidence is strong that a bleeding disorder exists, the cadre of traditional vWD tests may be indicated from the start, namely vWF:Ag, vWF:RCof, and factor VIII. Otherwise, these tests would be reserved for when the initial tests do not show any abnormality that suggests a different reason for the bleeding tendency, such as thrombocytopenia or liver disease. An isolated prolonged PTT that corrects upon mixing 1:1 with normal plasma, both immediately and after 1- or 2-hour incubation times (excluding possibility of a factor inhibitor present), may be consistent with hemophilia A or vWD, so additional vWD testing is warranted. Many physicians use low-resolution multimeric testing as a complement to the vWD tests, mainly to evaluate the possibility of types 2A, 2B, or 3 disease. Intermediate resolution multimer analysis presents the previously described advantage of detecting more subtle abnormalities associated with variants of type 1 disease (such as type 2A[IIE] described later) and types 2M and 2N, but it is not readily commercially available. A similar scheme incorporates the use of the vWF:CB assay instead of the vWF:RCof assay, but in terms of standardized classification, there is much less experience with the vWF:CB assay, and neither has fully validated strict criteria in terms of functional to antigen ratios that can classify with high enough accuracy. The question of when to use PFA-100, particularly in screening, remains somewhat controversial, mainly because of the sensitivity and specificity issues.

In light of the diagnostic issues, standard criteria remain largely clinical and are based on the 2006 publication by the scientific and standardization committee of the International Society of Thrombosis and Haemostasis. A simplified diagnostic scheme is presented in **Fig. 5**. In general, it is useful to think of the bleeding history as being critical in the clinical evaluation of vWD. A high pretest probability improves significantly the ability of the tests to produce accurate results. Without it, results are prone to errors in diagnosis, classifying normal individuals with borderline levels of antigen as affected and missing affected at-risk patients who happen to have had a reactively high level at time of sampling.

Molecular Testing

Many molecular techniques have been used in the identification of vWD mutations, but gene sequencing using site-specific primers remains the gold standard. Unfortunately, there are significant drawbacks and pitfalls. At 178 kb, the gene is much too long to make DNA sequencing economically viable as a diagnostic test, even using the most modern techniques available. Polymorphisms are abundant, with more than 130 reported to date, which adds some challenges to the design of a simplified molecular diagnostic approach. The presence of a pseudogene on chromosome 22 further complicates analysis by creating a source of potential interference during isolation and detection, although it is relevant to note that mutations in the pseudogene can be introduced into the fully encoded gene, resulting in clinically significant disease in offspring.[56] Perhaps the greatest difficulties come from four properties of vWD mutations: (1) more than 200 mutations have been associated with vWD; (2) compound mutations occur with regularity; (3) many patients with vWD have normal vWF genes by sequencing; and (4) mutations and other factors contributing to vWD may be outside the vWF gene. A Web site at the University of Sheffield serves as repository of vWF mutations (http://www.vwf.group.shef.ac.uk/).

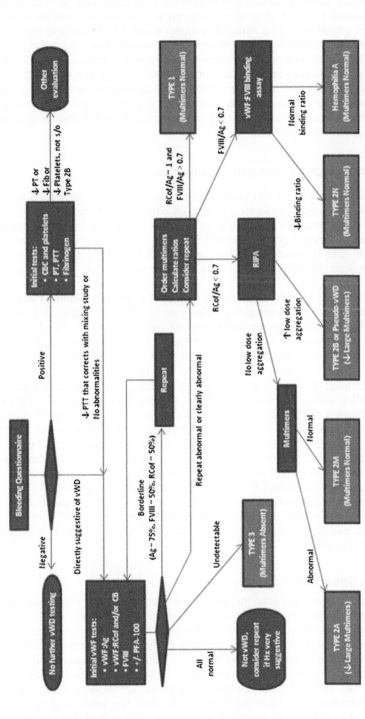

Fig. 5. General diagnostic scheme for vWD evaluation in a patient presenting with either personal or family history of bleeding or an abnormal coagulation test. Scheme is based on NHLBI guidelines[79] and Favoloro.[31]

When molecular testing is performed (primarily for research studies), an approach is to sequence exons 1 and 18 to 52 using polymerase chain reaction amplification with site-specific primer sets. If no mutation is found, exons 2 to 18 are also sequenced. Alternatively, all the exons are sequenced. Unfortunately, exon sequencing misses many of the possible mutations that occur in the intervening regions, especially splice sites, and in the gene regulatory regions upstream from the protein encoding portion. Parenthetically, intron 40 has polymorphism and heterozygosity with potential for paternity and other forensic testing as reported recently.[57] vWF gene properties make it difficult to come up with a cost-effective and efficient molecular diagnostic test strategy for vWD, however.

MECHANISTIC- AND GENOTYPIC-BASED CLASSIFICATION

With all these caveats, we can begin to undertake the task of identifying patterns in genotype/phenotype correlations to help us better predict clinical behavior. The current favored classification scheme as described follows a traditional designation of types 1, 2 and 3 corresponding to (1) type 1: decrease in overall multimers with normal ratio of activity (vWF:RCof or vWF:CB) to antigen; (2) type 2: qualitative deficiencies of vWF; and (3) type 3: Absence or near absence of vWF multimers.

A basic rationale for this classification exists in the use of a standard laboratory medicine designation of quantitative defects as type 1 and qualitative defects as type 2. Severity of bleeding symptoms generally increases as one goes from type 1 to type 3, and prevalence decreases from type 1 to type 3. Type 2 is subdivided into types 2A, 2B, 2N, and 2M on the basis of differing test results and multimer patterns with the associated etiologies. The old 1987 classification used further subcategorization of type 2A into subclasses IIA through IIE (with case reports for IIF through II-I), which many in the field continue to use. Causally, they seem to correspond to different identifiable mechanisms, but currently this distinction is not easily achieved. The research work that has evolved in the past few years has identified molecular mechanisms associated with genetic mutations in many of these subtypes, some of which were classified as type 1 using standard testing, which contributes to the confusion in vWD classification. An important result of the genotypic classification work being undertaken is that it can start to assign potential mechanistic causes for the more subdivided classification work summarized in the 1987 classification by Ruggieri. In the future, we may return to that more detailed scheme, particularly if we can reorganize it mechanistically and genotypically to create a more accurate picture of abnormalities in vWF.

Type 1 and Type Vincenza

Several mechanisms have been identified or postulated as being responsible for the various forms of vWD that result in what is currently classified as type 1, including (1) decreased synthesis, (2) decreased secretion, (3) increased clearance, and (4) increased cleavage. Most of the studies have focused on evaluating these mechanisms in patients who have identified mutations. A significant proportion of patients (approximately 30%–35% of patients with type 1), however, do not have identifiable mutations with standard gene sequencing techniques.[58–60] As a result, the large cohort studies that have been published in the past few years tend to separate patients on the basis of (1) presence or absence of mutations and (2) normal or abnormal multimer patterns on intermediate- to high-resolution gel electrophoresis.

One of these studies[58] observed that bleeding symptoms as determined by bleeding scores correlate to these categories:

Type 1/Abnormal multimers/No mutations: rare/only slightly abnormal bleeding scores

Type 1/Normal multimers/0, 1, or >1 mutation: moderately elevated bleeding scores

Type 1/Abnormal multimers/1 mutation: high bleeding scores

Type 1/Abnormal multimers/ >1 mutation: highest bleeding scores

Conceptually at least, it seems that identifiable abnormalities on multimer distribution by intermediate- or high-resolution electrophoresis have the most bearing on the predictable risk for bleeding. The presence of detectable mutations is less relevant, but compound mutations can have a significant cumulative effect. From the clinical laboratory point of view, one may consider that intermediate- or high-resolution gel electrophoresis is superior in terms of bleeding risk assessment in vWD. There also seems to be a rare but distinct subset of patients with abnormal multimers who have only slightly increased risk of bleeding. This group could have non-vWF gene-related reasons for the abnormal multimer distribution or result from intron abnormalities with normal residual capacity to respond appropriately to bleeding injury.

Increased Clearance

The bulk of the vWF gene mutations that have been associated with reduced survival of circulating vWF are located in the D3 region, including mutations such as C1130G, C1130F, C1130R, and W1144G. The D3 region is associated with multimerization, but its specific role in clearance has not been elucidated. D4 region defects also have been linked to shortened survival, namely S2179F. Some of these D3 and D4 defects are associated with decreased satellite band intensity. In many cases, there is a concomitant minimal decrease in large multimers, the basis for categorization as type 2A, subclass IIE. Absence or decrease of these satellite bands and the minimal large multimer decrease would not be detected in low-resolution gel electrophoresis, leading to a diagnosis of type 1 vWD. Patients with these mutations also have been shown to have increased ratio of vWF propeptide to mature antigen ratio. The mature vWF half-life in these patients has been measured to be roughly 3.5 hours, significantly shorter than the normal patient approximations of 8 to 12 hours[40] (possibly even longer in persons with non-blood type O).[50] These patients are reported to have a marked increase in vWF:Ag in response to DDAVP, which lends credence to the theory that their vWF synthesis is unaffected. The shortened half-life abnormality is usually reflected in DDAVP challenge tests. The many-fold increases in antigen level tend to require sample draws at 30 minutes to 1 hour after infusion, however.

A related mutation in the D3 region that results in increased clearance is R1250H, which carries the designation of vWD-Vincenza. The R1205H mutation of vWD Vincenza results in a pronounced increase in clearance of vWF multimers. Genetic penetrance is high and is associated with an especially severe bleeding diathesis for a "type 1" disorder. Some have classified Vincenza as a type 2M vWD variant, based partly on the decreased RIPA and the decreased Ag/RCof ratio (although normal on some studies) observed in this disorder. The subtleness of the multimer abnormalities in vWD Vincenza often leads to characterization as type 1 using routine testing. Although originally thought to also correspond to increased ultra-large vWF multimers, this observation is now believed to represent a second associated abnormality. In some studies, the R1205H has been linked to a M740I mutation, especially among those from the Vincenza region, but no specific phenotypic characteristic has been attributed to this genetic feature. Like the other rapid clearance mutations, there is a pronounced response to DDAVP followed by a markedly shortened vWF:Ag survival, and the propeptide ratio is elevated.

Based on the available data, the grouping of these abnormalities into an increased clearance category seems reasonable, particularly because there are distinct phenotypic characteristics with clinical implications. When suspected and possible, it may also warrant genetic analysis, although the main practical use at this time is in genetic counseling.

Other Mechanisms in Type 1

At least one other subgroup of type 1 patients as defined by current criteria likely deserves a special designation. A subset of type 1 patients seems to have a moderate to high risk of bleeding, normal or near normal multimer distribution, and lower responses to DDAVP. Some of these cases correspond to the originally identified group of patients with low platelet vWF (type I platelet low), which when combined with the low DDAVP response suggests a synthesis defect in megakaryocytes and endothelial cells. An example mechanism was described in a case that demonstrated a mutation in the D3 region that resulted in an abnormal monomer that can incorporate itself during the multimer assembly and prevent multimer transport out of the ER.[61] These patients and other "severe" type 1 patients are not adequately managed with DDAVP and require factor concentrate infusions or platelet transfusions during bleeding episodes. They are also characterized by markedly low vWF:Ag levels but visible multimers on gel electrophoresis, which reinforces the view that antigen levels less than 20 or 30 IU/dL in type 1 disease increases the likelihood of detectable mutations and more significant disease. These cases also support the idea that risk in type 1 disease still needs to be evaluated on a case-by-case basis.

Other type 1 vWD cases are not as easily characterized. Nearly every region in the vWF gene has been associated with type 1 vWD, despite the strong association between certain regions and specific vWD subtypes. We may speculate that some of these mutations result in mild structural abnormalities with subtle effects in any of the synthesis, secretion, and degradations steps of the vWF life-cycle, and that, in combination, they result in decreased steady state or decreased responsiveness to injury and a bleeding diathesis. The continuing long-term studies of type 1 patients in Europe, Canada, and the United States should help us focus on the variables with the highest impact, but other than antigen levels and the DDAVP challenge, there is insufficient information to currently allow for the routine standardized identification of the highest risk type 1 patients.

Type 2A

Type 2A vWD patients share characteristics such as decreased functional/antigen ratio, reduced response to DDAVP, abnormalities in the multimer pattern, and increased risk of bleeding. They are probably the most common type of non-type 1 vWD; however, like type 1, type 2A represents a heterogeneous group of disorders with several different underlying mechanisms[62] (**Table 2**). Of type 2A cases, the sub-subtype originally designated as IIA is generally considered the most common. It is caused by dominant mutations in the A2 domain (or the adjacent N terminal portion of the A3 domain) that create folding instability of the mature vWF protein such that mechanical unfolding is not needed to expose the nearby ADAMTS-13 cleaving site. As a result, increased proteolysis manifests on gel electrophoresis as a decrease in large multimers and increase in the proportion of the intermediate degradation products seen as satellite bands (see **Fig. 3**). The severity of the abnormality and resulting bleeding phenotype depends on the specific amino acid substitution because different degrees of instability can modulate susceptibility to cleaving and the ability to sustain large multimer assembly. Although there is insufficient evidence to fully support using the specific multimer pattern as a prognostic indicator in these cases, it seems logical that the proportional reduction in large multimers corresponds to the degree to which the mutation in a specific case is hampering normal clotting function.

Several other rarer type 2A subtypes have mechanisms that have been at least partially elucidated and generate distinct multimer patterns that are readily recognizable. The originally designated type IIC results from mutations in the D2 propeptide region that impair its ability to promote multimer assembly in the golgi, resulting in abnormally small multimers that adopt conformations resistant to ADAMTS-13–mediated proteolysis. Multimer profiles include only the smallest multimers and are devoid of satellite bands, yielding a characteristically clean gel pattern (see **Fig. 3**). Although sometimes touted as representative of type 2 disease on gel electrophoresis, only homozygous mutations result in the clearly identifiable phenotype, which makes this abnormality uncommon and somewhat unique.

Subtype IIE in the older classifications is another uncommon but distinct 2A subtype that may be labeled as type 1 based on low-resolution multimer analysis. In the variant that is currently classifiable as type 2A, the abnormality stems from mutations in the D3 domain that impair disulfide bond formation necessary for normal multimer assembly. Some decrease in the largest multimers reflects this impaired assembly, but the impairment is too subtle to be detected with most gels. The vWF:Rcof/vWF:Ag ratio may be near the normal range, but the more sensitive vWF:CB seems to be more clearly abnormal in these cases. Intermediate- and high-resolution gels also identify the reduced satellite band intensity, the cause of which remains unknown but which is possibly related to increased clearance, as seen with other D3 mutations that result in Vincenza-like phenotypes. The two may represent varying degrees of impairment of the same processes based on the specifics of the conformational abnormalities.

Yet another subtype of type 2A vWD, originally known as IID, involves the impaired dimerization of vWF monomers in the endoplasmic reticulum caused by mutations in the CK portion of the molecule. Monomeric proteins can later become incorporated during multimerization, in effect serving as chain terminators. The multimer pattern has a significant reduction in large multimers but also is notable for intermediate bands seen on intermediate- and high-resolution gels that represent odd-numbered multimers. When heterozygous, the phenotype is of a moderate bleeding tendency. When homozygous, the severity increases. Fortunately, the mutation is rare.

A few other type 2A subtypes have been reported, known as IIF, IIG, IIH, and II-I, but they are case report material. Less is known about the molecular basis of these abnormalities. Still they satisfy the general criteria for qualification as general type 2A. In most of these and the other type 2A cases, DDAVP is inadequate as hemostatic therapy, and purified vWF is recommended for treatment or prophylaxis in the event of a planned surgical intervention. Cases previously classified variably as type Ib, type I platelet discordant, and currently a subset of 2A, seem to fit best under a subclass of severe type 2M (discussed later).

Type 2B

Mutations in the A1 and proximal A2 domain may cause increased binding to GPIbα.[63] The mutant vWF, especially the largest multimers, bind platelets without the need for shear stresses that normally unravel vWF at sites of injury. Coated platelets may get

Table 2
Evolution of vWD classification scheme with distinguishing features and representative mechanisms and mutations

2006	1994	1987	Multimers on Gel	DDAVP Response	Rcof:Ag Ratio	Inheritance	Mechanism	Bleeding Risk	Representative Mutations
1	1	IA, I Platelet normal, I-2	All present but↓	Good	Normal	Autosomal dominant		Mild to moderate	Upstream regulatory region, D1,D2,D'/D3,A1,A2,A3,D4, B2,B3,C1,C2,CK
		I-3	All present	Good	Normal	Autosomal dominant	Normal plasma vWF-Ag, low in platelets		
		I Platelet low, I-1	All present but↓	Poor	Normal	Autosomal dominant	Impaired intracell transport, heterodimers		D'/D3-C1149R
1	2M	Unclassified, I Vincenza	Large↑ (Variable)/ large mildly↓ with satellite ↓(C1130)	Pronounced immediate but shortened half-life	Usually low (normal on some studies)	Autosomal dominant	Increased clearance, ↓RIPA	Moderate	D'/D3-R1205H or C1130F/ G/R, W1144G

2A									
2A	IB, I Platelet discordant	Large, mildly↓	Poor–variable	Low	Autosomal dominant	Same as severe type 2M?		A1-R1374C/H?
	IIA (IIA-1, IIA-2, IIA-3)	Large and intermediate↓/ satellite bands↑↑	Poor–variable	Low	Autosomal dominant	Increased ADAMTS13 susceptibility	Mild to moderate	A2/A3 - C1272S, G1505R, S1506L, M1528V, R1569dl, R1597W, V1607DM G1609R, I1628T, G1629E, G1631D, E1638K, P1648S
	IIC	Larger↓↓/ satellite↓↓	Poor	Low	Recessive–rare	Propeptide mutations impair Golgi multimer assembly and make resistant to ADAMTS13		D2
	IID	Larger↓↓/ abnormal satellite↓↓/ old numbered multimers	Poor	Low	Autosomal dominant–rare	Impaired dimerization in ER → Monomers become chain terminators	Hetero, moderate; homozyogous, severe	CK-C2010R
	IIE	Larger↓/ satellite↓ (Smeary)	Poor	Low	Autosomal dominant–rare	Impaired assembly at disulfide bonds	Mild to moderate	D3-Y1146C, C1153Y, T1107C
	IIF, IIG, IIH, II-I	Larger↓/ satellite↓ abnormalities	Poor	Low	Rare	Case reports		

(continued on next page)

Table 2
(continued)

2006	1994	1987	Multimers on Gel	DDAVP Response	Rcof:Ag Ratio	Inheritance	Mechanism	Bleeding Risk	Representative Mutations
2B	2B	IIB	Large ± intermediate/ satellite bands↑↑	Contraindicated but increase in response	Often low (Ag normal, borderline RCof)	Autosomal dominant	↑GPIb binding leads to platelet aggregation and clearance = ↑RIPA, periodic ↓plts	Variable, correlates with thrombocytopenia	A1/A2-C1272G/R, M1304Insm, R1306W/Q/L, I1309V, S1310F, W1313C, V1314F/L/P, V1316M, H1268D, P1337L, R1306W, R1341Q/W/L, R1308C/P, L1460V, A1461V
		I New York, Malmö	Near normal	Good	Usually normal	Autosomal dominant	Increased RIPA but apparently normal function in vivo	Low to none - usually no thrombocytopenia	A1-P1266L/ Q, R1308L

Type	Multimer structure	Multimer gel	RIPA	Inheritance	Mechanism	Severity	Mutations
2M							
2M	All present but↓	Poor–variable	Low	Autosomal dominant	Impaired binding to GPIb	Variable- R1374C/H more severe	A1-Y1321D, G1324A/S, E1359K, K1362T, F1369I, R1374C/H, R1394I, K148del, I1425F, I1526T
Type B							B2-C2362F
IC	Smaller/Satellite bands↓	Hetero–good	Normal	Recessive	Decreased proteolysis	Heter, mild; homozygous, severe	
ID	All↓/satellite bands↓	Good	Low	Autosomal dominant?	Decreased RIPA May be a Vicenza analog		
2N Normandy	Normal	Not indicated	Normal	Recessive	Impaired binding to factor VIII cause increased FVIII degradation	Severity depends on mutation. Mimicks mild hemophilia A	D'/D3-R854G= milder disease. Others include P812, R816W, R854Q, R1035
3 III	Absent or nearly absent	None	Unmeasurable	Recessive		High	Nonsense, frameshift, deletions, unique

Differences	Mutation Locus	Type 1 Criteria
1994	Only vWF gene	Decreased vWF:Ag but no multimer abnormalities
2006	Not restricted	Decreased vWF:Ag normal multimer distribution, may have satellite band abnormalities, normal activity-to-antigen ratio

Data are compiled from multiple references as listed in the text.

cleared, presumably by the reticuloendothelial system, which reduces the availability of large multimers and periodically causes thrombocytopenia, particularly in response to conditions that increase circulating vWF (eg, pregnancy, trauma). Recent evidence points to at least two distinct groups within vWD type 2B: the type formerly known as IIB and the type formerly known as type I New York/Malmö. The latter is a mild condition associated with specific mutations in the A1 domain (P1266L/Q or R1308L) that give normal antigen and activity levels, nearly normal multimer distributions by gel electrophoresis, mild to no bleeding symptoms, and absence of thrombocytopenia. It is recognizable as type 2B merely by the increased RIPA, but probably in the future should be classified separately, especially because patients do not seem to respond adversely to therapy with DDAVP, unlike patients with the classic IIB.

The IIB cases are heterogeneous in and of themselves. There is a spectrum of symptoms and laboratory findings ranging from mild bleeding tendencies, mild multimer abnormalities, and mild thrombocytopenia, to severe phenotypes. Recent evidence points to a correlation between the degree of observed thrombocytopenia and bleeding symptoms with few findings when platelet counts remain above 140 k/μL.[64] Baseline studies in the more significant cases tend to show fewer circulating large and intermediate sized multimers on electrophoresis, more reduced activity levels, and increased GPIb binding by immunoassay. Satellite bands may become pronounced in gel electrophoresis, probably because of the proteolysis of multimers attached to platelets that enriches the circulating degraded pool and resembles closely type 2A (IIA). Making the distinction may be difficult even with higher resolution gels. The differentiation with RIPA may become clinically important because DDAVP use is contraindicated in patients with 2B because it results in increased platelet clearance, which causes or worsens thrombocytopenia. Curiously, a detailed analysis of the specific 2B mutation R1308P has shown an associated abnormal megakaryocyte maturation in these patients that contributes to the severe thrombocytopenia observed in affected families, which, in effect, makes it a variant of familial thrombocytopenia.[65]

Type 2M

Subtype 2M (for multimer or miscellaneous) in its classic form is akin to type 2B (IIB) because it is also the result of mutations in the A1 domain that affect GPIbα binding, but in this case, diminishing the vWF affinity for the receptor. Again, functional platelet aggregation is impaired disproportionately to the concentration of vWF, manifesting as a reduced RCof activity/Ag ratio. The impaired GPIbα binding also results in reduced overall antigen levels, but multimer distribution is preserved, implying that synthesis and proteolytic mechanisms are unaffected. The discordant normal multimer distribution with markedly low functional levels using GPIbα based assays should prompt consideration of type 2M versus type 2A. The response to DDAVP in these patients is characterized by normalization of Ag levels and vWF:CB based function but persistently low RCof activity, which distinguishes these patients from patients with type 1. Markedly decreased RIPA seems to be an invariant feature of type 2M cases as well.

A subset of these 2M patients manifests a more severe bleeding phenotype. Gene analysis has identified that R1374-C and H are A1 region mutations that reduce GPIbα binding but tend to demonstrate a slight reduction in large multimers and lower total antigen levels in addition to the markedly decreased to absent RIPA.[62] It seems that patients with these mutations have been variably categorized as belonging to type I platelet discordant, type Ib, or type 2A, but the mechanism, mutation location, RIPA results, DDAVP response, and multimer pattern suggest that a special 2M designation is warranted.

Additional rare mutations are currently classified as type 2M, although their mechanism of action does not involve GPIbα binding. Decreased proteolysis that results from a mutation in the B2 domain is an example.[66] The multimer pattern in the mild heterozygous form shows an unusual proportional decrease in smaller multimers and reduced satellite bands. The homozygous condition in the case reported has low levels of vWF with a severe bleeding diathesis. The preservation of the larger multimers with a decreased RIPA may prompt consideration of 2M, but the heterozygous cases described demonstrate a proportional decrease in RCof and Ag levels. In the homozygous state, the disease is more likely to be deemed a severe type 1 disorder on the basis of the relatively preserved multimer distribution at low levels, but the increase in largest multimers without satellite bands should alert one to the possibility of this variant.

Type 2N

Of all the vWD subtypes, type 2N (for Normandy) is perhaps the one that has remained most unchanged over the years. It has been long noted that the disorder stems from a defect in binding of soluble coagulation factor VIII, which is rapidly degraded when not in the protected bound conformation with vWF. As anticipated, mutations giving rise to this variant occur mainly in the factor VIII binding region of the molecule – D'/D3,[62] although a few have been identified outside this region, probably resulting in alterations of the three-dimensional structure of the binding site. The phenotype is of a recessive condition that mimics mild hemophilia A. Some mutations result in more severe bleeding, but the mutation R854G is one that is singled out as being significantly milder. There are no telltale signs of vWD type 2N on routine diagnostic testing because, like in hemophilia A, there is reduced factor VIII, normal vWF:Ag, normal vWF:RCof, normal vWF:CB, normal RIPA, and normal multimer patterns. When factor VIII levels are above 5 IU/dL, it should be considered, but the more severe cases have levels around 1 IU/dL and can only be confirmed by measuring bound factor VIII:vWFB.

Type 3

More than 70 different mutations have been related to the severe vWF deficiency known as vWD type 3.[56,67] Although originally reported as a complete absence of vWF, some cases of severe deficiency of vWF do demonstrate low levels of antigen with the use of sensitive techniques. The mutations range from single point/frame-shift mutations causing unstable mRNA or incomplete vWF monomers to large deletions of gene sections. In a study of 40 patients with type 3, most mutations identified resulted in null alleles. Homozygosity and compound heterozygosity are the most common genetic mechanism, but the incorporation of the pseudogene in substitution of a normal allele by homologous conversion occurs with surprising frequency in these patients.

As a result of the congenital near absence of vWF, these patients are at risk for developing inhibitors that can complicate replacement therapy in a manner analogous to that seen in hemophilia. Fortunately, based on published case series, clinically significant antibodies to vWF in type 3 vWD do not seem to be a frequent occurrence. The potential to reconstitute vWF in transformed cells has been explored by gene therapy investigators who have reported some success with experimental systems.[68]

Platelet Type von Willebrand Disease (Pseudo-von Willebrand Disease)

The abnormality associated with type 2B vWD that causes increased binding of vWF to GPIbα by means of mutations in the region encoding the vWF receptor binding site also can be caused analogously by abnormalities in the GPIbα itself. A total of four mutations in the *GPIBA* gene on chromosome 17 have been identified to cause this mild to moderate bleeding diathesis.[69] Like type 2B, DDAVP treatment can cause or exacerbate thrombocytopenia in platelet type vWD. The distinction from type 2B is clinically relevant in that recombinant vWF or cryoprecipitate is not adequate therapy for such patients during a bleeding episode. These patients are best treated with platelet transfusion. One laboratory test devised to differentiate between the two types involves manually mixing combinations of platelet and plasma fractions from patient and control with measurement of RIPA (see the section on RIPA). Another involves RIPA measurements with diluting cryoprecipitate in an attempt to overwhelm the endogenous defective vWF in type 2B disease. The remainder of the clinical and laboratory phenotype is similar, leading to the speculation that platelet type vWD is often misdiagnosed.

Acquired von Willebrand Disease

Low levels of circulating and functional vWF caused by mechanisms that are not congenital are known as acquired vWD. A variety of conditions not directly related to the normal life-cycle of the protein are believed to be responsible.[70] Some cases of acquired vWD involve the development of antibodies to vWF (or less often to factor VIII-vWF in a complex) as described in the original case report of a patient with lupus. In lymphoproliferative disorders and plasma cell dyscrasias, malignant cells may target adsorption and ingestion, increasing clearance rates. In hypothyroidism, decreased synthesis is likely responsible. In cardiovascular disease, platelet activation with increased clearance and mechanical vWF damage have been suggested. Drug-related clearance or increased proteolysis of vWF also has been reported. Myeloproliferative disorders apparently may induce ADAMTS-13–mediated proteolytic degradation of vWF. Impaired ADAMTS-13 activity also has been associated with malignancy, resulting in multimer abnormalities analogous to those seen in TTP[71] (see later discussion). On the other hand, mechanisms in association with Wilm's tumor and other malignancies remain unclear. Importantly, the incidence of acquired vWD is unknown and is felt to be vastly underestimated, particularly in patients with hematologic malignancies who often suffer problems with coagulation, many of whom could have acquired vWD.

One reason for the postulated frequency of missed diagnosis is the lack of adequate available diagnostic tests. Dilutional assessment of RCof activity, collagen binding assays, and RIPA as done for inhibitor titers of factor levels are the methods most commonly used, but their sensitivity and specificity are unproven. The fact that the assays involve the use of site-specific antibodies to a large multicomponent protein presents the likely theoretical possibility that the offending antibody binding at a different site may not be detected. The development of more accessible and practical tests for determination of vWF degradation, clearance, and antibody binding is needed to further characterize the incidence and significance of this potentially important vWD variant.

VON WILLEBRAND FACTOR TESTING IN THROMBOTIC THROMBOCYTOPENIA PURPURA

Tests for evaluation of TTP have evolved from monitoring of degradation by ADAMTS-13 with a time-series of gel electrophoresis assays in high urea to more specific

ADAMTS-13 activity and inhibitor measurements. Despite the pathogenesis currently understood as a deficiency of the cleaving protease leading to increased amounts of the more physiologically active multimers, the measures of circulating multimers show uncleaved ultra-large multimers only in cases of chronic relapsing TTP. Total antigen levels may be reduced, normal, or increased in acute episodes of sporadic TTP, but multimer analysis in these cases suggests that most tend to have somewhat high antigen levels with abnormal degradation that results in relative decreases of large multimers and relative increases in intermediate sized multimers.[72] This is consistent with the interpretation that vWF cleaving protease deficiency in TTP is associated with increased secretion of ultra-large active multimers that remain adherent to endothelial surfaces, where they cause unmitigated platelet activation and from which pieces break off into circulation. Regardless of mechanism, in one small study, the vWF:CB assay showed relatively good sensitivity for the multimer abnormalities noted in TTP.[73] The RCof/Ag ratio may be abnormal as well. The potential for improved diagnosis and surveillance in this disorder rests on the further development of an understanding of the pathogenesis and increasing availability of tests for ADAMTS-13 and multimer distribution assessment.

VON WILLEBRAND FACTOR IN COMMON DISORDERS, THROMBOSIS, AND FUTURE PROSPECTS

Apart from the variety of diseases associated with TTP, abnormalities in vWF have been identified in a whole host of common clinical conditions, many of which are characterized by frequent and clinically significant hypercoagulability. Diabetes, heart disease, postcoronary bypass states, malignancies, chronic inflammatory diseases, obesity, and hepatic and renal disease are associated with chronically elevated vWF levels.[74,75] The direct association of venous and arterial thrombotic risk with elevated vWF is more tenuous than that with chronically elevated factor VIII, but studies have supported an important link.[76–78] It is possible that undetermined qualities of vWF in these conditions contribute to the clotting abnormalities commonly seen in such patients. As vWD testing continues to demonstrate, vWF antigen concentration is merely one component of vWF function. An important long-term goal continues to be to gain sufficient insight into the interplay of coagulation components that contribute to bleeding and clotting complications that arise in these common clinical conditions so that tests to evaluate and better manage risk can be developed.

This article is a laboratory perspective on the diagnostic tests routinely used in the diagnosis of vWD and the emerging tools that seek to aid in the categorization of disease variants. There is continuously updated progress in the identification of genetic abnormalities and the corresponding molecular mechanisms thought to be causal in vWD, which are relevant to the eventual goal of reducing coagulation complications in vWD patients. This progress is reflected in the visible trend to further subcategorize vWD, in many ways returning to the older classification systems. Still, the available evidence has to be interpreted with the understanding that coagulation is a carefully coordinated process with many actors, complicating attempts at simple categorization based on identified mutations. Scientific progress has begun to provide a stronger basis for a more complete understanding of the processes that contribute to abnormalities in vWF, and it is hoped that we can begin to use this knowledge to tailor our management of individual patients.

REFERENCES

1. Zimmerman TS, Ruggeri ZM. von Willebrand disease. Hum Pathol 1987;18(2): 140–52.

2. Schneider SW, Nuschele S, Wixforth A, et al. Shear-induced unfolding triggers adhesion of von Willebrand factor fibers. Proc Natl Acad Sci U S A 2007; 104(19):7899–903.
3. Tsai H-M. Shear stress and von Willebrand factor in health and disease. Semin Thromb Hemost 2003;29(5):479–88.
4. Reininger AJ. VWF attributes—impact on thrombus formation. Thromb Res 2008; 122(Suppl 4):S9–13.
5. Watson SP, Auger JM, McCarty OJ, et al. GPVI and integrin alphaIIb/beta3 signaling in platelets. Thromb Haemost 2005;3:1752–62.
6. Shattil SJ, Newman PJ. Integrins: dynamic scaffolds for adhesion and signaling in platelets. Blood 2004;104:1606–15.
7. Wagner DD. Cell biology of von Willebrand factor. Annu Rev Cell Biol 1990;6: 217–46.
8. de Wit TR, van Mourik JA. Biosynthesis, processing and secretion of von Willebrand factor: biological implications. Baillieres Best Pract Res Clin Haematol 2001;14(2):241–55.
9. Michaux G, Abbitt KB, Collinson LM, et al. The physiological function of von Willebrand's factor depends on its tubular storage in endothelial Weibel-Palade bodies. Dev Cell 2006;10(2):223–32.
10. Ruggeri ZM. Structure of von Willebrand factor and its function in platelet adhesion and thrombus formation. Baillieres Best Pract Res Clin Haematol 2001;14(2): 257–79.
11. Singh I, Shankaran H, Beauharnois ME, et al. Solution structure of human von Willebrand factor studied using small angle neutron scattering. J Biol Chem 2006; 281(50):38266–75.
12. Metcalf DJ, Nightingale TD, Zenner HL, et al. Formation and function of Weibel-Palade bodies. J Cell Sci 2008;121(Pt 1):19–27.
13. Haberichter SL, Shi Q, Montgomery RR. Regulated release of VWF and FVIII and the biologic implications. Pediatr Blood Cancer 2006;46(5):547–53.
14. Borchiellini A, Fijnvandraat K, Wouter ten Cate J, et al. Quantitative analysis of von Willebrand factor propeptide release in vivo: effect of experimental endotoxemia and administration of I-Deamino-8-DArginine vasopressin in humans. Blood 1996;88:2951–8.
15. Giblin JP, Hewlett LJ, Hannah MJ. Basal secretion of von Willebrand factor from human endothelial cells [see comment]. Blood 2008;112(4):957–64.
16. Blann AD. Plasma von Willebrand factor, thrombosis, and the endothelium: the first 30 years. Thromb Haemost 2006;95(1):49–55.
17. Mohlke KL, Ginsburg D. von Willebrand disease and quantitative variation in von Willebrand factor [see comment]. J Lab Clin Med 1997;130(3):252–61.
18. Denis CV, Christophe OD, Oortwijn BD, et al. Clearance of von Willebrand factor. Thromb Haemost 2008;99(2):271–8.
19. Kaufmann JE, Oksche A, Wollheim CB, et al. Vasopressin-induced von Willebrand factor secretion from endothelial cells involves V2 receptors and cAMP. J Clin Invest 2000;106(1):107–16.
20. Ruggeri ZM, Zimmerman TS. von Willebrand factor and von Willebrand disease [erratum appears in Blood 1988 Mar;71(3):830]. Blood 1987;70(4): 895–904.
21. Sadler JE. A revised classification of von Willebrand disease. For the Subcommittee on von Willebrand Factor of the Scientific and Standardization Committee of the International Society on Thrombosis and Haemostasis. Thromb Haemost 1994;71(4):520–5.

22. Sadler JE, Budde U, Eikenboom JCJ, et al. Update on the pathophysiology and classification of von Willebrand disease: a report of the Subcommittee on von Willebrand factor [see comment]. J Thromb Haemost 2006;4(10):2103–14.

23. Schlammadinger A, Vanhoorelbeke K, Laszlo P, et al. von Willebrand factor antigen latex immunoassays are affected to a different extent by rheumatoid factor. Clin Appl Thromb Hemost 2006;12(2):242–3.

24. Hubbard AR, Heath AB. Standardization of factor VIII and von Willebrand factor in plasma: calibration of the WHO 5th International Standard (02/150). J Thromb Haemost 2004;2(8):1380–4.

25. Salem RO, Van Cott EM. A new automated screening assay for the diagnosis of von Willebrand disease. Am J Clin Pathol 2007;127(5):730–5.

26. De Vleeschauwer A, Devreese K. Comparison of a new automated von Willebrand factor activity assay with an aggregation von Willebrand ristocetin cofactor activity assay for the diagnosis of von Willebrand disease. Blood Coagul Fibrinolysis 2006;17(5):353–8.

27. Pinol M, Sales M, Costa M, et al. Evaluation of a new turbidimetric assay for von Willebrand factor activity useful in the general screening of von Willebrand disease. Haematologica 2007;92(5):712–3.

28. Federici AB, Canciani MT, Forza I, et al. A sensitive ristocetin co-factor activity assay with recombinant glycoprotein Ibalpha for the diagnosis of patients with low von Willebrand factor levels. Haematologica 2004;89(1):77–85.

29. Budde U, Pieconka A, Will K, et al. Laboratory testing for von Willebrand disease: contribution of multimer analysis to diagnosis and classification. Semin Thromb Hemost 2006;32(5):514–21.

30. Smejkal GB, Shainoff JR, Kottke-Marchant KM. Rapid high-resolution electrophoresis of multimeric von Willebrand Factor using a thermopiloted gel apparatus [erratum appears in Electrophoresis 2003 May;24(9):1482]. Electrophoresis 2003;24(4):582–7.

31. Favaloro EJ. An update on the von Willebrand factor collagen binding assay: 21 years of age and beyond adolescence but not yet a mature adult. Semin Thromb Hemost 2007;33(8):727–44.

32. Favaloro EJ. A better approach to monitoring of therapy in von Willebrand disease? [comment]. Thromb Haemost 2008;100(3):371–3.

33. Hayward CPM, Harrison P, Cattaneo M, et al. Platelet function analyzer (PFA)-100 closure time in the evaluation of platelet disorders and platelet function [see comment]. J Thromb Haemost 2006;4(2):312–9.

34. Favaloro EJ. Clinical utility of the PFA-100. Semin Thromb Hemost 2008;34(8):709–33.

35. van Vliet HHDM, Kappers-Klunne MC, Leebeek FWG, et al. PFA-100 monitoring of von Willebrand factor (VWF) responses to desmopressin (DDAVP) and factor VIII/VWF concentrate substitution in von Willebrand disease type 1 and 2 [see comment]. Thromb Haemost 2008;100(3):462–8.

36. Favaloro EJ, Patterson D, Denholm A, et al. Differential identification of a rare form of platelet-type (pseudo-) von Willebrand disease (VWD) from Type 2B VWD using a simplified ristocetin-induced-platelet-agglutination mixing assay and confirmed by genetic analysis [comment]. Br J Haematol 2007;139(4):623–6.

37. Miller JL, Kupinski JM, Castella A, et al. von Willebrand factor binds to platelets and induces aggregation in platelet-type but not type IIB von Willebrand disease. J Clin Invest 1983;72(5):1532–42.

38. Sztukowska M, Gallinaro L, Cattini MG, et al. Von Willebrand factor propeptide makes it easy to identify the shorter Von Willebrand factor survival in patients

with type 1 and type Vicenza von Willebrand disease. Br J Haematol 2008;143(1): 107–14.

39. Haberichter SL, Balistreri M, Christopherson P, et al. Assay of the von Willebrand factor (VWF) propeptide to identify patients with type 1 von Willebrand disease with decreased VWF survival. Blood 2006;108(10):3344–51.

40. Haberichter SL, Castaman G, Budde U, et al. Identification of type 1 von Willebrand disease patients with reduced von Willebrand factor survival by assay of the VWF propeptide in the European study: molecular and clinical markers for the diagnosis and management of type 1 VWD (MCMDM-1VWD). Blood 2008; 111(10):4979–85.

41. Chen D, Daigh CA, Hendricksen JI, et al. A highly-sensitive plasma von Willebrand factor ristocetin cofactor (VWF: RCo) activity assay by flow cytometry. J Thromb Haemost 2008;6(2):323–30.

42. Giannini S, Mezzasoma AM, Leone M, et al. Laboratory diagnosis and monitoring of desmopressin treatment of von Willebrand's disease by flow cytometry. Haematologica 2007;92(12):1647–54.

43. Kempfer AC, Silaf MR, Farias CE, et al. Binding of von Willebrand factor to collagen by flow cytometry. Am J Clin Pathol 1999;111(3):418–23.

44. Torres R, Levene M. Clinical multimer analysis of vWF by fluctuation spectroscopy, In: SPIE Photonics West; 24–29 January 2009; San Jose, CA, Photonics West 2009-BiOS: Biomedical Optics (Special Collection) Proceedings of SPIE Volume: CDS329, SPIE, Bellingham, WA, 2009. Abstract# 7186-15.

45. Gill JC, Endres-Brooks J, Bauer PJ, et al. The effect of ABO blood group on the diagnosis of von Willebrand disease. Blood 1987;69(6):1691–5.

46. Souto JC, Almasy L, Muniz-Diaz E, et al. Functional effects of the ABO locus polymorphism on plasma levels of von Willebrand factor, factor VIII, and activated partial thromboplastin time. Arterioscler Thromb Vasc Biol 2000;20(8): 2024–8.

47. Schleef M, Strobel E, Dick A, et al. Relationship between ABO and Secretor genotype with plasma levels of factor VIII and von Willebrand factor in thrombosis patients and control individuals. Br J Haematol 2005;128(1):100–7.

48. Davies JA, Collins PW, Hathaway LS, et al. Effect of von Willebrand factor Y/C1584 on in vivo protein level and function and interaction with ABO blood group. Blood 2007;109(7):2840–6.

49. Miller CH, Haff E, Platt SJ, et al. Measurement of von Willebrand factor activity: relative effects of ABO blood type and race. J Thromb Haemost 2003;1(10): 2191–7.

50. Gallinaro L, Cattini MG, Sztukowska M, et al. A shorter von Willebrand factor survival in O blood group subjects explains how ABO determinants influence plasma von Willebrand factor. Blood 2008;111(7):3540–5.

51. Jenkins PV, O'Donnell JS. ABO blood group determines plasma von Willebrand factor levels: a biologic function after all? Transfusion 2006;46(10):1836–44.

52. Popov J, Zhukov O, Ruden S, et al. Performance and clinical utility of a commercial von Willebrand factor collagen binding assay for laboratory diagnosis of von Willebrand disease. Clin Chem 2006;52(10):1965–7.

53. Casonato A, Pontara E, Bertomoro A, et al. Fainting induces an acute increase in the concentration of plasma factor VIII and von Willebrand factor. Haematologica 2003;88(6):688–93.

54. Tosetto A, Rodeghiero F, Castaman G, et al. A quantitative analysis of bleeding symptoms in type 1 von Willebrand disease: results from a multicenter European study (MCMDM-1 VWD). J Thromb Haemost 2006;4(4):766–73.

55. Bowman M, Mundell G, Grabell J, et al. Generation and validation of the Condensed MCMDM-1VWD Bleeding Questionnaire for von Willebrand disease. Thromb Haemost 2008;6:2062–6.
56. Gupta PK, Saxena R, Adamtziki E, et al. Genetic defects in von Willebrand disease type 3 in Indian and Greek patients. Blood Cells Mol Dis 2008;41(2): 219–22.
57. Tamura A, Iwata M, Fukunishi S, et al. Identification of newly polymorphic intron 40 markers of the von Willebrand factor gene in a Japanese population. Legal Medicine, in press. doi:10.1016/j.legalmed.2008.11.004.
58. Goodeve A, Eikenboom J, Castaman G, et al. Phenotype and genotype of a cohort of families historically diagnosed with type 1 von Willebrand disease in the European study, Molecular and Clinical Markers for the Diagnosis and Management of Type 1 von Willebrand Disease (MCMDM-1VWD) [erratum appears in Blood 2008 Mar 15;111(6):3299–300]. Blood 2007;109(1):112–21.
59. James PD, Notley C, Hegadorn C, et al. The mutational spectrum of type 1 von Willebrand disease: results from a Canadian cohort study. Blood 2007;109(1):145–54.
60. Budde U, Schneppenheim R, Eikenboom J, et al. Detailed von Willebrand factor multimer analysis in patients with von Willebrand disease in the European study, molecular and clinical markers for the diagnosis and management of type 1 von Willebrand disease (MCMDM-1VWD) [see comment]. J Thromb Haemost 2008; 6(5):762–71.
61. Tjernberg P, Vos HL, Castaman G, et al. Dimerization and multimerization defects of von Willebrand factor due to mutated cysteine residues. J Thromb Haemost 2004;2(2):257–65.
62. Michiels JJ, Berneman Z, Gadisseur A, et al. Classification and characterization of hereditary types 2A, 2B, 2C, 2D, 2E, 2M, 2N, and 2U (unclassifiable) von Willebrand disease. Clin Appl Thromb Hemost 2006;12(4):397–420.
63. Victor M, Rugeri L, Nougier C, et al. Contribution of genetical analysis for diagnosis of von Willebrand's disease type 2B. Haemophilia 2009;15:610–2.
64. Federici A, Mannucci PM, Castaman G, et al. Clinical and molecular predictors of thrombocytopenia and risk of bleeding in patients with von Willebrand disease type 2B: a cohort study of 67 patients. Blood (online prepublication Sep 19, 2008). doi:10.1182/blood-2008-04-152280.
65. Nurden P, Debili N, Vainchenker W, et al. Impaired megakaryocytopoiesis in type 2B von Willebrand disease with severe thrombocytopenia. Blood 2006;108(8): 2587–95.
66. Casonato A, De Marco L, Gallinaro L, et al. Altered von Willebrand factor subunit proteolysis and multimer processing associated with the Cys2362Phe mutation in the B2 domain. Thromb Haemost 2007;97(4):527–33.
67. Baronciani L, Cozzi G, Canciani MT, et al. Molecular defects in type 3 von Willebrand disease: updated results from 40 multiethnic patients. Blood Cells Mol Dis 2003;30(3):264–70.
68. Laje P, Shang D, Cao W, et al. Correction of murine ADAMTS13 deficiency by hematopoietic progenitor cell-mediated gene therapy. Blood 2009;113(10):2172–80.
69. Franchini M, Montagnana M, Lippi G. Clinical, laboratory and therapeutic aspects of platelet-type von Willebrand disease. Int J Lab Hematol 2008;30(2):91–4.
70. Franchini M, Lippi G. Acquired von Willebrand syndrome: an update. Am J Hematol 2007;82(5):368–75.
71. Koo B-H, Oh D, Chung SY, et al. Deficiency of von Willebrand factor-cleaving protease activity in the plasma of malignant patients. Thromb Res 2002;105(6): 471–6.

72. Galbusera M, Noris M, Rossi C, et al. Increased fragmentation of von Willebrand factor, due to abnormal cleavage of the subunit, parallels disease activity in recurrent hemolytic uremic syndrome and thrombotic thrombocytopenic purpura and discloses predisposition in families. The Italian Registry of Familial and Recurrent HUS/TTP. Blood 1999;94(2):610–20.

73. Casonato A, Fabris F, Pontara E, et al. Diagnosis and follow-up of thrombotic thrombocytopenic purpura by means of von Willebrand factor collagen binding assay. Clin Appl Thromb Hemost 2006;12(3):296–304.

74. Martinelli I. von Willebrand factor and factor VIII as risk factors for arterial and venous thrombosis. Semin Hematol 2005;42(1):49–55.

75. Franchini M, Lippi G. Von Willebrand factor and thrombosis. Ann Hematol 2006; 85(7):415–23.

76. Bongers TN, de Maat MPM, van Goor M-LPJ, et al. High von Willebrand factor levels increase the risk of first ischemic stroke: influence of ADAMTS13, inflammation, and genetic variability. Stroke 2006;37(11):2672–7.

77. Folsom AR, Rosamond WD, Shahar E, et al. Prospective study of markers of hemostatic function with risk of ischemic stroke. The Atherosclerosis Risk in Communities (ARIC) Study Investigators. Circulation 1999;100(7):736–42.

78. Tsai AW, Cushman M, Rosamond WD, et al. Coagulation factors, inflammation markers, and venous thromboembolism: the longitudinal investigation of thromboembolism etiology (LITE) [see comment]. Am J Med 2002;113(8):636–42.

79. Nichols WL, Hultin MB, James AH, et al. von Willebrand disease (VWD): evidence-based diagnosis and management guidelines, the National Heart, Lung, and Blood Institute (NHLBI) Expert Panel report (USA) [see comment]. Haemophilia 2008;14(2):171–232.

The Laboratory Approach to Inherited and Acquired Coagulation Factor Deficiencies

Benjamin L. Wagenman, MD[a,c], Kelly T. Townsend, BS, MT(ASCP) SH[a],
Prasad Mathew, MD, FAAP[b], Kendall P. Crookston, MD, PhD, FCAP[a,c,*]

KEYWORDS

- Hemophilia • Coagulation factor deficiency
- Hypoprothrombinemia • Hemostasis • Prothrombin time
- Activated partial thromboplastin time • Pre-analytical variables
- Bleeding • Coagulation factor inhibitors

Coagulation factors are usually either enzymes (eg, F9, F2) or cofactors (eg, F5, F8) that circulate at varying concentrations in the blood. Rather than reporting the absolute concentration of the circulating factors (as is done with most chemistry analytes), the clinical laboratory reports *activities* for most coagulation factors (ie, the functional activity of the factor in the patient's plasma compared with that of calibrator or a standard plasma, the latter with a defined assayed activity of 100%).

Factor deficiencies traditionally are classified as type 1 or type 2. In type 1 deficiency, the protein structure of the factor is normal, but there is a decreased concentration in the circulation, so the activity level is decreased. This can be caused by increased clearance or decreased production of the factor. Essentially all acquired and many inherited disorders fall into this category. In type 2 deficiencies, there is a normal or nearly normal concentration of a circulating protein that is intrinsically defective and therefore also demonstrates a lower overall activity level. Either type

This work was supported in part by a grant from Blood Systems Inc.

Note: Although Roman numerals traditionally are used to identify coagulation factors (eg, FIX, FVII), Arabic numerals will be used in this discussion (eg, F9, F7) as the latter are less confusing for the learner and also for an international audience.

[a] Department of Pathology, University of New Mexico, TriCore Reference Laboratories, 915 Camino de Salud NE, Albuquerque, NM 87102, USA

[b] Department of Pediatrics, and the Ted R. Montoya Hemophilia Program, University of New Mexico, 2211 Lomas Boulevard NE, Albuquerque, NM 87106, USA

[c] United Blood Service of New Mexico, 1515 University Avenue, NE, Albuquerque, NM 87102, USA

* Corresponding author.

E-mail address: kcrookston@salud.unm.edu (K.P. Crookston).

Clin Lab Med 29 (2009) 229–252
doi:10.1016/j.cll.2009.04.002
0272-2712/09/$ – see front matter
labmed.theclinics.com

of deficiency will show decreased activity when measured by laboratory assays. When measuring the protein itself using an antigen assay, type 2 deficiencies show a relative preservation of the antigen level in relation to the activity level, while type 1 deficiency also shows decreased antigen. This situation is illustrated best in von Willebrand disease (vWD) (see article by Torres in this issue).

A brief survey of the clinical aspects of the inherited and acquired factor deficiencies is presented first, followed by a discussion of the laboratory considerations in evaluating patients who have possible factor deficiencies. **Table 1** and **Box 1** illustrate the etiologies, relative incidence, and other characteristics of the various factor deficiencies discussed. Some deficiencies of proteins involved in hemostatic regulation also will lead to bleeding diatheses (eg, alpha-2-antiplasmin); however, these abnormalities are not within the scope of this article.

INHERITED FACTOR DEFICIENCIES

Inherited bleeding disorders have been recognized since ancient times, often caused by severe bleeding with circumcision or minor trauma. Severe hemophilia A and B, and severe F11 deficiency typically prolong the patient's activated partial thromboplastin time (aPTT), but this abnormality is not always overwhelming. Many patients present with an aPTT between the upper end of the normal reference range and the middle of the typical aPTT heparin reference range. Deficiencies of the contact factors—most commonly F12—can prolong the aPTT more significantly, similar to what is seen with a high level of therapeutic heparin or heparin contamination after blood is drawn through a heparinized line. Hemophilia A (F8 deficiency) and B (F9 deficiency) are the only factor deficiencies typically inherited in a sex-linked pattern.

Sufficient hemostasis often can be achieved despite having coagulation factor levels below the normal laboratory reference ranges. Similarly, a modest increase in the endogenous circulating factor activity level (eg, from 0.5% to 5%) in hemophilia can have major clinical implications, essentially converting a severe to a mild phenotype. This provides hope to researchers working to use gene therapy as a possible treatment of inherited hemophilia.[1]

Factor 8 Deficiency (Hemophilia A)

Hemophilia A[2] is the most common inherited factor deficiency. This X-linked disorder is caused by a deficiency of F8. F8 is the cofactor that works with F9 to activate F10, increasing the reaction rate by several orders of magnitude. Older nomenclature calls the F8 *coagulant* activity "VIII:C" and the measurement of the *antigen* "VIII:Ag." The F8 molecule usually circulates in the bloodstream, protected from degradation by forming a stable complex with von Willebrand factor (vWF). Deficiency of vWF leads to increased clearance of F8 from the circulation; therefore, F8 activity typically is included in screening panels for vWD.

Many different genetic mutations have been classified in various hemophilia A pedigrees.[3,4] Mild and moderate hemophilias typically are caused by one of many missense mutations induced by single base pair substitutions. Severe hemophilia A, by contrast, is caused more often by larger gene defects, including inversions (intron 22), large deletions, and insertions. Thus, both activity and antigenic protein measures are typically very low. Intrachromosomal intron–exon recombinations of the X chromosome account for about half of the severe forms. For the prenatal genetic diagnosis of known males to be effective, family studies must identify the mutation particular to that pedigree. There is a high sporadic occurrence (high spontaneous mutation rate), however, of hemophilia also; thus, about 30% of newly diagnosed severe hemophilia

Table 1
Congenital factor deficiencies

Factor Deficiency	Estimated Incidence	Inheritance Pattern/Genes Involved	Bleeding Severity
F8 (hemophilia A)	1:10,000	X-linked recessive (Xq28)	Mild >5% Moderate (1% to 5%) Severe (<1%)
F9 (hemophilia B)	1:30,000	X-linked recessive (Xq27)	Mild to severe
F11	Rare, 5% in Ashkenazi Jews	Autosomal recessive (4q32q3)	Mild to severe
F2 (prothrombin)	Rare	Autosomal recessive (11p11–q12)	Mild to moderate
F5	1:1 million	Autosomal recessive (1q21–q25)	Mild to moderate
F7	1:500,000	Autosomal recessive (13q34)	Mild to severe
F10	1:500,000	Autosomal recessive (13q34)	Mild to severe
F12	Rare	Autosomal recessive 5q33	No bleeding
Other contact factors (including prekallikrein, high molecular weight kininogen)	Rare, unknown	Autosomal recessive (various genes)	No bleeding
F13	<1:1 million	A subunit: 6p24-p25 B subunit: 1q31-q32	Moderate to severe; postoperative
Afibrinogenemia	Rare	Autosomal dominant (various mutations at 4q31)	Variable
Dysfibrinogenemia	Rare	Autosomal dominant (various mutations at 4q31)	Variable—may be asymptomatic
Hypofibrinogenemia	Rare	Autosomal dominant (various mutations at 4q31)	Variable
Combined F5 and F8	Rare	Autosomal recessive (18q21, 2p21)	Variable
Combined F2, F7, F9, & F10	Rare	—	Variable

Box 1
Acquired factor deficiencies

Immune-mediated factor deficiencies

Alloantibody factor inhibitors in hereditary hemophilia patients

F8 inhibitors in hemophilia A patients on factor replacement therapy (incidence = 24% of hemophilia A patients)

F9 inhibitors in hemophilia B patients on factor replacement therapy (incidence = 1.5–3% of hemophilia B patients)

Autoantibodies causing acquired hemophilia

Acquired hemophilia A (most common, may cause severe bleeding)

Prothrombin deficiency complicating the antiphospholipid syndrome (rare)

Acquired F5 deficiency (from antibodies to bovine thrombin preparation used in certain fibrin glues, uncommon)

Nonimmune-mediated

Increased destruction

Disseminated intravascular coagulation (DIC)

Extracorporeal membrane oxygenation (ECMO)

Fibrinolytic drugs in thrombolytic therapy (eg, tissue plasminogen activator)

Decreased production

Liver disease

Abnormal production

Warfarin use

Other causes of vitamin K deficiency

Loss and sequestration

Nephrotic syndrome

Acquired F10 deficiency associated with light chain amyloidosis (accelerated removal of F10 caused by adsorption of the factor to the amyloid fibrils); 8.7% of amyloidosis patients had F10 levels less than 50% of normal; 56% of these had bleeding complications if F10 less 25% of normal; can be fatal

Plasma exchange apheresis (particularly decreased fibrinogen)

Inactivation

Direct thrombin inhibitor use (eg, hirudin, argatroban)

---

patients may not have a family history. Activity assays sometimes are performed on cord blood from male newborns delivered to a known carrier in a family with severe hemophilia. This is of particular interest in premature infants, as there is increased risk of intracranial bleeding.[5] It is an important caveat that such results must be interpreted with caution, as cord blood is not an optimal specimen for coagulation testing. This is because activation of clotting in cord blood often occurs during the delivery and subsequent blood collection processes, and cord blood samples are clotted commonly, at least partially. In addition, maturation of the hemostatic system occurs during childhood, such that newborns generally have lower levels of some factors than adults. For example, the mean F9 in newborns has been reported at only 53% for full-term and 35% for healthy premature infants, with F11 at 38% and 30%, respectively. Exceptions to this maturation are F8 and vWF levels, which are typically greater than or equal to100% in both full-term and healthy premature infants.[6] Testing of boys from families that have milder forms of the disease typically can be performed later in child-hood, preferably before they begin learning to walk.

The clinical manifestations of hemophilia A usually correlate with the severity of the deficiency measured in the laboratory. Because the difference between severe (less than 1% F8 activity) and moderate hemophilia (1 to 5%) is clinically significant, labo-ratory assays should have linearity down to less than 1%. In recent decades, there has been dramatic improvement in long-term treatment using both plasma-derived factor concentrates and recombinant factors. Today, because of prophylactic regimens and early treatment of bleeding episodes, many young adult males who have severe hemophilia A do not exhibit some of the classical clinical manifestations that include joint arthropathy from repeated bleeding into joints, contractures of musculature from frequent muscle and joint involvement, hemorrhage from mild trauma, and even central nervous system (CNS) bleeds.

Severe cases often receive prophylactic factor administration, either primary prophylaxis, before development of any joint bleeding (a hallmark of hemophilia), or secondary prophylaxis, after a significant bleed into a vital organ, or after development of a target joint. The US Centers for Disease Control and Prevention definition of a target joint is that a minimum of four bleeds must have occurred in that joint within a consecutive 6-month period. Cryoprecipitate and fresh-frozen plasma revolution-ized the treatment of hemophilia A about 50 years ago. The ease of use and safety of purified factor concentrates and their recombinant counterparts, however, have replaced these blood products for hemophilia therapy in industrialized nations. Cryo-precipitate and plasma, however, remain the mainstays of treatment for bleeding in economically challenged countries around the world.

Infusion of factor at home has also revolutionized management of these patients. Home treatment allows for early institution of replacement products at the first sign of a bleed, which decreases the morbidity of these bleeds significantly. In patients who have mild deficiency, DDAVP can be used as an alternative to factor, either intra-venously or by nasal spray. DDAVP increases both F8 and vWF and thus aids hemo-stasis in those hemophiliacs who are mildly affected. However, before its use, each patient should be evaluated for their response to DDAVP. In addition, antifibrinolytic agents can be used as adjunct therapies, especially for mucosal bleeding.

Female carriers of hemophilia typically have low-normal to moderately decreased factor levels, but have been reported as low as 5%. As many as 10% of carriers will have levels less than 30%. Some carriers, therefore, may have a mild-to-moderate bleeding phenotype, particularly with major hemostatic challenges such as surgery, and their factor levels will need to be monitored for such procedures.

In addition to using factor activity assays to diagnose deficiency, a significant part of the coagulation laboratory workload is to monitor hemophilia treatment and to screen for increased clearance of administered factor caused by possible inhibitor formation.

Factor 9 Deficiency (Hemophilia B)

Sometimes known as Christmas disease (after the surname of the first patient diag-nosed with this disorder), hemophilia B is caused by a deficiency of F9, an enzyme rather than a cofactor, which activates F10. Hemophilia B is analogous to hemophilia A in many aspects. It is only about one-fifth as common, but follows similar clinical patterns in disease manifestation and severity. Although also X-linked, hemophilia B shows tremendous heterogeneity at the molecular level, making genetic screening much more difficult. The F9 mutation unique to each family needs to be identified before prenatal or other genetic screening can be performed.

Cryoprecipitate does not contain significant amounts of F9 and therefore cannot be used to treat this disease. Prothrombin complex concentrates once were used to treat the disease before specific factor products became available (both plasma-based and recombinant). It is important to note that some patients who have hemophilia B will develop allergic reactions to the infusion of these factors, including anaphylaxis. Hence, the first 10 to 15 infusions usually are administered in a clinic or hospital setting. As in hemophilia A, home therapy is an effective strategy in reducing the morbidity of bleeding in these patients. Patients who have mild hemophilia B may have normal or near-normal aPTT results. Therefore, specific factor assays should be performed in working up undiagnosed mild bleeding disorders, even if the aPTT is within the normal range.

Factor 11 Deficiency

In contrast to hemophilias A and B, F11 deficiency (which used to be termed hemophilia C)[7,8] is an autosomal disorder with variable penetrance. The gene is located on chromosome 4 (4q35.2). In addition, the bleeding manifestations are heterogeneous in relation to the factor activity levels (ie, there is a poor correlation between bleeding manifestations and the baseline F11 clotting activity, unlike hemophilia A and B). Thus, separation of patients into distinct clinical phenotypes is less clear-cut than in other bleeding disorders. Many patients do not exhibit bleeding until challenged with trauma or surgery; unlike hemophilia A and B, bleeding in F11 deficiency is often mucosal. Patients who have severe deficiency (levels less than 15% to 20%) have a high probability of postoperative bleeding. This, however, is not a uniform finding, and some may not bleed at all. Yet, patients who have mild deficiency may have severe bleeding when hemostatically challenged (eg, by platelet-inhibitory drugs). The reason for this discrepancy is unclear, but one possible explanation may be the coexistence of other bleeding disorders like vWD, which could contribute to the bleeding risk in these mildly deficient patients. Hence, it is important from a laboratory standpoint to consider testing for coinheritance of other bleeding disorders. Because many of these patients are asymptomatic until challenged by surgery or trauma, the diagnosis often is made in late childhood or early adulthood. Over half of the cases are diagnosed in patients of Ashkenazi Jewish descent. In this group, it is estimated that one in eight individuals are heterozygous for a gene defect, and 1 in 190 are homozygous.

Generally, screening coagulation tests will reveal an isolated prolonged aPTT with F11 deficiency. Because different partial thromboplastin reagents vary in sensitivity to F11, reference ranges should be established in each local laboratory. F11 assays should be performed based on clinical suspicion. Most identified mutations cause type 1 deficiency, with reduced amounts of normal F11 antigen leading to a lower concentration of the protein in the plasma. Because F11 antigen measurements correlate with activity levels, determination of antigen levels is not recommended routinely as part of the testing process. Given the poor correlation of F11 activity levels and bleeding risk, researchers are looking into global tests of hemostasis (thrombin generation, thromboelastography) to understand the role of F11 in hemostasis (see article by Teruya in this issue). Specific F11 replacement concentrates are available in the European Union and experimentally in the United States. Fresh-frozen plasma remains the mainstay of treatment in the United States, along with adjunct therapies like antifibrinolytic agents.

Other Inherited Factor Deficiencies

Genetic mutations may occur in any of the proteins involved in the formation of the fibrin clot or in regulation of the coagulation pathways. Deficiencies of some of these, such as tissue factor, do not appear to be compatible with life. Mutations of factors other than 8, 9, and 11 are typically very rare, and these are especially heterogeneous with respect to the range of bleeding symptoms (from none to severe).[9]

Deficiencies of factor 12 and other contact factors

Deficiencies of factors in the contact pathway of coagulation are typically autosomal recessive and include F12, prekallikrein (Fletcher factor), and high molecular weight kininogen. These coagulation curiosities produce a markedly prolonged aPTT in the test tube, but cause no bleeding diatheses. This is likely because the contact factors lack a major role in the in vivo clotting process (see article by Kriz and colleagues, elsewhere in this issue). F12 deficiency is the most common cause of an isolated and significantly prolonged aPTT in a nonbleeding patient, after ruling out heparin contamination and lupus anticoagulant (LA). Severe F12 deficiency is rare, and patients may never be identified unless an aPTT is performed for another indication. Although there are few if any clinical consequences, the patient, laboratory, and clinical care team should be aware of the situation so that unnecessary concern is avoided in the future if an aPTT is ordered again by an unknowing caregiver. Deficiencies of the other contact factors are much less common, and confirmation of these deficiencies may be performed by reference coagulation laboratories.

Deficiencies of factors 2 (prothrombin), 5, 7, and 10

In contrast to contact factor deficiencies, decreased activity of factors 2, 5, 7, and 10 often lead to bleeding disorders of varying severity.[10–14] These are all very infrequent, autosomal recessive disorders (incidence of less than 1 in 500,000).

Prothrombin deficiency is not always severe, because there is normally a large molar excess of F2 over the minimum needed to prevent bleeding. Bleeding is seen predominantly in homozygous or compound heterozygous individuals, and can be moderate to severe. In the laboratory, prothrombin deficiency is characterized by both a prolonged PT and aPTT. If clinical suspicion warrants, an F2 activity assay should be performed. Activity testing most often is performed using a one-stage assay. The prothrombin gene is found on chromosome 11p11.2. More than 40 different mutations have been identified in this deficiency. Given the rarity of this disorder, a clear genotype/phenotype correlation is difficult to ascertain, but the lower the levels, the greater the severity of bleeding; symptoms include mucosal bleeding, surgical and trauma related hemorrhage, hemarthroses, and intracranial bleeding. Treatment of bleeding episodes usually is accomplished by use of plasma or prothrombin complex concentrate (PCC), which contains F2, F7, F9, and F10. The exact amount of F2 in these products is unknown. PCC usually is dosed based on the F9 units in each lot. Hence, the dose of PCC will vary from product to product and may lead to supratherapeutic levels of the other transfused factors; this may increase the risk of thrombosis. Thus, PCC dosing is limited to less than 200 U/kg/d. Monitoring of this therapy is done by following the PT/aPTT or by specific F2 assays.

The clinical variability of F5 deficiency is complicated by the fact that F5 is found within platelet alpha-granules and in plasma. Aside from mutations that give rise to inherited F5 deficiency, deficiencies of F5 also can be acquired secondary to F5 inhibitors that result from exposure to bovine thrombin. Activated F5 serves as a cofactor in the prothrombinase complex (like F8 in the tenase complex) that cleaves and activates F2. Like F11, the F5 activity level has limited correlation with the severity of bleeding, but the lower the level, the greater the severity of bleeding. Patients who are seen clinically for bleeding usually have levels less than 5%. Data from the bleeding registries suggest that these patients usually present with skin and mucosal bleeding, but the more severely affected may present with CNS bleeds, hemarthrosis, or muscular bleeds, which explains why F5 deficiency has been termed parahemophilia. The gene for F5 is located on chromosome 1q23. More than 60 mutations associated with F5 deficiency have been identified. Similar to F2 deficiency, F5 deficiency is characterized by prolongation of both the PT and aPTT. If a low F5 is found, then inherited F5 deficiency must be distinguished from DIC, liver disease, combined deficiencies, or an acquired inhibitor. Plasma is the mainstay of therapy in these patients; however, platelet transfusions also may be beneficial in resistant bleeding cases and for outpatient therapy.

F7 deficiency is the most frequent among the more rare congenital bleeding disorders, characterized by an isolated prolongation of the PT. The gene is located on the long arm of chromosome 13. To date, more than 130 mutations have been reported. Similar to other rare bleeding disorders, bleeding in these patients is heterogeneous both in regards to site and severity, and the correlation between circulating F7 and clinical bleeding is not linear. Patients who present early in life (younger than 6 months) or have CNS or gastrointestinal (GI) hemorrhage or hemarthrosis, however, are clearly considered to be severe cases. The F7-dependent PT clotting assay is easily available, but nuances in the influence of different thromboplastin reagents on the specific assay must be considered. For example, if the PT with a purified thromboplastin reagent is prolonged in an African American patient (especially without a history of clinical bleeding), a F7 polymorphism may be present that actually yields a normal PT result using recombinant human thromboplastin. Several F7 plasma-derived products are available in the European Union to treat severe bleeding cases, but therapy is complicated by the short in vivo half-life of F7, especially in children who are the most severely affected. Hence, these products have to administered frequently. In addition to plasma-derived F7 products, the recombinant form of activated F7 is also available (NovoSeven, Novo Nordisk, Bagsvaerd, Denmark) worldwide.

F10 is a liver-produced serine protease that serves a pivotal role as the first enzyme in the common pathway of clot formation. Patients who have severe deficiency tend to have the most severe symptoms, and patients are classified similar to hemophilia as severe (less than 1% of F10 clotting activity), moderate (1% to 5%), and mild (6% to 10%). Severe F10 deficiency is one of the most rare disorders. The gene for F10 is located on chromosome 13q34-ter. More than 80 different mutations have been identified thus far. In contrast to F8 and F9 deficiency, the most frequent bleeding manifestations are mucocutaneous, including severe menorrhagia. Hemarthrosis also has been reported in rare patients. Patients who have severe deficiency may present in the newborn period with bleeding after circumcision, from the umbilical stump, or with GI or CNS hemorrhage. The diagnosis should be suspected when both the PT and aPTT are prolonged; the F10 functional assay will reveal the deficiency. Like F11, F10 levels are lower at birth, and do not approximate adult values till after 6 months of age. F10 replacement therapy is achieved with plasma or PCC (dosing is again by F9 units).

Deficiencies of factors 1 (fibrinogen) and 13

Fibrinogen (F1) is neither a cofactor nor an enzyme, but a glycoprotein produced in the liver that serves as a substrate to make fibrin clots. Unlike factor assays, which generally are reported as activity, the laboratory typically reports fibrinogen *concentration*, rather than activity. Prothrombin (F2) cleaves two small fibrinopeptides from fibrinogen, allowing it to spontaneously aggregate. In normal physiology, these cleavage products polymerize noncovalently to form a fibrin clot that subsequently is cross-linked covalently by

F13. It is one of these covalent bonds between the D regions of two fibrin molecules that produces the D-dimers measured in the laboratory after degradation of the clot during fibrinolysis. Fibrinogen contains many specific binding sites and plays other adhesive roles in addition to that of a substrate in secondary hemostasis. Fibrinogen interacts with platelet GPIIb-IIIa, fibronectin, and collagen in cell-based hemostasis. Inherited disorders can manifest as quantitative defects (afibrinogenemia/hypofibrinogenemia) or qualitative defects (dysfibrinogenemia), and clinical manifestations vary from asymptomatic to life-threatening bleeds, and paradoxically even to thromboembolic events.

Afibrinogenemia often is diagnosed in the newborn period with umbilical cord bleeding or other severe life- or limb-threatening bleeding. Hypofibrinogenemia presents with lesser bleeding episodes and usually is diagnosed after a challenge to the hemostatic system, while dysfibrinogenemia is diagnosed commonly during adulthood and also may be acquired with liver disease. In afibrinogenemia, all coagulation tests that depend on fibrin as the endpoint (PT, aPTT, thrombin time, reptilase time) are prolonged infinitely, and fibrinogen is undetectable by both functional (von Clauss) and antigenic assays. A fibrinogen level less than 100 mg/dL often will translate to prolonged PT and aPTT. In hypofibrinogenemia, the thrombin time is a very sensitive test, and is confirmed by an abnormal reptilase time. In dysfibrinogenemia, there is usually a discrepancy between clottable protein and antigenically measured fibrinogen. Replacement therapy is generally effective in treating bleeding episodes caused by any of the fibrinogen disorders, including cryoprecipitate and plasma-derived fibrinogen concentrate (RiaSTAP, CSL Behring, King of Prussia, PA, recently approved by the US Food and Drug Administration).

Inherited dysfibrinogenemia is an autosomal-dominant type 2 defect, with several identified mutations. The thrombin and reptilase times are prolonged. The former is assayed after the addition of thrombin to patient plasma, directly converting fibrinogen to fibrin. The thrombin time is sensitive to any deficiency of functional fibrinogen but is also very sensitive to heparin, which greatly increases the inhibition of added thrombin by endogenous antithrombin. The reptilase time is also sensitive to fibrinogen deficiencies. Reptilase is a thrombin-like molecule derived from snake venom that directly cleaves fibrinogen and allows clot formation, but is not affected by heparin, as reptilase is not inhibited by antithrombin.

Deficiency of F13[15] leads to an unstable clot that may be dissolved or dislodged by trauma. The short life of the uncross-linked clot leads to symptoms of delayed bleeding, often presenting as late umbilical cord bleeding (and poor wound healing). A specific F13 activity level is performed by some reference laboratories, but the most common test used to screen for homozygous (severe) F13 deficiency is urea clot lysis. Urea is a chaotropic agent that enhances the dissociation of the uncross-linked fibrin molecules in patients who have severe F13 deficiency. This test involves clotting the plasma, adding 5 mol/L urea, then assessing the time to clot dissolution. The thromboelastograph also can be used to diagnose F13 deficiency as evidenced by reduced maximal amplitude and a rapid decrease in clot size and strength (see article by Teruya in this issue). Plasma F13 is a heterotetramer (FXIII-A2B2). The gene coding for FXIII-A subunit is on chromosome 6p24-25, while that for the FXIII-B subunit is on chromosome 1q31-32.1. Congenital deficiency can be caused by defects in either FXIII-A (type 2 defect), usually resulting in clinical bleeding, or FXIII-B (type 1 defect), where bleeding occurs infrequently. More than 70 subunit gene mutations have been identified (67 in subunit A, only 4 thus far in subunit B). In those homozygous patients with levels that are either absent or less than 5% (variability caused by assay inaccuracy), F13 deficiency is associated with severe bleeding, spontaneous intracranial hemorrhages, poor wound healing, and spontaneous abortions.

Heterozygotes are usually asymptomatic. Replacement therapy includes cryoprecipitate and a plasma-derived FXIII concentrate (Fibrogammin, ZLB Behring, Marburg, Germany) approved in the European Union, but also available on a compassionate basis in the United States at the time of this writing.

Combined factor deficiencies

Many rare combined factor deficiencies have been identified in various pedigrees (see **Table 1** for examples). In the laboratory, if a single factor deficiency is diagnosed but does not explain all of the abnormal screening tests, the presence of an additional deficiency should be considered. Combined deficiency of both F5 and F8 can result from mutations in either the LMAN1 (located on chromosome 18q21) or MCFD2 (located on chromosome 2p21) genes encoding proteins that shuttle these factors from the endoplasmic reticulum to the Golgi complex. The deficiency is characterized by concomitant low levels (usually 5% to 20%) of both F5 and F8, and it is associated with mild-to-moderate bleeding. Treatment requires both F5 and F8 replacement. Combined deficiency of F7 and F10 has been reported with 13q deletions; the two genes are located very close to each other. Combined deficiencies of the vitamin K-dependent proteins 2, 7, 9, 10 can occur when there is an abnormality in the gamma–glutamyl carboxylase gene or the vitamin K epoxide reductase complex.

ACQUIRED FACTOR DEFICIENCIES

In contrast to the rare inherited deficiencies, coagulation factor deficiencies are acquired commonly.[16] These include deficiencies secondary to autoantibody formation leading to neutralization of factor activity or rarely, accelerated clearance from the circulation.[17] Other acquired causes include decreased production (eg, liver disease), impaired synthesis (eg, vitamin K deficiency), and increased destruction (disseminated intravascular coagulation and thrombolytic therapy).

Immune-mediated Acquired Factor Deficiencies

A complex interaction of several variables leads to inhibitor formation in congenital hemophilia, while acquired hemophilia in genetically normal individuals represents a failure of immune tolerance mechanisms.[18] The development of inhibitor antibodies is perhaps the most serious complication of coagulation factor replacement therapy in congenital hemophilia, while acquired hemophilia represents an uncommon disorder in older adults that is generally responsive to current immunosuppressive regimens.

Alloantibody factor inhibitors in hereditary hemophilia

Inhibitors of congenital hemophilia are alloantibodies stimulated by infusion of exogenous factor that contains epitopes that may not be present on the mutated endogenous factor.[3,17,19] These antibodies complicate the treatment of bleeding, because they bind and inactivate infused factor, or occasionally accelerate its clearance, often rendering standard factor replacement therapy ineffective. Approximately 20 to 30% of severe hemophilia A patients develop inhibitors, and this incidence is even higher in children who have large deletions or inversions. Inhibitors are far less common in moderate and mild hemophilia A and in severe hemophilia B (less than 5% in the latter). Inhibitors cause management of these patients to become more difficult and costly. The antibodies not only neutralize the infused factor but also may cross-react with endogenous factor, sometimes resulting in the conversion of moderate hemophilia to a severe phenotype.

Coagulation laboratories supporting hemophilia centers typically quantitate the titer of inhibitor (Bethesda units (BU)/mL) present using a series of F8 assays that have been modified to show neutralization of human F8 (**Fig. 1**). In patients who have high inhibitor levels (greater than 5 BU/mL) and severe bleeding, therapies to bypass the defect in the coagulation cascade must be used, because the antibody simply neutralizes the large amounts of factor that are infused. Recombinant activated F7 (rVIIa, Novoseven) and activated prothrombin complex concentrates (FEIBA, Baxter Healthcare, Westlake Village, CA, USA) are the most commonly used bypass drugs.[20] These agents directly stimulate F10 activation without involvement of the missing intermediaries (F8 or F9). The coagulation laboratory should be informed if bypass agents have been administered before any coagulation testing, as these may alter the results and clinical interpretation dramatically.

Autoantibodies causing acquired hemophilia

The laboratory diagnosis of acquired hemophilia typically is made when an isolated factor deficiency is identified in a patient with clinically significant bleeding who has

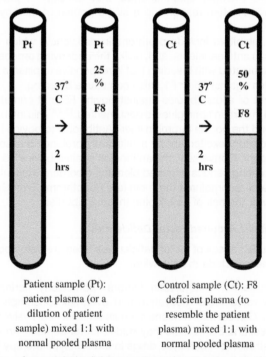

Patient sample (Pt): patient plasma (or a dilution of patient sample) mixed 1:1 with normal pooled plasma

Control sample (Ct): F8 deficient plasma (to resemble the patient plasma) mixed 1:1 with normal pooled plasma

Fig. 1. To quantitate a factor 8 (F8) inhibitor, patient plasma is incubated with a source of F8 (normal pooled plasma) at 37°C for 2 hours. A control (F8 deficient plasma + normal pooled plasma) is also incubated at 37°C for 2 hours. Residual F8 activity is then measured on both mixtures. The residual F8 activity of the patient mixture is compared to that of the control mixture (patient/control). If the resulting ratio is <0.40, the patient sample will need to be diluted in either buffer (Bethesda assay) or F8 deficient plasma (Nijmegen modification). The reciprocal dilution of patient plasma that results in a F8 activity that is 50% of that of the control mixture is defined as one Bethesda unit (BU). The stronger the inhibitor, the greater the dilution required to allow for expression of the F8 activity. In this example, after incubation, the patient's sample had a residual F8 activity of 25% compared to the 50% seen in the control (ratio of patient/control = 0.50). This patient has a 1 BU inhibitor. If the ratio of patient to control is >80%, this suggests no inhibitor (or a clinically insignificant inhibitor).

a negative personal and family history of a bleeding disorder. The most common entities caused by autoantibodies to coagulation factors are acquired hemophilia A,[21,22] followed by prothrombin deficiency complicating the antiphospholipid syndrome, and acquired F5 deficiency after surgical use of bovine thrombin. These coagulation factor deficiencies are uncommon acquired conditions that can lead to serious hemorrhage. Acquired hemophilia A typically presents in older patients who have no prior history of a bleeding disorder; about one-third of these patients will

have underlying disorders (autoimmune diseases such as systemic lupus erythematosus or rheumatoid arthritis), have lymphoproliferative disorders such as chronic lymphocytic leukemia,

be peripartum,

or have been treated with drugs such as penicillin and sulfonamides.

Whereas inhibitors that occur with inherited hemophilia A may be treated with heavy immunosuppressive therapy, autoantibodies that develop in patients who have acquired hemophilia A often respond to a single course of therapy (eg, anti-CD20 [rituximab]).[22]

Other acquired inhibitors include prothrombin deficiency, which typically occurs with persistent lupus anticoagulants, and, unlike the underlying procoagulant disorder, F2 deficiency is associated with bleeding that is responsive to plasma or PCC therapy. Rare autoantibodies against F5 or F13 also can cause bleeding.

The development of alloantibodies against bovine F5 that contaminate thrombin preparations used in certain fibrin glues is documented.[11,23] This inhibitor is in addition to antibodies toward the bovine thrombin itself. Antibodies to bovine F2 generally only create in vitro laboratory excitement by significantly prolonging assays using bovine thrombin as a reagent. Conversely, the antibodies against bovine F5 can cross-react with human F5, creating serious acquired bleeding disorders. Recent preparations of fibrin glue and use of recombinant thrombin (eg, Recothrom, ZymoGenetics, Seattle, WA, USA) may lower the risk of developing these antibodies.

Nonimmune-mediated Acquired Factor Deficiencies

Acquired nonimmune causes of factor deficiencies often are detected in the coagulation laboratory. These include the following:

Increased destruction. Coagulation factors—particularly fibrinogen— may be depleted by rapid factor activation and eventual consumption in conditions such as DIC. Clinical interventions such as artificial heart valves, left ventricular assist devices, and ECMO also may lead to factor depletion in varying degrees. The administration of fibrinolytic drugs in thrombolytic therapy (eg, tissue plasminogen activator) also decreases some factor levels.

Decreased production. Conditions that lead to decreased production of coagulation factors are seen commonly in the hospital laboratory. A common example of this is liver disease (see article by Ng in this issue).

Abnormal production. In addition to decreased production, abnormal production of coagulation proteins also is seen in liver disease. Posttranslational modification of fibrinogen, which is detrimental to its function (dysfibrinogenemia), occurs in patients who have liver disease, and also may be seen in the fetus or newborn. Yet, the prime example of abnormal coagulation factor production is iatrogenic and caused by warfarin (Coumadin) therapy. Warfarin removes the ability of the vitamin K-dependent factors (2, 7, 9, 10, and proteins C and S) to bind to the surfaces where coagulation reactions occur. Warfarin acts by interfering with the vitamin K-dependent gamma carboxylation of these particular factors, resulting in the formation of protein induced by vitamin K absence or antagonists (PIVKA). These modified factors are unable to bind calcium and therefore cannot be anchored to the phospholipid membrane (see article by Ng in this issue). As the proteins cannot bind to the areas of active clotting, the effective concentrations are decreased greatly.

Loss and sequestration. Proteins lost in conditions like nephrotic syndrome include some involved in hemostasis regulation, such as antithrombin. Acquired F10 deficiency is rare; it usually is associated with light chain amyloidosis as a result of accelerated removal of F10 by adsorption onto the amyloid fibrils.[24] An iatrogenic source of factor loss is plasmapheresis, which will lower the coagulation factors by straightforward plasma removal, unless the treatment indication requires plasma replacement (plasma exchange). If plasma is not used as a replacement fluid, fibrinogen (F1) deficiency commonly will limit the frequency of exchanges.

Inactivation. It must not be overlooked that many pharmacologic inhibitors to coagulation factors are entering the clinical arena rapidly. These include the direct thrombin inhibitors (DTI) such as hirudin and argatroban. As might be imagined, inhibition of one of the key factors in the coagulation cascade wreaks havoc upon all of the clot-based assays used in the coagulation laboratory. It is critical that the laboratory be informed when such agents are in therapeutic use to have a reasonable interpretation of coagulation results, including factor assays. A normal thrombin time result is useful in ruling out an effect of DTI.

THE LABORATORY EVALUATION OF FACTOR DEFICIENCY
Preanalytical Considerations

Any coagulation assay is only as good as the sample submitted. Although preanalytical variables can affect any laboratory test, coagulation testing is particularly influenced by collection and handling processes.[25] Inaccurate results caused by improper collection or handling may lead to inappropriate patient intervention and/or additional unnecessary testing. To ensure a quality sample, one must adhere to the current Clinical and Laboratory Standards Institute (CLSI) guidelines for collecting and handling light blue top tubes (H21-A5).[26] **Box 2** outlines a checklist of key preanalytical considerations.

The proper anticoagulant is 3.2% (109 mmol/L) buffered trisodium citrate (light blue top tubes). This blue-top tube is required for most coagulation tests performed by the laboratory. The citrate anticoagulant chelates calcium, thus preventing the sample from clotting. For accurate results, a blood-to-anticoagulant ratio of 9:1 must be maintained. If the patient has a hematocrit of greater than 55% and thus a significantly reduced plasma volume, the amount of citrate must be reduced similarly to prevent falsely prolonged clotting times because of a relative excess of citrate. Too little citrate (as seen when the hematocrit is less than 20%) may not prevent factor activation or clotting in the tube. For this reason, it is recommended that patient samples should be checked for a clot whenever clotting times are inexplicably longer or shorter than either the reference or therapeutic range.

If the sample is collected using a winged blood collection set (ie, butterfly) and a vacuum tube, a discard tube should be drawn first to prevent underfilling of the tube because of the extra air within the collection set. Drawing a discard tube first is also advisable when drawing samples for any coagulation assay beyond routine PT and aPTT testing, although there are no current studies proving this is necessary.

Box 2
Preanalytical checklist. These questions should be asked as part of the preanalytical checklist to determine sample integrity

Was the specimen collected in the correct anticoagulant?

Are the tubes properly filled?

Was the sample collected through a venous access device?

Is the hematocrit less than 55%?

Is the sample already clotted?

Is the plasma platelet-poor?

Is the sample hemolyzed?

Is the sample lipemic or icteric?

Has the sample been maintained either at room temperature or frozen?

Has the sample age exceeded the stability limit?

Within 4 hours of collection, (1 hour for assays evaluating heparin), the blood must be centrifuged and plasma processed for testing or freezing. A two-spin centrifugation method will ensure that the resulting plasma is truly platelet-poor, because phospholipid from residual platelets interferes with many coagulation assays. Plasma should be kept at room temperature until testing or freezing, because both vWF and F8 activity can be lost with 4°C storage. Frozen plasma must be stored at -20°C or lower (preferably -70°C), and avoiding the use of a frost-free freezer, as the periodic defrost cycles allow samples to partially thaw and then refreeze. Frozen plasma should be thawed at 37°C just before testing, avoiding any refreezing of plasma, as the coagulation proteins tend to denature with more than one freeze–thaw cycle.

Using the Prothrombin Time and Activated Partial Thromboplastin Time to Screen for Factor Deficiency

Establishing reference ranges

To successfully use the PT and aPTT as screening tests, the coagulation technologist needs to be very familiar with the characteristics of the reagent/instrument systems. Selecting a combination of coagulation reagents and analyzers that facilitate the identification of patients with factor deficiencies or inhibitors is critical. The aPTT reagents touting lupus anticoagulant sensitivity should be reserved for actual LA testing. For PT testing, it is preferable to use a low International Sensitivity Index (ISI) reagent containing a heparin neutralizer; the latter enables accurate PT results in patients who are receiving both warfarin and heparin. The neutralizer generally is effective when heparin levels are less than or equal to 1 U/mL, but can be overwhelmed by contaminant heparin when specimens are drawn from an indwelling line.

To establish a valid reference range for the PT and aPTT, a pool of normal subjects must be identified. These subjects should match the patient population as closely as possible. This may be difficult if the population includes pediatric patients. In the absence of a neonatal or pediatric pool of donors, one must rely on published reference ranges for children of various ages.[6,27] Adult outpatients can be used to establish ranges as long as they do not have orders for coagulation assays (suspected bleeding or clotting history) and additionally meet predefined criteria (**Box 3**). Historically, donors who were on oral contraceptives (OCPs) were excluded from the normal donor pool, but many sites now include them, because they constitute a large portion of the population to be tested,

---

Box 3
List of donor requirements for use as normal donor plasma. Criteria for inclusion in a normal reference range study

Not pregnant

Not taking anticoagulants

Not taking antibiotics

Not taking insulin

No history of a blood clot

No history of a bleeding disorder

No history of autoimmune disease (eg, lupus erythematosus, rheumatoid arthritis)

---

and newer OCPs contain less estrogen. Estrogen may increase ambient F8 and vWF levels, thus shortening the aPTT in affected patients. This is illustrated from data collected from students at the authors' institution, where the average aPTT of women using OCP was 27.6 seconds, n = 18, while for women not on OCP, the average aPTT was 29.5 seconds, n = 14, (P = .026). For men the average was 29.4 seconds, n = 18.

Ideally, donor samples should be collected and tested over a period of days or weeks. They should be centrifuged and analyzed in the same manner as patient samples. A bare minimum of 20 donors (10 male and 10 female) can be used to verify the reference range of a new lot of a current reagent; however, when changing type of reagent, at least 50 donors should be used. Statistical analysis also will determine the required geometric mean PT value for international normalized ratio (INR) calculation.

In order to interpret results of the PT and aPTT, it is helpful to know their sensitivity for factor deficiencies. To evaluate a reagent for factor sensitivity, one may dilute a pooled normal plasma into factor-deficient plasma to achieve factor activities of 60%, 50%, 40%, 30%, and 20%. The appropriate factor assay then is performed, as well as a standard PT and aPTT on each dilution (**Fig. 2**). The percent activity is plotted against the clotting time in seconds to determine what clotting time corresponds to a factor activity level of 30%, which generally is considered to be the minimum amount of factor activity needed for consistent hemostasis (**Table 2**).

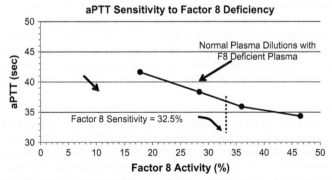

Fig. 2. Determining the upper limit of the activated partial thromboplastin time (aPTT) reference range is aided by measuring the factor 8 activity against the aPTT. Using dilutions of control plasma, a factor 8 activity of approximately 32.5% confirms the statistically-derived upper limit of normal of 37.0 seconds.

Table 2
Half-lives and hemostatic levels of coagulation factors

Factor	Category	Approximate Half-Life	Approximate Hemostatic Level
Fibrinogen	Substrate	96 hours	50 mg/dL
F2	Protease	72 hours	20%
F5	Cofactor	16 hours	25%
F7	Protease	4 hours	20%
F8	Cofactor	11 hours	30%
F9	Protease	22 hours	30%
F10	Protease	30 hours	25%
F11	Protease	60 hours	25%
F13	Transglutaminase	10 days	2% to 3%

Some table content courtesy of George Fritsma (www.fritsmafactor.com).

The reference ranges for both PT and aPTT should be established for each lot of reagent by examining both the statistical analyses and the results of the factor sensitivity studies. The upper and lower limits of normal should initially be set at the 95th percentile (mean plus or minus 2 SD). The upper limit can then be adjusted so that true factor deficiencies (less than or equal to 30%) will be detected. If possible, patient plasmas known to be mildly factor-deficient should be assayed to confirm that the reference ranges have been set correctly. This procedure is also useful in circumstances where the in vitro factor sensitivity curve looks relatively flat in the 30% range (eg, the F9 curve is relatively insensitive in some reagent systems). Plasma from patients with mild factor deficiencies should be frozen for future use in setting reference ranges. The factor sensitivity information should be supplied to hematologists, pathologists, and all other providers who routinely use the PT or aPTT for screening.

Mixing studies

To guide in the evaluation of a prolonged PT or aPTT, mixing studies can be employed to help discern the presence of factor inhibitors. In its simplest form, one part of patient plasma is mixed with one part of pooled normal plasma, and the clotting tests are repeated. Pooled normal plasma supplies the missing factor(s) and corrects the prolonged clotting times of patients who have factor deficiency. If a patient has an inhibitor (antibody) that interferes with factor activity, the prolonged clotting time should not correct with addition of normal pooled plasma. A 1- to 2-hour incubation at 37°C is needed for time- or temperature-dependent antibodies to exert their effect. A normal control must be used for interpretation, as extended incubation may prolong the clotting time of plasma because of factor degradation, without regard to inhibitors or deficiencies.

Exactly defining a mixing study correction can be difficult, and there are many opinions as to how this should be accomplished.[28,29] Some experts suggest that the result of the mix must correct to within the reference range, while others hold that correction occurs if the mix result is no greater than 5 seconds above the upper limit of the range. Others compare the results of the mix with a control of normal pooled plasma. Using various dilution ratios of patient plasma to pooled normal plasma or incorporating saline into the mix may increase the sensitivity of the study for an inhibitor.

In practice, in the authors' laboratories, mixing studies are often misleading.[28] Severe factor deficiencies may not correct even though factor levels have been restored to 50%, depending on where the reference ranges are set in relation to factor sensitivities. This is especially true with current PT reagents, which are very sensitive; restoring a factor level to 50% may yield a PT within the reference range. Mixing also may dilute a mild inhibitor sufficiently, such that clotting times correct. With a good clinical history and knowledge of one's laboratory test limits, an experienced coagulation laboratory may be able to determine the cause of a prolonged PT or aPTT without mixing studies.

Factor activity assays

Three types of assays can be used to measure factor activity: chromogenic, one-stage clotting, and two-stage clotting. Although expensive, chromogenic assays are superior for measuring factor activity in the presence of LA or heparin, in assigning factor concentrate potency, and for detecting mild F8 deficiencies that may be missed with a one-stage clotting assay.

Chromogenic assays are based upon the principle that clotting factors are proteinases that specifically cleave their natural substrates. By substituting a chromogenic substrate that gives off a color when cleaved, the reaction rate and the magnitude of color development are proportional to the factor activity. Each chromogenic assay is designed specifically for the factor being measured. For example, one method for F8 uses optimal amounts of Ca^{2+}, phospholipid, and activated F9, with an excess of F10, such that the rate of activation of F10 is related linearly to the amount of F8. F10 hydrolyzes the chromogenic substrate S-2765, thus liberating a chromophore. The color then is read photometrically at 405 nm. The intensity of color is proportional to the amount of S-2765 cleaved by F10 and thus yields the F8 activity in the sample.

Two-stage clotting assays are precise, insensitive to preanalytic factor activation, and superior at detecting mild F8 deficiency compared with the one-stage assay. Two-stage assays do not require the use of factor-deficient plasmas, but they are complicated and not automated easily. For this reason, they are not performed in many laboratories. In the two-stage method for F8, the patient plasma is treated with aluminum hydroxide to remove factors 2, 7, 9 and 10. This arrests the clotting process after formation of the prothrombinase complex. The treated patient's plasma then is mixed with activated serum, F5, calcium, and phospholipids to initiate coagulation and generate activated F10. After a defined period of incubation, one volume of this mixture is added to one volume of normal plasma, and the time to clot formation is measured. Clotting times of a calibrator or standard plasma are plotted, and the F8 level in the patient sample is read from the graph.

The one-stage clotting assay is the most commonly used method in clinical laboratories because of its simplicity and automation. Factors 8, 9, 11, and 12 typically are tested using a one-stage assay based on the aPTT. F7 is tested using an assay based on the PT, while factors 2, 5, and 10 can be assayed using either. The PT-based assay is preferred, however, because it is faster and less prone to interference by heparin and LA.

Regardless of whether a PT- or aPTT-based assay is used, a calibration curve first must be prepared. It is important to choose a good calibrator referenced to World Health Organization standards. The standard curve should be designed to contain enough points to extend below 1% (especially for factors 8, 9, and 11) so that severe hemophilia can be differentiated from moderate disease. Some automated coagulation analyzers require the use of a low curve to enhance sensitivity below 20% activity. The low curve is made by diluting the standard down to approximately 20% before loading it on the analyzer. The analyzer then can prepare dilutions to include a point at 1%.

To make factor assays more sensitive, patient and calibrator plasma first are diluted in buffer (longer times are more sensitive to small changes); then the diluted plasma is mixed 1:1 with factor deficient plasma. An aPTT or PT then is performed on the mix. Most automated coagulation analyzers prepare all patient and calibrator dilutions without technologist intervention.

Factor-deficient plasma is provided as a lyophilized powder or frozen plasma. Deficient plasma may originate from a single donor who is congenitally factor-deficient, or it may be prepared from pooled normal donor plasma by immunodepletion of the appropriate factor. If an immunodepleted plasma is used, it should be validated to ensure that only the factor under consideration has been removed. With F8-deficient plasma, it is important to know if vWF also has been removed, as the absence of vWF may affect the results of the factor activity assay.

To rule out interference from heparin, LA, or antibodies to another factor, each sample must be tested at a minimum of three dilutions. If the results, after correcting for the various dilutions, exhibit increasing activity with each subsequent greater dilution of the patient plasma, this is termed an inhibitor pattern (**Fig. 3**). It is important to note that an inhibitor pattern may not be observed when an antibody is directed specifically against the factor being tested. Specific factor inhibitors usually bind to the factor and completely interfere with its coagulation function, preventing it from being measured in an activity assay. Subsequent dilutions do not produce a rise in factor activity.

Heparin causes aPTT-based assays to have prolonged clotting times (and thus falsely low factor activity). When the patient plasma is diluted out, the heparin also is diluted, causing less interference in the assay and resulting in an apparent increase in factor activity. A prolonged thrombin time with a normal reptilase time (or measuring the actual heparin level) will confirm heparin as the cause of an inhibitor pattern.

LA may show an inhibitor pattern in a manner similar to heparin. The antibody interferes with phospholipid in the PT- or, most often, aPTT-based assays and leads to prolonged clotting times. As the patient plasma is diluted, the antibody also is diluted, causing less interference and thus higher—and more accurate—factor activity with

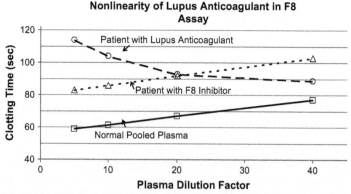

Fig. 3. Lupus anticoagulant (LA) pattern with serial plasma dilutions. The normal pooled plasma shows a straight-line pattern; by contrast, the lupus anticoagulant inhibitor line is nonlinear, with the clotting time shortening at a greater pace with increasing dilutions. This pattern suggests that the inhibitor effect is being diluted out. Note that the a patient with a factor 8 inhibitor generally runs parallel to the normal pooled control, though at an increased clotting time due to the low amount of factor 8.

each dilution. A positive dilute Russell viper venom test (DRVVT) will confirm the diagnosis of LA, but a negative DRVVT does not rule out its presence. A hexagonal phase phospholipid neutralization (eg, StaClot LA, Diagnostica Stago, Asnieres Sur Seine, France), platelet neutralization procedure, or other assays for LA may be needed to confirm the presence of a LA inhibitor.[30]

If a patient has an antibody to a factor other than the one being assayed, it may react with that factor which is present in the factor-deficient plasma and thereby cause prolongation of the PT- or aPTT-based factor assay. As the patient's plasma is diluted, the antibody also is diluted, resulting in less interference and a gain in factor activity with each subsequent dilution. This produces a nonlinear curve compared with the calibration curve.

Assays for detecting specific factor inhibitors

Bethesda-type assays (or its modification, the Nijmegan assay) can be employed to screen for inhibitors to factors.[31] Although predominantly used for F8 inhibitors, these assays can be adapted to detect any factor inhibitor. In a Bethesda assay, patient plasma is incubated with a source of factor (usually normal pooled plasma) for 2 hours at 37°C. Residual factor activity then is measured and compared with a control mixture. One Bethesda unit is defined as the amount of antibody that will inhibit 50% of the available factor in the normal pooled plasma. It may be necessary to dilute the patient plasma in buffer or factor-deficient plasma before incubation to achieve a mixture with the optimal range of 40% to 60% residual factor activity. The residual factor activity is converted to BUs by the use of a Bethesda graph and then multiplied by the dilution factor (see **Fig. 1**).[31]

The control mixture should mimic the patient mixture as closely as possible. If the patient has a low titer inhibitor (less than or equal to 1 BU), the control should be composed of normal pooled plasma and factor-deficient plasma. If the patient has to be diluted in buffer, the control should be made using normal pooled plasma and buffer. In the Nijmegan modification, the use of buffered normal pooled plasma stabilizes the pH, permitting more accurate measurement of low-titer inhibitors. Using the lowest possible patient dilution that gives a 40% to 60% residual factor activity prevents overestimation of inhibitors possessing complex kinetics.

The inhibitor testing protocol is accepted widely for use in patients who have no circulating factor activity (less than 1%). When the patient has measurable factor activity in the sample, however, there is less agreement on protocols. Although there is some evidence that heat-treating the plasma before incubation with normal pooled plasma will inactivate the patient's own factor, but not the antibody, the World Federation of Hemophilia Laboratory Manual recommends either adjusting the concentration of the control solution to match that of the patient or mathematically correcting for the baseline factor activity of the patient.[32]

Laboratory Evaluation of a Prolonged Prothrombin Time or Activated Partial Thromboplastin Time

Having access to the patient's clinical, medication, and transfusion history is one of the best coagulation screening tests, and often may eliminate the need for mixing studies to guide test selection.[33] Is the patient actively bleeding or bruising? Is the patient anemic? Is there any personal or family history of bleeding? If the answer to any of these questions is yes, it makes sense to look for factor deficiencies (either congenital or acquired) and vWD.

If there is a history consistent with clotting (eg, deep vein thrombosis, pulmonary embolism, stroke, or spontaneous abortion), or if the prolonged screening test is the only reason for workup in an asymptomatic patient, this favors LA testing.

Medication history will reveal if the patient is receiving warfarin or heparin or another anticoagulant such as a direct thrombin inhibitor. Does the patient have a venous access catheter? If so, screen for heparin or consider a dilution effect. If there is an isolated prolonged PT, one must ask: Has the patient been given vitamin K, been on antibiotic therapy, or taken any herbal or natural therapeutics? Although most clinicians expect a prolonged PT/INR in vitamin K depletion, an accompanying prolongation of the aPTT may surprise them and trigger a workup for prolonged aPTT. Most aPTT reagents are fairly sensitive to the low levels of F9 seen in vitamin K depletion, and the decreases in factors 2 and 10. Thus, it is not unusual for the aPTT to be somewhat prolonged with warfarin or other causes of vitamin K deficiency.

One always must investigate the patient's transfusion history. Has the patient received any plasma, cryoprecipitate, bypassing agents, or factor concentrates? If so, coagulation studies may be difficult to interpret. Bypassing agents contain activated F7, which can cause extremely short clotting times (and thus overestimation of factor activity levels).

Patients may have more than one coagulopathy. For instance, combined F5/F8 deficiency is a well-characterized familial defect. These patients will present with a prolonged PT and aPTT and usually will have bleeding symptoms when challenged.

Isolated prothrombin time elevation

Once heparin, warfarin, and other anticoagulants are ruled out, an isolated elevation of the PT/INR likely has one of several etiologies (**Table 3**):

> Vitamin K deficiency. The most frequent cause of an elevated PT is vitamin K deficiency. Some herbal or natural products also may induce vitamin K deficiency. Patients on antibiotics are susceptible to vitamin K deficiency, because the antibiotics may destroy gut bacteria that synthesize vitamin K. Because F5 is not

Table 3
Isolated prothrombin time elevation (assumes that heparin, warfarin, and other anticoagulants have been ruled out)

Differential Diagnosis	Tests to Run	Interpretation/Follow-up
Vitamin K deficiency Liver disease F7 deficiency (or inhibitor), Lupus anticoagulant	Factors 5, 7, and LA panel Recommend repeat draw to verify low factor levels	If both F5 and F7 are ↓, suspect liver involvement If only F7 is ↓, run at least one more vitamin K-dependent factor If ↓, suspect vitamin K deficiency If only F7 is ↓, suspect congenital deficiency or acquired inhibitor (rare) Consider Bethesda assay if no family history and recent onset of bleeding If lupus anticoagulant positive, repeat in 3 months to confirm persistence and therefore significance

vitamin K- dependent, assaying F5 along with one or several of the vitamin K dependent factors will help differentiate vitamin K deficiency from liver disease. It is helpful to be familiar with the half-lives of the various factors when interpreting results of coagulation assays (see **Table 2**). As a rule, the shorter the half-life, the faster the decrease in activity when starting warfarin, and the faster the recovery of activity when discontinuing warfarin. In early vitamin K deficiency, only the F7 may have fallen enough to prolong the PT. If inflammation is present, acute-phase elevations of F8 and fibrinogen often keep the aPTT from prolonging. Additionally, when more than one factor is decreased, the PT may prolong more than the single factor sensitivity studies would predict.

Factor 7 deficiency. The degree of correlation between the F7 activity level and patient bleeding varies depending on the type of tissue factor used in the F7 assay. An inhibitor to F7 is rare and is usually attributable to IgG autoantibodies. A Bethesda-type assay can be performed to confirm the presence of an F7 inhibitor.

Lupus anticoagulant. Although more commonly associated with an elevation of the aPTT, LA may produce an isolated elevated PT. The source of phospholipid and phospholipid content of the PT reagent will define how sensitive the reagent is to LA. Elevated F8 or fibrinogen may keep the aPTT from prolonging. One should consider LA testing on any sample with unexplained prolongation of the PT.

Isolated activated partial thromboplastin time elevation

After excluding LA, the clinical picture as well as the personal, family, and medication history (including anticoagulant therapy) will guide the workup of an isolated prolonged aPTT **(Table 4)**.[33] With a history of bleeding, assays for F8 activity, vWD, F9, and F11 are most informative. If any factor activity level is low, one should evaluate at least three patient dilutions for an inhibitor pattern. If any one factor shows very low activity that does not increase with patient dilution, a Bethesda-type assay is warranted. Patients also can have more than one disorder responsible for the prolonged aPTT (eg, F8 deficiency or F8 inhibitor with a LA). The presence of LA also can make it challenging to monitor replacement therapy with clot-based assays. A chromogenic F8 assay may give a more accurate factor result in the presence of LA.

Table 4
Isolated elevated activated partial thromboplastin time (aPTT) (assumes heparin and other anticoagulants have been ruled out)

Differential Diagnosis	Initial Tests to Run	Interpretation/Follow-Up
Von Willebrand disease (VWD) Factor deficiency Factor inhibitor Lupus anticoagulant (LA)	If positive history for bleeding or bruising do F8, then F9, then F11	If only F8 slightly ↓ to moderately ↓, then run von Willebrand factor antigen and activity If not vWD, do F8 inhibitor If F8, F9, or F11 is markedly ↓, do Bethesda assay for that factor
	If negative history for bleeding or bruising and • moderately ↑ aPTT, then do LA, then, F8, F9, F11 • markedly ↑↑ aPTT, then do F12, then consider other contact factors	If positive LA and factor activity does not normalize with additional dilutions, may need to do chromogenic assay If positive LA, repeat in 3 months to confirm persistence and therefore significance

If there is no history of bleeding, and LA is not present, assays for F12 and other contact factors may explain the elevated aPTT.

Combined elevated prothrombin time and activated partial thromboplastin time

Congenital deficiencies or acquired inhibitors of factors 2, 5, or 10 are rare. Laboratory workup should begin with testing the common pathway factor activities, as well as LA testing (**Table 5**). It is not uncommon for patients who have LA to produce antibodies to prothrombin, and approximately 30% of these will result in a prothrombin deficiency with some degree of bleeding. A laboratory phenomenon coined lupus cofactor effect frequently occurs in patients who have hypothrombinemia–lupus anticoagulant syndrome. When patient plasma is mixed with normal pooled plasma, the clotting time (PT, aPTT, DRVVT, or LA-PTT) actually prolongs to an even greater extent. When this phenomenon is noticed in LA testing, a F2 activity assay should be performed.

Decreased F5 activity is a good predictor of liver disease and is used commonly in evaluating liver toxicity in acetaminophen overdose. Because F8 and fibrinogen are acute phase reactants, they often are increased in liver disease, which may keep the aPTT from prolonging even with decreased synthesis of F2, F5, F9, and F10.

Each laboratory's approach to diagnosing factor deficiencies and inhibitors must be flexible. Not all patients have well-defined coagulopathies,[33] and many, especially hospitalized patients, have more than one issue at a time. For example, patients who have congenital or acquired hemophilia have been known to develop LA. Workups must be conducted as efficiently and timely as possible to be of help to the patient and clinician. Abnormal results should be verified on fresh samples (new draws if possible), as there is ample opportunity for preanalytical error.

The laboratory approach to inherited and acquired coagulation factor deficiencies requires active use of clinical information. The coagulation pathologist and hematologist should be familiar with the methods and capabilities of their laboratories. An understanding of the laboratory approach to evaluating factor deficiency not only

Table 5
Combined elevated prothrombin time and activated partial thromboplastin time (assumes heparin and other anticoagulants have been ruled out)

Differential Diagnosis	Initial Tests to Run	Interpretation/Follow-Up
Vitamin K deficiency	F2, F5, and LA	If only F2 ↓, with + LA, look for lupus cofactor effect
Liver disease		
Disseminated intravascular coagulation (DIC)		If LA-negative, rule out vitamin K deficiency
Lupus anticoagulant (LA) with hypoprothrombinemia		Do F7 or 10 and if normal test for F2 inhibitor
Congenital factor deficiency	F10	If only F5 ↓, do F5 inhibitor and do F8
Factor inhibitor		Rule out DIC
		If only F10↓, look for evidence of amyloidosis, respiratory infection, and malignancy
		Do F10 inhibitor
		If F7 and F2 are ↓ but F5 is normal, likely vitamin K deficiency/warfarin therapy
		If multiple factors are ↓, look for liver disease or DIC

will aid clinicians in obtaining a prompt diagnosis, but also avoid pitfalls for false diagnoses in coagulation testing.

ACKNOWLEDGEMENT

The authors wish to acknowledge the timely contributions of the Special Coagulation technologists at TriCore Reference Laboratories in preparing this manuscript: Pam Owens, Donna Rospopo, and Trish Lowery.

REFERENCES

1. High KA. Update on progress and hurdles in novel genetic therapies for hemophilia. Hematology Am Soc Hematol Educ Program 2007;2007:466–72.
2. Verbruggen B, Meijer P, Novakova I, et al. Diagnosis of factor VIII deficiency. Haemophilia 2008;14(Suppl 3):76–82.
3. Kempton CL, White GC 2nd. How we treat a hemophilia A patient with a factor VIII inhibitor. Blood 2009;113:11–7.
4. Peyvandi F, Jayandharan G, Chandy M, et al. Genetic diagnosis of haemophilia and other inherited bleeding disorders. Haemophilia 2006;12(Suppl 3):82–9.
5. Kulkarni R, Ponder KP, James AH, et al. Unresolved issues in diagnosis and management of inherited bleeding disorders in the perinatal period: a white paper of the Perinatal Task Force of the Medical and Scientific Advisory Council of the National Hemophilia Foundation, USA. Haemophilia 2006;12:205–11.
6. Williams MD, Chalmers EA, Gibson BE. The investigation and management of neonatal haemostasis and thrombosis. Br J Haematol 2002;119:295–309.
7. Gomez K, Bolton-Maggs P. Factor XI deficiency. Haemophilia 2008;14:1183–9.
8. Franchini M, Veneri D, Lippi G. Inherited factor XI deficiency: a concise review. Hematology 2006;11:307–9.
9. Peyvandi F, Kaufman RJ, Seligsohn U, et al. Rare bleeding disorders. Haemophilia 2006;12(Suppl 3):137–42.
10. Herrmann FH, Wulff K, Auerswald G, et al. Factor VII deficiency: clinical manifestation of 717 subjects from Europe and Latin America with mutations in the factor 7 gene. Haemophilia 2009;15:267–80.
11. Huang JN, Koerper MA. Factor V deficiency: a concise review. Haemophilia 2008;14:1164–9.
12. Lapecorella M, Mariani G. Factor VII deficiency: defining the clinical picture and optimizing therapeutic options. Haemophilia 2008;14:1170–5.
13. Brown DL, Kouides PA. Diagnosis and treatment of inherited factor X deficiency. Haemophilia 2008;14:1176–82.
14. Asselta R, Tenchini ML, Duga S. Inherited defects of coagulation factor V: the hemorrhagic side. J Thromb Haemost 2006;4:26–34.
15. Hsieh L, Nugent D. Factor XIII deficiency. Haemophilia 2008;14:1190–200.
16. Watson HG, Chee YL, Greaves M. Rare acquired bleeding disorders. Rev Clin Exp Hematol 2001;5:405–29.
17. Franchini M, Veneri D. Acquired coagulation inhibitor-associated bleeding disorders: an update. Hematology 2005;10:443–9.
18. Andre S, Meslier Y, Dimitrov JD, et al. A cellular viewpoint of anti-FVIII immune response in hemophilia A. Clin Rev Allergy Immunol 2009; in press.
19. Barnett B, Kruse-Jarres R, Leissinger CA. Current management of acquired factor VIII inhibitors. Curr Opin Hematol 2008;15:451–5.

20. Knight C, Dano AM, Kennedy-Martin T. Systematic review of efficacy of rFVIIa and aPCC treatment for hemophilia patients with inhibitors. Adv Ther 2009;26:68–88.
21. Collins P, Budde U, Rand JH, et al. Epidemiology and general guidelines of the management of acquired haemophilia and von Willebrand syndrome. Haemophilia 2008;14(Suppl 3):49–55.
22. Franchini M, Targher G, Montagnana M, et al. Laboratory, clinical and therapeutic aspects of acquired hemophilia A. Clin Chim Acta 2008;395:14–8.
23. Banninger H, Hardegger T, Tobler A, et al. Fibrin glue in surgery: frequent development of inhibitors of bovine thrombin and human factor V. Br J Haematol 1993; 85:528–32.
24. Choufani EB, Sanchorawala V, Ernst T, et al. Acquired factor X deficiency in patients with amyloid light-chain amyloidosis: incidence, bleeding manifestations, and response to high-dose chemotherapy. Blood 2001;97:1885–7.
25. Favaloro EJ, Lippi G, Adcock DM. Preanalytical and postanalytical variables: the leading causes of diagnostic error in hemostasis? Semin Thromb Hemost 2008; 34:612–34.
26. CLSI. Collection, transport, and processing of blood specimens for testing plasma-based coagulation assays and molecular hemostasis assays; approved guideline. 5th edition. 2008; CLSI document H21–A5.
27. Flanders MM, Crist RA, Roberts WL, et al. Pediatric reference intervals for seven common coagulation assays. Clin Chem 2005;51:1738–42.
28. Ledford-Kraemer M. All mixed up about mixing studies. In: Clot-Ed: coagulation, lysis, or thrombosis, an educational resource; 2004. p. 1–11.
29. Peterson P, Hayes TE, Arkin CF, et al. The preoperative bleeding time test lacks clinical benefit: College of American Pathologists' and American Society of Clinical Pathologists' position article. Arch Surg 1998;133:134–9.
30. Moffat KA, Ledford-Kraemer MR, Plumhoff EA, et al. Are laboratories following published recommendations for lupus anticoagulant testing? An international evaluation of practices. Thromb Haemost 2009;101:178–84.
31. Giles AR, Verbruggen B, Rivard GE, et al. A detailed comparison of the performance of the standard versus the Nijmegen modification of the Bethesda assay in detecting factor VIII: C inhibitors in the haemophilia A population of Canada. Thromb Haemost 1998;79:872–5.
32. McCraw A, Kitchen S. Diagnosis of haemophilia and other bleeding disorders— a laboratory manual. World Federation of Hemophilia; 2000.
33. Greaves M, Watson HG. Approach to the diagnosis and management of mild bleeding disorders. J Thromb Haemost 2007;5(Suppl 1):167–74.

Prothrombin Time and Partial Thromboplastin Time Assay Considerations

Valerie L. Ng, PhD, MD

KEYWORDS

- Prothrombin time • International normalized ratio
- Partial thromboplastin time • Thromboplastin • Reagent
- Partial thromboplastin • FVIII • Standardization

The prothrombin time (PT) and activated partial thromboplastin time (PTT) are commonly used screening tests. These tests assess the "global" function of the extrinsic (PT) or intrinsic (PTT) clotting pathways. The specific cause of an abnormal PT or PTT requires more specific and specialized coagulation tests.

PT and PTT testing first emerged in the early 1900s using manual coagulation test methods (ie, "tilt tube") and reagents meticulously and painstakingly prepared and used by individual laboratories. Over the past century, these have been supplanted with commercially available reagents and automated instrumentation.

As "global" tests of coagulation, PT and PTT results are highly dependent on the combination of reagent and instrumentation used. Results for the same specimen tested in multiple laboratories are variable, with much of the variability directly attributable to the specific reagent and to a lesser degree, the instrument. As for the thromboplastin (for PT) or partial thromboplastin (for PTT) reagents themselves, each lot of reagent—even from the same manufacturer—exhibits variable responses to factor deficiencies. Some reagents are less sensitive than others. To complicate matters further, reagent responses and PT or PTT results for specimens containing only a single-factor deficiency are often different than those for specimens with multiple mild factor deficiencies. The PT stands alone as the single coagulation test that has undergone the most extensive attempt at assay standardization. Notably, this

Professor Emeritus, Department of Laboratory Medicine, School of Medicine, University of California San Francisco; and Chairman, Department of Pathology & Laboratory Medicine, Alameda County Medical Center, Oakland, CA, USA
Department of Pathology, c/o Clinical Laboratory Room 3408, Highland General Hospital, 1411 East 31st Street, Oakland, CA 94602, USA
E-mail address: vang@acmedctr.org

Clin Lab Med 29 (2009) 253–263
doi:10.1016/j.cll.2009.05.002
0272-2712/09/$ – see front matter © 2009 Elsevier Inc. All rights reserved.

labmed.theclinics.com

standardization has been limited to only one clinical use of the PT: warfarin therapeutic monitoring.

PROTHROMBIN TIME

The PT measures the extrinsic coagulation pathway. It is most sensitive to factor VII (FVII) deficiencies. Because FVII has a short half-life and is decreased in patients with liver disease, PTs are often prolonged in patients with liver disease.

Thromboplastin reagents in clinical laboratories are typically changed yearly because of limitations in "batch" size and stability. When a reagent changeover is to occur, the proposed new thromboplastin reagent undergoes in-depth characterization within each clinical laboratory to assess how it will perform relative to the thromboplastin currently in use. This is undertaken with the goal of matching the two reagents as carefully as possible to minimize confusion and treatment changes resulting solely from reagent differences.

One of the many PT reagent characterizations performed is a thromboplastin dilution curve. A thromboplastin dilution curve is performed by diluting "normal" with saline- or clotting factor-deficient plasma and determining PTs for each dilution. The dilution at which the PT prolongs beyond the reference range determines the level of combined multiple-factor deficiencies at which the thromboplastin reagent under evaluation will yield a prolonged PT. Thromboplastin-dilution curves to characterize reagents have not been standardized.

The considerable variability of thromboplastin reagents in response to prothrombin deficiencies has been well recognized. This is most relevant for patients on chronic anticoagulation therapy (eg, warfarin). An early example of PT reagent variability to prothrombin dilutions is shown in this **Fig. 1**, from a 1949 publication.[1] This data was obtained in an era before thromboplastin reagents became commercially available and depicts the sensitivity of this particular "home-made" thromboplastin reagent to represent differences in clotting times relative to the "% prothrombin" between different "batches" of thromboplastin prepared from human brain and made within one laboratory.

Why is knowing your prothrombin reagent dilutional curve important? Because there are two related clinical questions: (i) What is the threshold of prothrombin deficiency at which a PT will prolong? and (ii) What is the threshold of PT prolongation beyond which a patient will bleed?

The answer to the second question is easiest: there is no definitive answer. The answer to the first question, however, depends on the PT reagent used. Differences in PT results related to differing thromboplastin reagent sensitivity have been well recognized since the 1940s. An example of this reagent variability was well demonstrated in one study demonstrating comparing eight different thromboplastin reagents for detecting FVII deficiency.[2] The actual test method itself—a manual tilt tube versus automated coagulometer, even if they are the same make and model—introduces additional variability in PT results.[3,4]

In the 1990s, it was recognized that tissue-based thromboplastin reagents were derived from a variety of tissues (eg, human brain, rabbit brain, rabbit brain and lung, human placenta, and so forth), and that the tissue of origin introduced variability in clotting times. One extreme example of variability introduced by specific animal species of thromboplastin origin and serious clinical impact is misdiagnosis of "FVII deficiency" because of FVII Padua in asymptomatic African Americans.[5,6] FVII Padua has a nucleotide substitution (R304Q) likely affecting FVII binding to tissue factor, and possibly also affecting FX binding. FVII Padua does not react with rabbit

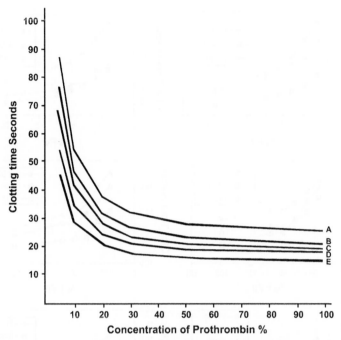

Fig. 1. Example of prothrombin dilution curves for five different "home-made" thrombo-plastin batches ("A", "B", "C", "D" and "E"). (*From* Biggs R, Macfarlane R. Estimation of prothrombin in dicoumarin therapy. J Clin Pathol 1949;2(1):37; with permission.)

thromboplastins, resulting in dramatically prolonged PTs and less than 1% measured FVII levels. Human-derived thromboplastins, however, react normally with FVII Padua, yielding normal PTs and FVII levels. The nonreactivity of FVII Padua with rabbit thrombo-plastins has led to incorrect diagnoses of FVII deficiency and unnecessary transfusions.[5,6]

A major effort was expended to develop recombinant thromboplastins for clinical laboratory use instead of tissue-derived thromboplastins, with the hope of providing a more standardized reagent with predictable characteristics. Unfortunately, use of a more homogeneous thromboplastin (ie, one recombinantly derived) did not eliminate the variability in PT reagent responsiveness. **Fig. 2** depicts the differences in PTs relative to specific single-procoagulant factor deficiencies for a variety of tissue-based or recombinant thromboplastin reagents.[7]

Notably, the impetus for PT reagent standardization was to improve therapy for one particular group of patients: those on chronic Vitamin K antagonist (VKA) therapy. This PT standardization was needed because of the narrow therapeutic index of warfarin and the high risk of bleeding or clotting if the dose was incorrect. It became clear that a system to normalize PTs and control for variations in clotting times attributable to a multitude of reagent-instrument combinations was necessary to effectively manage VKA therapy worldwide. The desire to standardize PTs started in the mid-1960s and progressed methodically through the 1970s and 1980s.[8–12] A seminal study highlighting the decreased warfarin dosing in countries using "sensitive" thrombo-plastin reagents and decreased incidence in bleeding dramatically accelerated the international interest to standardize PT results and the impetus for the rapid clinical adoption of the international normalized ratio (INR).[13]

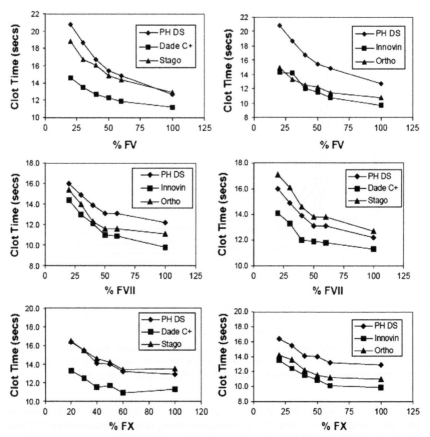

Fig. 2. Responsiveness of different thromboplastin reagents to specific individual procoagulant factor deficiencies (ie, deficiencies of FV, FVII, or FX) related to tissue of origin. Thromboplastin reagents assessed were derived from rabbit brain [Pacific Hemostasis Thromboplastin DS (PH DS), Stago Neoplastin CI Plus (Stago), Dade Thromboplastin C-Plus (Dade C+)] or recombinantly derived [Dade Innovin (Innovin) and Ortho Recombiplastin (Ortho)]. (*Courtesy of* L. Worfolk, PhD, Chantilly, VA.)

International Normalized Ratio

The INR was intended to be a reliable and accurate measure of VKA anticoagulation. At the time the INR was introduced, PT reagents in the United States (typically of rabbit origin) were relatively insensitive to factor deficiencies as compared with those used in Europe or Canada (typically of bovine or ovine origin). The INR was intended to "normalize" all PT reagents to a World Health Organization (WHO) reference thromboplastin preparation standard, such that a PT measured anywhere in the world would yield an INR value comparable to that which would have been obtained had the WHO reference thromboplastin been used. Thus, INRs generated from one laboratory would be comparable to that generated from any other laboratory in the world.[14]

The INR is calculated from the measured PT using the formula below:

$$INR = \left\{ \frac{PT_{,\,patient}}{PT_{,\,mean}} \right\}^{ISI}$$

Where

PT$_{,\,patient}$ = measured prothrombin time
PT$_{,\,mean}$ = geometric mean PT of the reference range
ISI = International Sensitivity Index, specific to each reagent-instrument combination

Every component of this equation has been reported as a source of error affecting the INR.[15] In addition, something as seemingly innocuous as collecting blood for INR determination in plastic versus glass tubes will affect the INR.[16] Finally and of note, assignment of the ISIs to individual reagents relative to international reference thromboplastin preparations (IRPs) ironically still relies on the "tilt tube" manual method of clotting,[11,17,18] not the most reproducible of clotting time methods nor representative of modern clotting time testing using automated coagulometers.

The following sections detail the many issues related to INR determination.

International Sensitivity Index assignment
The thromboplastin manufacturer assigns the International Sensitivity Index (ISI). Historically, ISIs were assigned for two broad categories: spectrophotometric coagulometers versus mechanical clot detection coagulometers. These general ISI assignments did not account for differences between individual instruments, even between the same models of the same make from the same manufacturer in each of these categories. Thus, the individual laboratory must verify the ISI assignment for its own unique reagent-instrument combination (local ISI).[19,20]

A second controversy regarding ISI assignment is the mathematical method (ie, orthogonal regression) used for ISI assignment.[21] Finally, standardization of INRs was speculated to be easier with high-sensitivity reagents (ie, low ISIs) given the historical observation of too high INR variability at a time when insensitive (ie, high ISI) thromboplastin reagents were in use. Unfortunately, high sensitivity (ie, low ISI) thromboplastins, either tissue- or recombinantly derived, did not improve INR precision or reproducibility between laboratories.[22]

One systematic evaluation of thromboplastin reagents has demonstrated increased sensitivity to coagulation factor deficiencies by simply increasing the phosphatidylserine content or decreasing the ionic strength.[23] Controlling for these two factors, however, did not completely eliminate the variability between thromboplastins in detecting deficiencies of individual coagulation factors FII, FV, FVII, or FX.[24]

Prothrombin Time, $_{mean}$
In determining an INR or establishing a local ISI, it is recommended that the PT, $_{mean}$ value be the geometric, not arithmetic, mean. This recommendation is based on the fact that PT values in a "normal" population are distributed log-normally.[18,25] Of note, this recommendation is somewhat controversial in at least two regards: how many specimens to use to determine the reference range and whether the geometric mean provides any benefit over the arithmetic mean.[15,26]

Local International Normalized Ratio calibration
The effect of unique instrument-reagent combinations on INR determinations has generated the development of "INR calibrators." These calibrators were intended

for use by individual laboratories to determine the "local ISI" to use with their unique instrument-reagent combination. Lyophilized plasmas intended for this INR calibration, however, have had only mixed success.[25,27–31]

When the International Normalized Ratio is Reliable

INRs are only reliable and reproducible between laboratories for patients stably anticoagulated with VKA therapy.[9,15,31] The reason why the INR is reproducible in this unique clinical setting was originally postulated to be because of the effect of "proteins induced by Vitamin K antagonists or absence" (PIVKA) on coagulation tests.[9,32]

PIVKAs are the precursors to coagulation factors. They lack the final Vitamin K-mediated gamma carboxylation posttranslational modification to create the active form of the clotting factor. PIVKAs have an inhibitory effect on in vitro clotting tests, prolonging clotting times. Unfortunately, the PIVKA inhibitory effect is variable, related to different thromboplastin reagent sensitivities to PIVKAs.[15] Talstad had recommended that INR standardization of thromboplastin reagents include correction for the PIVKA effect.[21]

When the International Normalized Ratio is not Reliable

INRs are not reliable or reproducible between laboratories for patients for whom VKA therapy has recently been initiated and the VKA effect not yet stabilized.[20,33,34]

INRs are not reliable or reproducible between laboratories for patients with prolonged PTs because of liver disease.[20,33–36] It is specifically recommended that PT values, in seconds, be used instead of the INR for expressing PT results for patients with liver disease.[37] Of note, the INR instead of the PT is incorporated into commonly used classification scores for classifying severity of liver disease (eg, Child-Turcotte-Pugh classification of liver disease, or the model for end-stage liver disease).[38] The reliance on the INR for these classifications has led Deitcher to speculate that patients assessed at transplant centers using thromboplastin reagents resulting in a higher INR for a given degree of hepatic dysfunction might have an inherent advantage over patients assessed at transplant centers using a different (and presumably less sensitive) thromboplastin.[36]

From these experiences, it is inferred that INRs are not reliable between laboratories for any other clinical conditions associated with a prolonged PT (eg, disseminated intravascular coagulation, congenital factor deficiencies, and other conditions) besides stable oral VKA therapy.

International Normalized Ratio Use in Clinical Settings Other Than Managing Vitamin K Antagonist Therapy

INRs are a simple mathematical transformation of PT ratios. Logically, INRs can be calculated for any PT. Reproducibility of INRs between laboratories, however, only occurs with specimens from that population stably anticoagulated with VKAs.

To minimize confusion regarding the clinical utility of INRs, some laboratories have limited INR reporting to only those patients being treated with VKAs. This has been accomplished by having INR as a separate, orderable test unique and distinct from a PT. Introduction of a separate INR test has to be accompanied by ample provider education to order an INR only for management of chronic VKA therapy and to order a PT for all other clinical situations.

In contrast, other laboratories report INRs for all PTs. This approach is typically undertaken because performing the mathematical transformation of a PT to an INR is faster and easier than verifying whether the patient has received VKA treatment and appropriateness of reporting an INR. This practice of reporting an INR with every PT has inadvertently led to an assumption that INRs must be reliable in all clinical situations because, after all, it is reported for all clinical situations.

For clinical conditions other than VKA therapy, INRs from the same laboratory can be used reliably to trend coagulation status for an individual patient treated within the facility served by that laboratory. As an example, INRs for a hospitalized patient could be trended over time for correction or worsening of coagulation status during the hospitalization. The INRs generated for a non-VKA treated patient by a single laboratory, however, cannot be assumed to be reproducible by a different laboratory. This is an important concept to grasp because if this hospitalized patient, after discharge, presented to an outpatient clinic served by a different laboratory, his or her INR generated by the laboratory providing services to the outpatient clinic may not match that from the hospital laboratory, and treatment decisions may differ accordingly.

PARTIAL THROMBOPLASTIN TIME

The PTT globally measures the effectiveness of the intrinsic coagulation pathway. The PTT has historically been regarded as a one-tailed or loss-of-function test; that is, only prolonged PTTs have clinical relevance as an indication of factor deficiency or presence of inhibitors (eg, heparin, lupus anticoagulants, coagulation factor-specific inhibitors, and so forth). The relatively recent clinical association of shortened PTTs with hypercoagulability, however, suggests a new use for the PTT: that is, a shortened PTT may have clinical utility for assessing risk of occurrence or recurrence of venous thrombosmbolisms.[39–43] Thus, the PTT may emerge in the future as a two-tailed test (ie, clinical significance attached to either prolonged or shortened values).

Partial Thromboplastin Time Reagent Considerations

PTT reagents vary in their sensitivity to coagulation factor deficiencies.[44–48] There are many similarities regarding PTT reagent sensitivities and variability as those discussed previously for the thromboplastin (PT) reagents. Unfortunately and in contrast to the longstanding international effort directed at PT reagent standardization for INR reporting, there has been little progress in the standardization of PTT reagents.[44,47,48]

Partial Thromboplastin Time Response to Single- versus Multiple-procoagulant Deficiencies is different

PTT reagents respond differently to single-factor deficiency than to multiple-factor deficiencies. Most laboratorians are familiar with PTT prolongation for a single-factor deficiency. Typically, the degree of PTT prolongation has a predictable relationship to the level of the individual factor level; in other words, there is a correlation between the degree of PTT prolongation and the level of the specific procoagulant factor. For multiple procoagulant deficiencies, however, the relationship between the degree of PTT prolongation and level of procoagulants is less predictable. In one study, prolongation of the PTT was observed to be paradoxically long relative to the mild reductions in individual procoagulant factors.[49] In this study, a mixture of plasmas yielding 75% of two and 100% of all other procoagulant factors yielded PTTs more prolonged than the PTTs obtained for plasmas with a 50% deficiency of only a single factor and 100% of all other procoagulant factors.[50] This means that patients with multiple, mild factor deficiencies (eg, patients with liver disease) may have PTTs prolonged disproportionate to the actual individual factor levels.

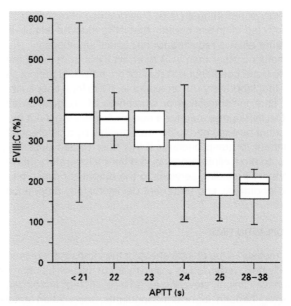

Fig. 3. Correlation of elevated FVIII procoagulant levels and PTT shortening. (*From* Ten Boekel E, Bartels P. Abnormally short activated partial thromboplastin times are related to elevated plasma levels of TAT, F1+2, D-dimer and FVIII: C. Pathophysiol Haemost Thromb 2002;32(3):140; with permission.)

Elevated FVIII Levels: Partial Thromboplastin Time Shortening is Linked to Clinical Hypercoagulability

Elevated FVIII levels have been linked with shortened PTTs and, more importantly, clinically relevant hypercoagulability.[41–43,51,52] One study assessing abnormally shortened PTTs (ie, PTTs below the reference range) identified an inverse relationship between PTT shortening and increasing FVIII levels (**Fig. 3**).[53] This same study demonstrated no relationship of the elevated FVIII levels with C-reactive protein. Because C-reactive protein is an acute phase reactant and is a surrogate for all acute phase reactants, the lack of correlation between C-reactive protein levels and PTT shortening excluded the presence of acute phase reactants as the cause of the shortened PTTs. The presence of Factor V Leiden or the prothrombin G20210A gene mutation was also not correlated with PTT shortening.[52,53] Plasmas with shortened PTTs and elevated FVIII levels also had elevated levels of thrombin-antithrombin-III complex, prothrombin fragment F1+2, and d-dimer, suggestive of increased thrombin generation, activation of the coagulation system, and a prothrombotic state.[54] Finally, one group noted shortened PTTs, if confirmed on repeated testing, was associated with a significantly increased risk of death, thrombosis, bleeding, and overall morbidity.[39] Notably (and hopefully of no surprise to the reader) different commercial PTT reagents exhibited different sensitivities for detecting shortened PTTs.[55]

SUMMARY

Significant interlaboratory variablity still exists for PT, INR, and PTT determinations. More information on the serious clinical impact of this variability is contained within the articles by Ng on "Liver disease, coagulation testing and hemostasis" and "Anticoagulant monitoring" elsewhere in this issue. Obviously, these laboratory coagulation-testing issues should be at the forefront of the reader's consciousness whenever critically evaluating and extrapolating published study conclusions reliant on PT, INR, or PTT results.

REFERENCES

1. Biggs R, Macfarlane R. Estimation of prothrombin in dicoumarin therapy. J Clin Pathol 1949;2:33–44.
2. Massignon D, Moulsma M, Bondon P, et al. Prothrombin time sensitivity and specificity to mild clotting factor deficiencies of the extrinsic pathway: evaluation of eight commercial thromboplastins. Thromb Haemost 1996;75(4):590–4.
3. Poggio M, van den Besselaar AM, van der Velde EA, et al. The effect of some instruments for prothrombin time testing on the International Sensitivity Index (ISI) of two rabbit tissue thromboplastin reagents. Thromb Haemost 1989;62(3): 868–74.
4. Thomson JM, Taberner DA, Poller L. Automation and prothrombin time: a United Kingdom field study of two widely used coagulometers. J Clin Pathol 1990;43(8): 679–84.
5. Triplett DA, Brandt JT, Batard MA, et al. Hereditary factor VII deficiency: heterogeneity defined by combined functional and immunochemical analysis. Blood 1985;66(6):1284–7.
6. Pollak ES, Russell TT, Ptashkin B, et al. Asymptomatic factor VII deficiency in African Americans. Am J Clin Pathol 2006;126(1):128–32.
7. Worfolk L. Thromboplastin correlation study. Available at: http://ekomed-diagnostic.com/pacific_hemostasis/PacifichemostasisPTkorrelasyonraporu.pdf. Accessed January 24, 2009.
8. Poller L. Standardization of anticoagulant control. Ric Clin Lab 1978;8(4):237–47.
9. Poller L. International Normalized Ratios (INR): the first 20 years. J Thromb Haemost 2004;2(6):849–60.
10. Poller L, Keown M, Chauhan N, et al. European concerted action on anticoagulation. Use of plasma samples to derive International Sensitivity Index for whole-blood prothrombin time monitors. Clin Chem 2002;48(2):255–60.
11. Thomson JM, Darby KV, Poller L. Calibration of BCT/441, the ICSH reference preparation for thromboplastin. Thromb Haemost 1986;55(3):379–82.
12. van den Besselaar AM. Standardization of the prothrombin time in oral anticoagulant control. Haemostasis 1985;15(4):271–7.
13. Hull R, Hirsh J, Jay R, et al. Different intensities of oral anticoagulant therapy in the treatment of proximal-vein thrombosis. N Engl J Med 1982;307(27):1676–81.
14. Kirkwood TB. Calibration of reference thromboplastins and standardisation of the prothrombin time ratio. Thromb Haemost 1983;49(3):238–44.
15. Favaloro EJ, Adcock DM. Standardization of the INR: how good is your laboratory's INR and can it be improved? Semin Thromb Hemost 2008;34(7):593–603.
16. Fiebig EW, Etzell JE, Ng VL. Clinically relevant differences in prothrombin time and INR values related to blood sample collection in plastic vs glass tubes. Am J Clin Pathol 2005;124(6):902–9.
17. Thomson JM, Tomenson JA, Poller L. The calibration of the second primary international reference preparation for thromboplastin (thromboplastin, human, plain, coded BCT/253). Thromb Haemost 1984;52(3):336–42.
18. WHO. WHO Expert Committee on biological standardization guidelines for thromboplastins and plasma used to control oral anticoagulant therapy. Geneva: WHO; 1999.

19. Ng VL, Levin J, Corash L, et al. Failure of the International Normalized Ratio to generate consistent results within a local medical community. Am J Clin Pathol 1993;99(6):689–94.

20. Ts'ao C, Neofotistos D. The use and limitations of the INR system. Am J Hematol 1994;47(1):21–6.

21. Talstad I. Why is the standardization of prothrombin time a problem? Haemostasis 2000;30(5):258–67.

22. Ng VL, Valdes-Camin R, Gottfried EL, et al. Highly sensitive thromboplastins do not improve INR precision. Am J Clin Pathol 1998;109(3):338–46.

23. Smith SA, Morrissey JH. Properties of recombinant human thromboplastin that determine the International Sensitivity Index (ISI). J Thromb Haemost 2004;2(9): 1610–6.

24. Smith SA, Comp PC, Morrissey JH. Phospholipid composition controls thromboplastin sensitivity to individual clotting factors. J Thromb Haemost 2006;4(4): 820–7.

25. Adcock D, Brien W, Duff S, et al. Procedures for validation of INR and local calibration of PT/INR systems; approved guideline. Wayne (PA): Clinical and Laboratory Standards Institute; 2005. p. H54-A.

26. Arkin C. Do we need the geometric mean as the mean normal value in INR determination? J Thromb Haemost 2005;3(Suppl 1) [abstract number: P1903].

27. van den Besselaar AM, Neuteboom J, Meeuwisse-Braun J, et al. Preparation of lyophilized partial thromboplastin time reagent composed of synthetic phospholipids: usefulness for monitoring heparin therapy. Clin Chem 1997;43(7):1215–22.

28. Leichsenring I, Plesch W, Unkrig V, et al. Multicentre ISI assignment and calibration of the INR measuring range of a new point-of-care system designed for home monitoring of oral anticoagulation therapy. Thromb Haemost 2007;97(5):856–61.

29. Critchfield GC, Bennett ST, Swaim WR. Calibration verification of the International Normalized Ratio. Am J Clin Pathol 1996;106(6):786–94.

30. Chantarangkul V, Frontoni R, Gresele P, et al. Usefulness of lyophilized calibration plasmas for International Normalized Ratio determination with the bovine combined thromboplastin (thrombotest): results of a collaborative study. Blood Coagul Fibrinolysis 2005;16(2):157–63.

31. Favaloro EJ, Hamdam S, McDonald J, et al. Time to think outside the box? Prothrombin time, international normalised ratio, International Sensitivity Index, mean normal prothrombin time and measurement of uncertainty: a novel approach to standardisation. Pathology 2008;40(3):277–87.

32. McKernan A, Thomson JM, Poller L. The reliability of international normalized ratios during short-term oral anticoagulant treatment. Clin Lab Haematol 1988; 10(1):63–71.

33. Bellest L, Eschwege V, Poupon R, et al. A modified international normalized ratio as an effective way of prothrombin time standardization in hepatology. Hepatology 2007;46(2):528–34.

34. Robert A, Chazouilleres O. Prothrombin time in liver failure: time, ratio, activity percentage, or international normalized ratio? Hepatology 1996;24(6):1392–4.

35. Kovacs MJ, Wong A, MacKinnon K, et al. Assessment of the validity of the INR system for patients with liver impairment. Thromb Haemost 1994;71(6):727–30.

36. Deitcher SR. Interpretation of the international normalised ratio in patients with liver disease. Lancet 2002;359(9300):47–8.

37. Dufour DR, Lott JA, Nolte FS, et al. Diagnosis and monitoring of hepatic injury. I. Performance characteristics of laboratory tests. Clin Chem 2000;46(12): 2027–49.

38. Cholongitas E, Papatheodoridis GV, Vangeli M, et al. Systematic review: the model for end-stage liver disease—should it replace Child-Pugh's classification for assessing prognosis in cirrhosis? Aliment Pharmacol Ther 2005;22(11–12): 1079–89.

39. Reddy NM, Hall SW, MacKintosh FR. Partial thromboplastin time: prediction of adverse events and poor prognosis by low abnormal values. Arch Intern Med 1999;159(22):2706–10.

40. Tripodi A, Mannucci PM. Activated partial thromboplastin time (APTT). New indications for an old test? J Thromb Haemost 2006;4(4):750–1.

41. Bobrow RS. Excess factor VIII: a common cause of hypercoagulability. J Am Board Fam Pract 2005;18(2):147–9.

42. Sauls DL, Banini AE, Boyd LC, et al. Elevated prothrombin level and shortened clotting times in subjects with type 2 diabetes. J Thromb Haemost 2007;5(3): 638–9.

43. Tripodi A, Chantarangkul V, Martinelli I, et al. A shortened activated partial thromboplastin time is associated with the risk of venous thromboembolism. Blood 2004;104(12):3631–4.

44. Brandt JT, Triplett DA. Laboratory monitoring of heparin. Effect of reagents and instruments on the activated partial thromboplastin time. Am J Clin Pathol 1981;76(Suppl 4):530–7.

45. D'Angelo A, Seveso MP, D'Angelo SV, et al. Effect of clot-detection methods and reagents on activated partial thromboplastin time (APTT). Implications in heparin monitoring by APTT. Am J Clin Pathol 1990;94(3):297–306.

46. Kitchen S, Jennings I, Woods TA, et al. Wide variability in the sensitivity of APTT reagents for monitoring of heparin dosage. J Clin Pathol 1996;49(1):10–4.

47. Brandt JT, Arkin CF, Bovill EG, et al. Evaluation of APTT reagent sensitivity to factor IX and factor IX assay performance. Results from the College of American Pathologists Survey Program. Arch Pathol Lab Med 1990;114(2):135–41.

48. Hales SC, Johnson GS, Wagner D. Comparison of six activated partial thromboplastin time reagents: intrinsic system factors' sensitivity and responsiveness. Clin Lab Sci 1990;3(3):194–6.

49. Sahud M. Coagulation tests in differential diagnosis. Clin Lab Haematol 2000; 22(Suppl 1):2–8 [discussion: 30–2].

50. Burns ER, Goldberg SN, Wenz B. Paradoxic effect of multiple mild coagulation factor deficiencies on the prothrombin time and activated partial thromboplastin time. Am J Clin Pathol 1993;100(2):94–8.

51. Korte W, Clarke S, Lefkowitz JB. Short activated partial thromboplastin times are related to increased thrombin generation and an increased risk for thromboembolism. Am J Clin Pathol 2000;113(1):123–7.

52. Hron G, Eichinger S, Weltermann A, et al. Prediction of recurrent venous thromboembolism by the activated partial thromboplastin time. J Thromb Haemost 2006;4(4):752–6.

53. Ten Boekel E, Bartels P. Abnormally short activated partial thromboplastin times are related to elevated plasma levels of TAT, F1+2, D-dimer and FVIII: C. Pathophysiol Haemost Thromb 2002;32(3):137–42.

54. Bick RL. Disseminated intravascular coagulation current concepts of etiology, pathophysiology, diagnosis, and treatment. Hematol Oncol Clin North Am 2003; 17(1):149–76.

55. Ten Boekel E, Bock M, Vrielink GJ, et al. Detection of shortened activated partial thromboplastin times: an evaluation of different commercial reagents. Thromb Res 2007;121(3):361–7.

Liver Disease, Coagulation Testing, and Hemostasis

Valerie L. Ng, PhD, MD

KEYWORDS

- Liver disease • Prothrombin time
- International normalized ratio • Fresh frozen plasma
- Transfusion

In vivo hemostasis results from the delicate balance and complex interplay of naturally occurring clotting factors (procoagulants), clotting inhibitors (anticoagulants), endothelial surface, and platelets. The most well known and researched entities in each of these individual categories are:

Procoagulants—fibrinogen, Factors II (prothrombin), V, VII, VIII, X, IX, XI, XII, and XIII
Vitamin K-dependent procoagulants—Factors II, VII, IX, X
    Anticoagulants—Proteins C, S, Z, antithrombin III (ATIII)
Vitamin K-dependent anticoagulants—Proteins C and S
Fibrinolytic agents—plasminogen, plasmin, plasminogen activators, plasminogen activator inhibitors
Products of fibrinolysis—fibrin degradation products (fdps), d-dimer
Platelets—number, qualitative function

Other coagulation tests (eg, ecarin clotting times, dilute Russell's viper venom time, lupus anticoagulant tests, tissue factor pathway inhibitor or thrombin-activatable fibrinolysis inhibitor, and so forth) have not yet been adopted widely in the clinical laboratory for care of patients with liver disease. These other tests are not addressed in this article.

In vitro clinical laboratory coagulation tests assess isolated clotting pathways (eg, extrinsic versus intrinsic pathway) under artificial in vitro conditions. Meanwhile, in vivo clotting involves near simultaneous activation and interplay of many of these pathways, and involve participation of the endothelium, a pathway and process not amenable to today's in vitro coagulation testing.[1,2] As a result, in vitro clotting tests do not correlate well with hemostasis in general.

A variety of clotting test abnormalities in three of the pathways for which in vitro tests exist (ie, procoagulants, anticoagulants, platelets) have been identified in patients with

Clinical Laboratory, Highland General Hospital, 1411 East 31st Street, Oakland, CA 94602, USA
E-mail address: vang@acmedctr.org

Clin Lab Med 29 (2009) 265–282
doi:10.1016/j.cll.2009.05.001
0272-2712/09/$ – see front matter © 2009 Elsevier Inc. All rights reserved.

labmed.theclinics.com

liver disease. In general, the more advanced the liver disease, the more abnormalities are present. Many excellent reviews on this subject have been published over the past few decades, with a general consensus that coagulation testing for patients with liver disease correlates poorly with clinical hemostasis.[3–8] This review will reiterate the common findings and provide relevant updates to coagulation abnormalities in patients with liver disease. Coagulation test and hemostasis considerations related to the anhepatic phase of liver transplantation are not be addressed in this review because they are substantially different and sufficiently complex to warrant a separate, independent, and focused discussion.[8,9]

COAGULATION TESTS IN LIVER DISEASE

It is important to acknowledge that liver disease is in fact a spectrum of diseases, ranging from minimal asymptomatic liver abnormalities to chronic stable liver disease to acute fulminant hepatic failure to absolute absence of liver function (ie, anhepatic phase of liver transplantation). This article focuses primarily on coagulation test abnormalities identified for patients with chronic stable liver disease.

An isolated prolonged prothrombin time (PT) is the most common coagulation test abnormality observed for patients with liver disease. As disease progresses, partial thromboplastin times (PTTs) often become prolonged. But what do these coagulation test prolongations mean clinically? Can they predict bleeding?

Procoagulant Levels in Patients with Liver Disease

The majority of procoagulants measured by the PT or PTT—fibrinogen, factors II, V, X, VII, VIII, IX, XI, XII—are synthesized in the liver. Notably, FVIII is also synthesized outside the liver by endothelial cells, thereby maintaining normal circulating levels in patients with liver disease. FV and FVII have the shortest in vivo half-lives (12 and 4–6 hours, respectively) and are the procoagulants most decreased in patients with liver disease. Because the PT is dependent on FVII levels and FVII has the shortest in vivo half-life, an isolated prolonged PT is common for patients with liver disease.

The effect of liver disease on procoagulant factor synthesis varies in proportion with the degree of liver failure. The important clinical issue is, however, whether the decreased procoagulant levels are still adequate for in vivo hemostasis. A related question is whether clinical bleeding can be predicted based on degree of prolongation of these various procoagulant laboratory tests.

Many studies to determine individual procoagulant levels in patients with liver disease were conducted many decades ago and, as such, many of these studies are not readily accessible. One of the retrievable studies assessed 30 well-characterized patients with advanced liver disease and biopsy-confirmed cirrhosis.[10] Only 18 of these patients had a documented bleeding history, consisting of melena or hematemesis or fecal occult blood. A variety of noncommercially available procoagulant tests were applied to plasmas obtained from this cohort. Tests performed included clotting time in glass and siliconized tubes, one-stage PT using an acetone extract of human brain, PT consumption index, factor V and VII activities, two-stage PT, thrombotest activity, thromboplastin generation test, fibrinogen concentration, or titer—Fibrindex.[10] Although this study was performed in 1968, findings from a few of these tests (eg, the clotting times in glass or siliconized tubes, one-stage PT, and fibrinogen concentration) are still relevant today because the test methodologies are relatively unchanged and the tests still in use. Notably, there were no consistent findings for the 30 patients. Of the patients, 17 of 30 (57%) had varying degrees of prolonged one-stage clotting times (either glass or silicone tubes). Factor V activity was decreased in only two patients, whereas FVII decreased in 10. Specimens with identified FV or FVII deficiencies did not correlate with prolonged one-stage PTs: that is, prolonged PTs were observed with specimens containing normal FV and FVII levels and vice versa.

From this study, the investigators concluded that bleeding or clotting times were of relatively little value.[10] They noted that hemorrhage could occur despite apparently normal coagulation and that clotting factor deficiencies did not have a clear relationship with causation or severity of bleeding. The investigators commented that despite abnormalities in one or more clotting tests, none of the patients had abnormal bleeding after percutaneous liver biopsy.

Similar lack of correlation between coagulation tests and bleeding in patients with liver diseases were obtained by Spector and Corn.[11] In their study, bleeding was defined as that requiring blood transfusion and included a mixture of anatomic versus microvascular bleeding manifestations (ie, esophageal varices, gastritis, gastric ulcer, hemorrhoids, persistent skin bleeding after biopsy, and marked menorrhagia).

A similar study was undertaken in the early 1990s.[12] The impetus for the study was the use of a thromboplastin reagent insensitive to FVII deficiency. This particular PT reagent resulted in PT prolongation beyond 1.5x midpoint of the PT reference range only when FVII levels were less than 15%. The investigators were concerned that patients with PT ratios less than 1.5x undergoing invasive procedures might have inadequate procoagulant levels for adequate hemostasis. (The PT ratio is the PT of the patient specimen divided by the PT value at the arithmetic midpoint of the PT reference range, expressed as an "x" of the midpoint of the PT reference range.) Three laboratories were involved, two using the same reagent but different coagulometers (laboratories A and C), and one using a different reagent and a different coagulometer (laboratory B). Specimens from 29 patients with chronic liver disease and prolonged PTs were obtained from patients attending a specialized clinic treating those awaiting liver transplantation. Specimens from all patients were aliquoted within 4 hours of obtaining the specimen, stored at −70°C, and thawed immediately before until evaluation in all three laboratories. Specimens underwent only one freeze–thaw cycle. PT ratios and levels of FII, FV, FVII, and FX were determined. Laboratories A and C, using the same thromboplastin reagent, noted PT prolongation most closely correlated with FVII levels (**Table 1**). For laboratory B, using a different thromboplastin reagent and coagulometer, no individual procoagulant factor was less than 25% for PT ratios of 1.3x to 1.9x.

This simple study once again demonstrated variability in PT reagent sensitivity to procoagulant factor deficiencies, and that the degree of PT prolongation was not well correlated with actual procoagulant factor levels.

How Much of Each Procoagulant Do you Need for in Vivo Hemostasis?

In general, there is no definitive answer to the question as to how much procoagulant is needed for in vivo hemostatis, let alone an answer specific for patients with liver disease. Insight into the answer to this question is provided from the study of the hemophilias.

The heritable single-factor deficiencies, hemophilias A and B (ie, factor VIII and IX deficiencies, respectively) have defined the minimum level of clotting factor for patients with a single-factor deficiency and for varying degrees of hemostasis. The hemophilia A and B diseases are categorized into three categories of severity: mild (6%–30% factor level), moderate (1%–5%), and severe (<1%). Mild hemophiliacs bleed only after external trauma or surgery, moderate hemophiliacs will bleed with relatively minor trauma or after surgical procedures, and severe hemophiliacs often

Table 1
PT ratios and levels of FII, FV, FVII, and FX

PT Ratio (Laboratories A and C)	1.2×	1.3×	1.4×	1.5×	1.6×	1.8×	2.0×
No. patients	5	8	8	2	2	1	3
PT (seconds)	15.2–15.5	16.8–17.5	17.4–18.7	19.7, 20.0	19.9, 20.2	22.8	26.0–27.1
FII activity (%)	29–67	18–62	21–46	22, 31	29, 50	24	10–25
FV activity (%)	37–48	17–69	20–46	32, 33	20, 40	27	10–20
FVII activity (%)	26–57	15–43	13–32	13, 15	10, 16	9	7–20
FX activity (%)	53–83	20–63	36–57	38, 51	40, 42	40	9–31

bleed spontaneously into joints or muscles after trivial trauma multiple times yearly. Current factor replacement recommendations to prophylax against spontaneous bleeding or hemarthrosis in severe hemophiliacs is to maintain trough levels greater than 1% for the relevant clotting factor.[13] If this hemophilia natural history data is extrapolated to patients with liver disease, one would infer that 6% to 30% of any single coagulation factor should be adequate for hemostasis in the absence of external trauma or surgery.

However, patients with liver disease usually have multiple coagulation-factor deficiencies. Thus, the single factor-deficient hemophilias may not be an appropriate analogy to apply to patients with liver disease. Instead, the rare familial, multiple congenital-factor deficiencies may provide the needed insight into hemostasis in the setting of multiple clotting-factor deficiencies.

There are at least seven types of these inherited multiple-factor deficiency disorders.[14] Only two of the most common entities within this disorder have been researched adequately to extrapolate the findings to liver disease.

Combined deficiency of FV and FVIII (F5F8D) is caused by autosomal-recessive inheritance of mutations in the *LMAN1* (lectin mannose binding protein, formerly known as the *ERGIC*-53 gene) or *MCFD2* (multiple coagulation-factor deficiency-2) genes.[15] The normal *LMAN1* or *MCFD2* gene products are responsible for intracellular trafficking of proteins from the endoplasmic reticulum and Golgi apparatus.[16] While these gene mutations would be expected to affect a wide range of secretory proteins that move between these intracellular compartments, surprisingly the only clinical manifestation observed to date has been bleeding associated with decreased FV and FVIII levels.[16] Affected individuals had plasma levels of FV and FVIII ranging from 5% to 30% for each individual factor. Epistaxis and bleeding after dental extractions were the most commonly observed bleeding tendencies. There were also histories of menorrhagia (for females), gastrointestinal bleeding, hemarthroses, hematomas, postcircumcision (for males), or postoperative or postpartum bleeding for a smaller subset of F5F8D patients. Bleeding tendencies and related decreases in FV or FVIII levels were of the same magnitude as those of patients with isolated FV or FVIII deficiency.[15,16] One study assessing the bleeding history of a relatively homogeneous group of F5F8D patients noted they did not have more severe bleeding symptoms when two, instead of one, clotting factors were concomitantly decreased.[17] In other words—and the important point from this study—multiple coagulation-factor deficiencies in this disorder did not have additive or multiplicative effects on bleeding; that is, affected individuals do not have an increased tendency to bleed when two instead of just one clotting factor is deficient. Therefore, if we are to extrapolate the findings from F5F8D to patients with liver disease, multiple factor deficiencies by themselves do not predispose to a greater risk of bleeding than the risk conferred from a single factor deficiency.

Another very rare heritable multiple coagulation-factor deficiency condition is that of combined deficiency of vitamin K-dependent clotting factors (VKCFD). This deficiency arises primarily from mutations in two different genes: VKCFD1, by point mutations in the genes coding for the γ-carboxylase gene (*GGCX*), and VKCFD2, by point mutations in the vitamin K epoxide reductase gene (*VKOR*).[16] Affected individuals have decreased levels of active vitamin K-dependent clotting factors (ie, FII, FVII, FIX, FX) because of their inability to γ-carboxylate glutamate residues of the clotting factor precursors to yield active clotting factors. Reported bleeding manifestations were variable and did not always correlate with clotting factor levels.[18–23] The natural history of this disorder suggests factors other than simple coagulation-factor deficiencies alone predispose to bleeding.

Patients with liver disease have deficiencies in the vitamin K-dependent coagulation factors, analogous to patients with VKCFD. If one were to extrapolate the findings from VKCFD patients to those with liver disease, one would conclude that bleeding in patients with liver disease is not related solely to multiple coagulation-factor deficiencies, nor can be reliably predicted based on procoagulant factor levels alone.

Vitamin K Deficiency is Uncommon in Patients with Liver Disease

Vitamin K is commonly given to patients with liver disease to augment synthesis of vitamin K-dependent clotting factors. This is undertaken because of the misconception that a prolonged PT in a patient with liver disease, presumably because of multiple coagulation-factor deficiencies, is associated with an increased risk of bleeding, and giving vitamin K will help by increasing vitamin K-dependent clotting factors. Vitamin K is a fat-soluble vitamin. Absorption of vitamin K (as well as the other fat-soluble vitamins A, D, and E) is dependent on bile production.

There are at least three reasons why patients with liver disease can have vitamin K deficiency: poor nutrition (especially for those for whom chronic alcohol intake is the cause of their liver disease), malabsorption because of decreased bile production caused by liver disease, and biliary obstruction because of liver disease and preventing bile release to the intestines.

But how vitamin K-deficient are patients with liver disease? It turns out that the answer depends on the laboratory method used to assay for vitamin K deficiency. Using PT prolongation as a surrogate measure for vitamin K deficiency, three studies demonstrated only 8 of 52 (15.4%),[24] 1 of 45 (2.2%),[25] or 14 of 170 (7.8%)[26] patients with histologically confirmed cirrhosis were vitamin K-deficient. In contrast, Kowdley and colleagues[27] used reverse-phase high performance liquid chromatography to measure and compare plasma vitamin K_1 levels in 77 patients with histologically confirmed primary biliary cirrhosis and 255 "healthy elderly subjects residing the in Boston metropolitan region, who had normal nutritional status and no chronic illness." Of patients with primary biliary cirrhosis, 18 of 77 (23.3%) had plasma vitamin K_1 levels below the reference range, but only 1 of the 18 (5.5%) had a prolonged PT.[27] Within the group of patients with primary biliary cirrhosis, the investigators noted no correlation between vitamin K_1 level and PT and no difference in the mean PT between groups with low or normal vitamin K_1 levels.[27]

From these studies, vitamin K deficiency in patients with liver disease—as defined by laboratory tests—ranges from 2% to 23%. Clinically evident coagulopathy, manifesting as prolonged PTs or clinical bleeding, however, was rare.[4,26,27]

A note about the laboratory methods used to assess vitamin K deficiency: in three of these four studies, "PT prolongation" was used as a surrogate for vitamin K deficiency. The rarity of PT prolongation, despite laboratory evidence of vitamin K deficiency (ie, high-performance liquid chromatography measurement of plasma vitamin K_1 levels), led to the conclusion that the PT was relatively insensitive for detecting procoagulant-factor deficiencies related to vitamin K deficiency. This is true (see "Procoagulant levels in patients with liver disease" section, above). The fourth study defined the surrogate measure for vitamin K deficiency "as a prothrombin time > 12.6 s which accounts for any calibration error in measurement."[26] (As an aside, this latter definition is baffling in that there are no commercially available PT "calibrators," not at the time this study was performed nor even today.)

FVIII, von Willebrand Factor, and Liver Disease

FVIII and von Willebrand Factor (vWF) are synthesized by both the liver and endothelial cells. Both are also "acute phase reactants;" that is, levels are increased during "acute" disease. Normal or elevated FVIII and vWF levels are typically observed in patients with liver disease because of (i) continued endothelial cell FVIII production despite decreased hepatic FVIII production, and (ii) increased synthesis because of acute disease or inflammation.[8,28–31]

One group compared FVIII, low-density lipoprotein receptor-related protein (LRP) and vWF mRNA levels and protein expression in tissue obtained from patients with cirrhosis versus noncirrhotic liver disease. (LRP binds a variety of ligands and is involved in a variety of physiologic processes. Thrombin-activated FVIII, through its light chain, binds to LRP in a dose-dependent manner and the complex is cleared from the circulation by endocytosis.[32]) They observed that FVIII and LRP mRNAs were decreased in liver tissue obtained from cirrhotics. In contrast, vWF mRNA and vWF protein expression was increased in liver tissue obtained from cirrhotics.[33] They concluded elevated circulating FVIII levels in patients with liver disease was not a result of increased FVIII synthesis, but was instead caused by increased hepatic synthesis of vWF and decreased synthesis of LRP.[33]

Many patients with liver disease have normal PTTs, a rather surprising result from a theoretical perspective; mild baseline deficiencies of multiple procoagulants should affect the PTT. Moreover, the normal PTT in liver disease is contradictory to the finding that multiple mild deficiencies of clotting factors disproportionately prolong the PTT (see the section "PTT response to single versus multiple procoagulant deficiencies is different" in the article "Prothrombin time and partial thromboplastin time assay considerations" by Ng, elsewhere in this issue for more detail). Because patients with liver disease often have elevated FVIII levels, it has been speculated that a "normal" PTT may actually reflect two separate but intertwined processes: a prolonged PTT because of multiple procoagulant deficiencies, and a shortened PTT because of elevated FVIII levels (see the section "Elevated FVIII levels and PTT shortening" section in the article "Prothrombin time and partial thromboplastin time assay considerations" by Ng, elsewhere in this issue).[3] The relative contributions of these opposing effects cannot be determined nor predicted, given the loose inverse relationship between increasing FVIII levels and PTT shortening.[34]

Disseminated Intravascular Coagulation Versus Hyperfibrinolysis in Patients with Liver Disease

Patients with liver disease have laboratory evidence of a consumptive coagulopathy. There has been longstanding controversy, however, as to whether the consumptive coagulopathy is indicative of disseminated intravascular coagulation (DIC) or of hyperfibrinolysis.[3,35,36] Inherent to this controversy is the fundamental difficulty of establishing a diagnosis of either DIC or fibrinolysis, given that many of the same tests are used to diagnose either entity.[35,37] This issue is much too complicated for adequate discussion or conclusions in this article, and the reader is referred to excellent reviews on these subjects for further reading.[3,35,36]

Factor VIII Levels Cannot Diagnose or Exclude Disseminated Intravascular Coagulation

A common clinical question for acutely ill patients with liver disease is whether concurrent DIC is present. FVIII levels are often requested, with the expectation that if the FVIII levels are normal (or elevated), DIC can be excluded. There are two flaws in this logic. The first flaw is the fact that a single FVIII level does not reveal the relative extent of the opposing rates of FVIII synthesis versus consumption (**Fig. 1**). In **Fig. 1**, note the two different scenarios of combined liver disease and DIC. In scenario one, the net measured FVIII activity exceeds the reference range because FVIII production

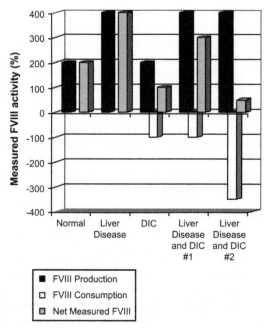

Fig. 1. Net measured FVIII levels in various clinical scenarios.

exceeds consumption. This scenario points out the fallacy of excluding DIC in a patient with liver disease even when a high FVIII activity level is determined. In scenario two, FVIII consumption outpaces production and the net measured FVIII activity is low. This scenario suggests that a low FVIII level in a patient with liver disease may be useful as evidence of FVIII consumption outpacing FVIII production, and thus be supportive evidence of concurrent DIC. The reality, however, is that patients with liver disease and an acute illness are likely to have elevated FVIII levels for at least two reasons—liver disease alone and acute illness—such that FVIII consumption does not outpace FVIII production and scenario two does not occur.

The second flaw in this logic is related to how FVIII levels are actually measured in the laboratory. Most laboratories use a PTT-derived assay and factor-deficient plasma substrates to determine procoagulant factor activity levels. In fulminant DIC, activated clotting factors—especially FXa, FIXa, and thrombin—are circulating and present in plasma specimens submitted for coagulation testing. Any FXa in the plasma specimen will bypass the need for FVIII for clotting in the PTT assay.[35] The FXa itself, without assistance from FVIII, will rapidly trigger fibrinogen to fibrin conversion, will result in an overall short clotting time, and will translate to a high FVIII level when the FVIII activity is interpolated from the short clotting time to a corresponding FVIII activity level using a "standard curve."[35] For this reason, "coagulation factor assays provide little, if any, measurement information in patients with DIC."[35]

Fibrinogen and Dysfibrinogen

Fibrinogen is also an acute-phase reactant, so levels would be expected to be increased during episodes of acute disease. In patients with liver disease, fibrinogen levels are typically normal or increased. Decreased levels are observed only in severe liver disease, and even in this situation fibrinogen levels are usually greater than 100 mg/dL.[38]

Approximately two-thirds of patients with liver disease have structurally abnormal fibrinogen ("dysfibrinogen"). These dysfibrinogens are typically fibrinogen with increased sialic acid residues caused by increased sialyl-transferase activity in immature hepatocytes in response to liver injury.[8,39]

The following sections explore what is known about other parts of the coagulation system for patients with liver disease.

Anticoagulant Levels are Decreased in Patients with Advanced Liver Disease

There is relatively scant literature on the subject of anticoagulant levels decreasing in patients with advanced liver disease. The predominant findings for patients with liver disease have been decreased levels of proteins C, S, and antithrombin.[3,8,40]

Proteins C and S are vitamin-K-dependent proteins synthesized by hepatocytes. In one study, protein C was decreased to the lower end of the reference range ($\sim 70\% \pm 10\%$ activity) but not to levels observed with inherited heterozygous deficiencies.[29] Protein C, protein S, and antithrombin deficiencies observed in patients with liver disease have been attributed to decreased hepatocyte function, increased consumption (because of DIC or hyperfibrinolysis, see above sections) and vitamin K deficiency.[3,8,41,42] (Note the previous section in this article debunking the myth of vitamin K deficiency in patients with liver disease.)

Hypercoagulability in Patients with Advanced Liver Disease?

Although bleeding is the most common concern for patients with liver disease, hypercoagulabilty is also observed, the most significant being portal vein thrombosis, clotting of extracorporeal circulation devices, and thrombotic occlusion of intrahepatic blood vessels further damaging the liver. Factors contributing to the hypercoagulability of liver disease include underlying DIC/hyperfibrinolysis and decreased levels of the natural anticoagulants.[3,8,41]

Other Coagulation Tests in Liver Disease

Much of this article so far has emphasized significant intra- and interlaboratory variability in conventional coagulation reagents and testing methods. More recent studies assessing coagulation disorders in patients with liver disease have applied newer tests assessing coagulation factors or assays of contemporary interest (eg, thrombin activatable fibrinolyis inhibitor, plasminogen activator inhibitor 1, tissue factor, tissue plasminogen activator, thrombomodulin, interleukin 11, tissue necrosis factor alpha, activated protein C-protein C inhibitor, thromboelastography, and so forth. Suffice it to say that there are no definitive conclusions for these newer coagulation factors or assays and patients with liver disease.[3-8]

Platelet Abnormalities in Patients with Advanced Liver Disease

Platelet abnormalities have been grouped into two major categories: quantitative versus qualitative abnormalities.

Quantitative platelet abnormalities

Thrombocytopenia, defined as a peripheral blood platelet count less than 150,000/mcL, is present in two-thirds of patients with liver disease.[43] The more severe the liver disease, the lower the platelet count. The platelet count in patients with liver disease rarely declines below 30,000/mcL. Thrombocytopenia in patients with liver disease is not associated with an increased risk of variceal bleeding or spontaneous bleeding.[3,8] There are many causes for the thrombocytopenia, including: (*i*) splenic enlargement because of portal hypertension and platelet sequestration, (*ii*) impaired platelet production because of a relative deficiency of thrombopoietin, and (*iii*) increased destruction by immune and nonimmune mechanisms.[8]

Qualitative platelet abnormalities

Platelets from patients with liver disease have abnormal platelet aggregometry results, with the abnormalities proportional to the severity of liver disease.[3,8] There are multiple causes for these abnormal results, including the presence of circulating inhibitors (d-dimers, dysfibrinogens), degradation of platelet receptors by plasmin, increased nitric oxide, defects in signal transduction pathways, and so forth.[44,45] None of these causes for qualitative platelet abnormalities, however, occur consistently in patients with liver disease.[3]

Summary of Coagulation Test Abnormalities in Liver Disease and Hemostasis

Coagulation test abnormalities for patients with liver disease are quite common and the underlying causes quite complex. Many of the documented coagulation test abnormalities, summarized in **Fig. 2**, are associated with contradictory hemostatic risks for bleeding or clotting. In addition, some of the coagulation test abnormalities have no definitive risk associated with bleeding or clotting. Given the complexity of the clotting system and hemostasis, coupled with the many coagulation test abnormalities observed in liver disease, it must be once again reemphasized that coagulation test results cannot reliably predict bleeding or clotting.[5–7]

WHEN TO TREAT COAGULATION ABNORMALITIES IN LIVER DISEASE

The most commonly used coagulation screening tests are the PT/international normalized ratio (INR) and the PTT. Note that these tests only assess the procoagulant arm of

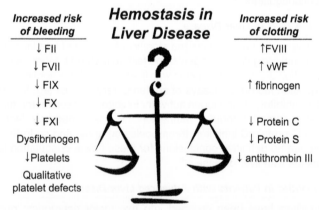

Fig. 2. Compilation of coagulation factor abnormalities identified for patients with liver disease and associated hemostasis risks (bleeding versus clotting). Note the contradictory risks for those clotting factors for which the hemostatic risk is known, as well as the numerous clotting factor abnormalities for which the risk of bleeding or clotting is unknown.

hemostasis. A prolonged PT/INR or PTT in patients with liver disease, without full recognition of the many variables causing these coagulation test prolongations, is often interpreted simplistically as evidence of procoagulant deficiency.

A common clinical reaction to a prolonged PT/INR or PTT is to administer a blood product or blood products, such as fresh frozen plasma (FFP) or frozen plasma (FP), capable of providing clotting factors in the hopes of correcting the clotting time prolongation and preventing bleeding. This clinical reaction is based on a simplistic interpretation of a prolonged clotting-time test representing clotting-factor deficiency only. It ignores evidence demonstrating adequate coagulation factor levels in patients with liver disease who have prolonged PT/INRs.[10,12,46] It also fails to consider circulating inhibitors (eg, dysfibrinogens, d-dimers) and not clotting-factor deficiencies as the cause of the clotting-test prolongation in patients with liver disease. Finally, it ignores the evidence that prolonged clotting times in patients with liver disease does not correlate with nor predict bleeding.

Despite this flawed logic, it is helpful to examine the efficacy of coagulation factor replacement or hemostatic agent administration on correcting coagulation test prolongations in patients with liver disease.

Prothrombin Time Ratios and International Normalized Ratio Threshold for Frozen Plasma Administration

A brief review is warranted of the history of PT—and subsequently INR—thresholds for coagulation factor replacement via FFP/FP administration in patients with liver disease.

In 1982, an National Institutes of Health (NIH) panel was convened to address the increasing use of FFP/FP in the absence of convincing evidence of efficacy.[47] Of the many FFP/FP recommendations made, one was a recommendation for FFP/FP use "for patients with multiple coagulation defects as in liver disease …"[47] This recommendation prompted studies to define a PT prolongation threshold, above which FFP/FP would be effective in correcting PT prolongation and maintaining adequate hemostasis. The studies divided this overarching question into two subordinate questions: What is the evidence that FFP/FP administration corrects prolonged PTs? What is the evidence that prophylactic FFP/FP administration to correct prolonged PTs prevents bleeding?

Origins of the 1.5× PT Threshold for Coagulation Factor Replacement in Liver Disease

Two major professional societies promulgated FFP/FP transfusion threshold recommendations. In 1992, the British Committee for Standards in Haematology, Working Party of the Blood Transfusion Task Force acknowledged lack of evidence for their recommendation of "a PT of 1.6–1.8 times the control value is probably realistic."[48] In 1996, the American Society of Anesthesiologists Task Force on Blood Component Therapy recommended FFP/FP for patients with "microvascular bleeding or hemorrhage who are massively transfused if the PT/PTT values exceed 1.5 times the laboratory's normal values."[49]

A series of studies were undertaken shortly after the NIH panel consensus recommendations to determine a PT "threshold" at which bleeding could be predicted. These studies was not restricted to just patients with liver disease; patients with other underlying diseases were also included. In all of these studies, PT thresholds were defined as a multiple ("×") of the arithmetic midpoint of the reference range (PT ratio). In some studies, PTT prolongation was also included with, unfortunately, different definitions of PTT ratios (ie, multiple of the arithmetic midpoint of the reference range versus multiple of the upper boundary of the reference range).

Recent reviews of these studies have been published,[50–52] with the same conclusions: there is insufficient evidence to conclude abnormal laboratory tests predict bleeding, support prophylactic use of FFP/FP to prevent bleeding, and accurately weigh the risks associated with the clinical benefits of FFP/FP transfusion. Furthermore, analysis of the various national FFP/FP transfusion guidelines has demonstrated significant lack of agreement of a FFP/FP transfusion threshold because of lack of supportive evidence.[53] Regardless, a common FFP/FP transfusion threshold in many clinical settings today, regardless of underlying disease condition, is 1.5× PT.

Validity of the 1.5× Prothrombin Time Threshold

Three studies by Toy and colleagues[54,55] deserve special mention in considering the validity of the 1.5× PT threshold for FFP/FP administration. All three of these studies were published around the time of the earliest guidelines for PT-based FFP/FP transfusion thresholds.[48,53] In one study, no increased risk of bleeding was observed for patients undergoing percutaneous thoracentesis or paracentesis if the PT (or PTT ratio) was less than or equal to 2.0×.[55] In the second study, there was no increased risk of bleeding from percutaneous liver biopsy if the PT ratio was less than or equal to 1.5×.[54] Both of these studies included a wide diversity of clinical conditions, of which patients with liver disease comprised a significant proportion. A criticism of these two studies was their definition of "bleed" as a drop in hemoglobin of greater than or equal to 2 gm/dL following the procedure, as bleeds less than or equal to 2 gm/dL could be clinically significant but not captured in the studies.

A third study by this group assessed patients who had received massive transfusion (> 10 units red blood cells within 24 hours) and determined PTs and PTTs were consistently prolonged greater than or equal to 1.5× when at least 12 units of plasma-free red blood cells had been given.[56] The investigators cautioned another prospective study was necessary to determine the relationship of the observed abnormal coagulation tests with clinical bleeding.

At the time these clinical studies were undertaken, the thromboplastin reagent in use had an International Sensitivity Index (ISI) greater than or equal to 2.0. (VL Ng, Personal communication, 2008) This means that mathematical transformation of the PT ratio into an INR would correspond to INR thresholds of 2.25 (1.5× PT threshold for significant bleeding observed in the study of percutaneous liver biopsy associated bleeding) to 4.0 (2.0× PT threshold associated with significant bleeding in the study of paracentesis or thoracentesis-associated bleeding).

How the 1.5× Prothrombin Time Threshold Incorrectly Morphed into the International Normalized Ratio = 1.5 Threshold

Studies assessing the relationship of PT prolongation with clinical bleeding were occurring simultaneously with the thromboplastin manufacturers shift towards producing more sensitive (lower ISI) thromboplastin reagents to improve interlaboratory INR reproducibility for vitamin K antagonist anticoagulation therapy monitoring (see the related article on "Anticoagulant monitoring" by Ng, elsewhere in this issue). The PT-ratio literature had not historically taken into account differing thromboplastin reagent sensitivities to factor deficiencies. As a result and as the commercial thromboplastin reagent ISIs trended down towards 1.0 to improve INR standardization, the 1.5× PT ratio threshold for FFP/FP administration incorrectly became an INR threshold of 1.5.

Evidence-based 1.5× Prothrombin Time Threshold is Actually the International Normalized Ratio = 2.25 to 4.0 Threshold for Increased Risk of Bleeding from Percutaneous Procedures in Patients with Liver Disease

While the calculated INR of 1.5 mathematically corresponds to a PT ratio of 1.5× for thromboplastin reagents with ISIs of approximately 1.0, it ignores the historical evidence from studies in which PTs were generated less sensitive thromboplastins (ISIs ≥ 2.0).[6] When using the true ISIs of the less sensitive thromboplastins in use at the time of these studies, the corresponding INRs would be 2.25 to 4.0.

Fresh Frozen Plasma/Frozen Plasma Does Not Correct Minimally Prolonged PTs/INRs

General studies to assess FFP/FP correction of prolonged PT/INRs did not selectively focus on patients with liver disease and prolonged PTs/INRs. With this caveat, two major studies demonstrated minimal if any effect of FFP/FP on correcting minimally prolonged PT/INRs. Of note, patients with liver disease were included in these studies, but data specific to this clinical condition were not separately analyzed.

Holland and colleagues assessed pre-and posttransfusion INRs for 90 patients who received FFP/FP.[57] The thromboplastin reagent in use had an ISI of 1.01, making the INR essentially identical to the PT ratio. In addition, their institutional INR threshold for FFP/FP transfusion was INR greater than 1.6. Of the 90 patients for whom 68 units of FFP/FP were requested and transfused, 22 had INRs less than 1.6 and did not meet criteria for appropriate FFP/FP transfusion. For these 22 patients, the mean change in posttransfusion INRs was 0.03 INR per unit of FFP/FP.

The group also determined an average INR of the FFP/FP units themselves of 1.1 (range 0.9–1.3). The investigators commented on the fact that FFP/FP INRs can be as high as 1.3, making any difference in coagulation activity between FFP/FP units and the plasma of patients with minimally prolonged PT/INRs too small to have an effect on the INR. In support of this, INR correction with FFP/FP administration for 10 control patients with more significantly prolonged INRs (ie, INRs prolonged > 1.6) was proportional to the degree of INR prolongation.

Abdel-Wahab and colleagues[58] conducted a prospective audit of 1,091 FFP/FP transfusions to patients with minimally prolonged PT/INRs. Minimally prolonged PT/INRs were defined as PTs between 13.1 and 17 seconds and corresponding INRs of 1.1 to 1.85. Three hundred and twenty-four units of FFP/FP administered to 121 patients met the study inclusion criteria: patients having a minimally prolonged PT/INR, and posttransfusion PT/INR available within 8 hours of FFP/FP transfusion. The median decrease was 0.2 seconds (95% confidence interval, 0.1–0.4) for the PT and 0.07 for the INR. Notably, only 0.8% of patients achieved correction of the INR to an INR less than 1.1 ("complete correction"). Stated differently, PT correction did not occur for 99% of patients. Only 15% achieved PT/INR correction at least halfway to the reference range. There was no obvious dose-response effect (ie, more FFP/FP units transfused did not correlate with greater PT-INR correction), and no difference dependent on when the PT/INR posttransfusion value was obtained (ie, posttransfusion PT/INRs obtained 1 hour versus more than 4 hours after FFP/FP transfusion). Finally, the investigators did not find a relationship between pretransfusion PT/INR and estimated red blood cell loss.[58] The investigators concluded, "regardless of the number of FFP units transfused or the number of hours after FFP transfusion, FFP resulted in only trivial decrements of the PT."[58] The investigators commented that given the exponential relationship of coagulation factors on the PT, transfusion of one to four units of FFP would contribute insufficient coagulation factors to correct the PT/INR by 50% for minimally prolonged PTs/INRs.[58]

Fresh Frozen Plasma/Frozen Plasma Does Not Correct Prolonged Prothrombin Time/International Normalized Ratios in Patients with Liver Disease

Many of the studies discussed earlier studied a diverse patient population. While patients with liver disease were included in the study population, data specific to patients with liver disease were not separately analyzed.

Only a few studies have specifically focused on the effect of transfusion on prolonged PTs/INRs in patients with liver disease. Early studies used nonstandardized coagulation tests, many of which are no longer in use.[59,60] Nonetheless, these studies did not demonstrate a consistent beneficial effect of blood or plasma transfusion on prolonged PT/INR correction.

More recently, Youssef and colleagues[61] reproduced these findings for 100 patients with cirrhosis. Briefly, all patients had stable chronic liver disease and prolonged PTs unresponsive to vitamin K injections; 80 patients were part of a retrospective review and 20 patients part of a prospective study. Two to four units of FFP were administered with the goal being PT correction to within 3 seconds of the control time. Only approximately 10% (prospective study) or 12.5% (retrospective study) of patients showed PT correction to within 3 seconds of the control time. The investigators concluded the benefits of FFP administration were "uncertain" and stated current FFP volumes administered "infrequently correct the coagulopathy of liver disease."[61] The investigators commented on an observed trend towards higher than the usual two to four volumes of FFP linked with PT correction, with the cautionary note that many patients cannot tolerate this higher fluid and volume load.[61] They also noted that many patients whose PT did not correct actually received sufficient FFP to correct prolonged PTs based on a published formula for FFP/FP administration to correct prolonged PTs.[61]

No Evidence for Increased Bleeding Related to Percutaneous Liver Biopsy for Patients with Prolonged Prothrombin Time/International Normalized Ratios

Prophylaxis against bleeding from a percutaneous liver biopsy is one of the most common justifications for which FFP is given for patients with liver disease and a prolonged PT/INR. What is the evidence linking prolonged PT/INRs with bleeding following this procedure? It is not compelling.

Grant and Neuberger reviewed the literature and identified three studies failing to demonstrate an increased risk of bleeding from percutaneous liver biopsy when the PT was less than or equal to 4 seconds above controls.[62] They identified a single study having the same lack of association with bleeding when the PT was less than or equal to 7 seconds above control values.[62]

A large study of 1,500 liver biopsy outcomes from 189 health districts in England and Wales identified an increased trend towards bleeding with increasing INRs; specifically, 3.3% of patients with an INR ranging from 1.3 to 1.5 had a significant bleed, and 7.1% when the INR was greater than 1.5.[63] Another way to look at this data, however, is that the vast majority (89.6%) of bleeding complications arose in patients with normal INRs (ie, INRs <1.3).[62]

Of interest and for FFP correction of prolonged INRs prior to percutaneous liver biopsy, the British Committee for Standards in Haematology recommends FFP administration if the PT is greater than or equal to four times the normal value (with an accompanying note of "results unpredictable"), the Canadian Members of the Expert

Working group recommends FFP if the INR greater than 2, and the corresponding French, Australasian, and American guidelines have no recommendations.[53]

SUMMARY

Coagulation tests for patients with liver disease do not correlate with hemostasis. The risk of bleeding cannot be correlated with the degree of coagulation test prolongation.

Prolonged PTs/INRs cannot be reliably corrected with FFP/FP administration.

An increased risk of bleeding from percutaneous procedures (liver biopsy, thoracentesis, paracentesis) occurs when the PT ratio greater than 1.5 (corresponding INR = 2.0–4.5), but

The majority of bleeding from percutaneous liver biopsy occurs in patients with normal coagulation tests (INRs <1.3).

REFERENCES

1. Hoffman M. Remodeling the blood coagulation cascade. J Thromb Thrombolysis 2003;16(1–2):17–20.
2. Furie B, Furie BC. Thrombus formation in vivo. J Clin Invest 2005;115(12): 3355–62.
3. Kujovich JL. Hemostatic defects in end stage liver disease. Crit Care Clin 2005; 21(3):563–87.
4. Trotter JF. Coagulation abnormalities in patients who have liver disease. Clin Liver Dis 2006;10(3):665–78, x–xi.
5. Mannucci PM. Abnormal hemostasis tests and bleeding in chronic liver disease: are they related? No. J Thromb Haemost 2006;4(4):721–3.
6. Thachil J. Relevance of clotting tests in liver disease. Postgrad Med J 2008; 84(990):177–81.
7. Tripodi A. Hemostasis abnormalities in liver cirrhosis: myth or reality? Pol Arch Med Wewn 2008;118(7–8):445–8.
8. Senzolo M, Burra P, Cholongitas E, et al. New insights into the coagulopathy of liver disease and liver transplantation. World J Gastroenterol 2006;12(48):7725–36.
9. Hambleton J, Leung LL, Levi M. Coagulation: consultative hemostasis. Hematology Am Soc Hematol Educ Program 2002;335–52.
10. Donaldson GW, Davies SH, Darg A, et al. Coagulation factors in chronic liver disease. J Clin Pathol 1969;22(2):199–204.
11. Spector I, Corn M. Laboratory tests of hemostasis. The relation to hemorrhage in liver disease. Arch Intern Med 1967;119(6):577–82.
12. Viele M, Atwater SP, Pham DT, et al. Revisiting fresh frozen plasma transfusion guidelines: correlation of prothrombin time with individual coagulation factor levels is reagent dependent. Blood 1995;86(Suppl):355a.
13. Medical and Scientific Advisory Committee, National Hemophilia Foundation, NHF. MASAC Recommendation Concerning Prophylaxis (Regular Administration of Clotting Factor Concentrate to Prevent Bleeding, 2006). Available at http://www. hemophilia.org/NHFWeb/Resource/StaticPages/menu0/menu5/menu57/170.pdf. Accessed June 18, 2009.
14. Roberts HR, Escobar MA. Chapter 118. Other clotting factor deficiencies. In: Hoffman R, Benz EJ Jr, Shattil SJ, et al, editors. Hematology. Basic principles and practice. 4th edition. Philadelphia: Elseviers Churchill Livingston; 2005. p. 2081–95.

15. Zhang B, Spreafico M, Zheng C, et al. Genotype-phenotype correlation in combined deficiency of factor V and factor VIII. Blood 2008;111(12):5592–600.
16. Zhang B, Ginsburg D. Familial multiple coagulation factor deficiencies: new biologic insight from rare genetic bleeding disorders. J Thromb Haemost 2004;2(9): 1564–72.
17. Peyvandi F, Tuddenham EG, Akhtari AM, et al. Bleeding symptoms in 27 Iranian patients with the combined deficiency of factor V and factor VIII. Br J Haematol 1998;100(4):773–6.
18. Pauli RM, Lian JB, Mosher DF, et al. Association of congenital deficiency of multiple vitamin K-dependent coagulation factors and the phenotype of the warfarin embryopathy: clues to the mechanism of teratogenicity of coumarin derivatives. Am J Hum Genet 1987;41(4):566–83.
19. Johnson CA, Chung KS, McGrath KM, et al. Characterization of a variant prothrombin in a patient congenitally deficient in factors II, VII, IX and X. Br J Haematol 1980;44(3):461–9.
20. Goldsmith GH Jr, Pence RE, Ratnoff OD, et al. Studies on a family with combined functional deficiencies of vitamin K-dependent coagulation factors. J Clin Invest 1982;69(6):1253–60.
21. Brenner B, Tavori S, Zivelin A, et al. Hereditary deficiency of all vitamin K-dependent procoagulants and anticoagulants. Br J Haematol 1990;75(4):537–42.
22. McMahon MJ, James AH. Combined deficiency of factors II, VII, IX, and X (Borg-schulte-Grigsby deficiency) in pregnancy. Obstet Gynecol 2001;97(5 Pt 2): 808–9.
23. Chung KS, Bezeaud A, Goldsmith JC, et al. Congenital deficiency of blood clotting factors II, VII, IX, and X. Blood 1979;53(4):776–87.
24. Kaplan MM, Elta GH, Furie B, et al. Fat-soluble vitamin nutriture in primary biliary cirrhosis. Gastroenterology 1988;95(3):787–92.
25. Munoz SJ, Heubi JE, Balistreri WF, et al. Vitamin E deficiency in primary biliary cirrhosis: gastrointestinal malabsorption, frequency and relationship to other lipid-soluble vitamins. Hepatology 1989;9(4):525–31.
26. Phillips JR, Angulo P, Petterson T, et al. Fat-soluble vitamin levels in patients with primary biliary cirrhosis. Am J Gastroenterol 2001;96(9):2745–50.
27. Kowdley KV, Emond MJ, Sadowski JA, et al. Plasma vitamin K1 level is decreased in primary biliary cirrhosis. Am J Gastroenterol 1997;92(11):2059–61.
28. McPherson R. Specific proteins. In: McPherson R, Pincus M, editors. Henry's clincial diagnosis and management by laboratory methods. 21st edition: Chapter 19. Philadelphia: Saunders Elsevier; 2007. p. 231–44.
29. Kelly DA, O'Brien FJ, Hutton RA, et al. The effect of liver disease on factors V, VIII and protein C. Br J Haematol 1985;61(3):541–8.
30. Langley PG, Hughes RD, Williams R. Increased factor VIII complex in fulminant hepatic failure. Thromb Haemost 1985;54(3):693–6.
31. Maisonneuve P, Sultan Y. Modification of factor VIII complex properties in patients with liver disease. J Clin Pathol 1977;30(3):221–7.
32. Schwarz HP, Lenting PJ, Binder B, et al. Involvement of low-density lipoprotein receptor-related protein (LRP) in the clearance of factor VIII in von Willebrand factor-deficient mice. Blood 2000;95(5):1703–8.
33. Hollestelle MJ, Geertzen HG, Straatsburg IH, et al. Factor VIII expression in liver disease. Thromb Haemost 2004;91(2):267–75.
34. Ten Boekel E, Bartels P. Abnormally short activated partial thromboplastin times are related to elevated plasma levels of TAT, F1+2, D-dimer and FVIII: C. Pathophysiol Haemost Thromb 2002;32(3):137–42.

35. Bick RL. Disseminated intravascular coagulation current concepts of etiology, pathophysiology, diagnosis, and treatment. Hematol Oncol Clin North Am 2003; 17(1):149–76.
36. Ferro D, Celestini A, Violi F. Hyperfibrinolysis in liver disease. Clin Liver Dis 2009; 13:21–31.
37. Joist JH. AICF and DIC in liver cirrhosis: expressions of a hypercoagulable state. Am J Gastroenterol 1999;94(10):2801–3.
38. Lechner K, Niessner H, Thaler E. Coagulation abnormalities in liver disease. Semin Thromb Hemost 1977;4(1):40–56.
39. Francis JL, Armstrong DJ. Fibrinogen-bound sialic acid levels in the dysfibrinogenaemia of liver disease. Haemostasis 1982;11(4):215–22.
40. Mannucci PM, Vigano S. Deficiencies of protein C, an inhibitor of blood coagulation. Lancet 1982;2(8296):463–7.
41. Northup PG, Sundaram V, Fallon MB, et al. Hypercoagulation and thrombophilia in liver disease. J Thromb Haemost 2008;6(1):2–9.
42. Yamaguchi M, Gabazza EC, Taguchi O, et al. Decreased protein C activation in patients with fulminant hepatic failure. Scand J Gastroenterol 2006;41(3):331–7.
43. Bashour FN, Teran JC, Mullen KD. Prevalence of peripheral blood cytopenias (hypersplenism) in patients with nonalcoholic chronic liver disease. Am J Gastroenterol 2000;95(10):2936–9.
44. Escolar G, Cases A, Vinas M, et al. Evaluation of acquired platelet dysfunctions in uremic and cirrhotic patients using the platelet function analyzer (PFA-100): influence of hematocrit elevation. Haematologica 1999;84(7):614–9.
45. Witters P, Freson K, Verslype C, et al. Review article: blood platelet number and function in chronic liver disease and cirrhosis. Aliment Pharmacol Ther 2008; 27(11):1017–29.
46. Deitcher SR. Interpretation of the international normalised ratio in patients with liver disease. Lancet 2002;359(9300):47–8.
47. Fresh frozen plasma: indications and risks. National Institutes of Health Consensus Development Conference Statement. Natl Inst Health Consens Dev Conf Consens Statement 1984;5(5):4.
48. Contreras M, Ala FA, Greaves M, et al. Guidelines for the use of fresh frozen plasma. British Committee for Standards in Haematology, Working Party of the Blood Transfusion Task Force. Transfus Med 1992;2(1):57–63.
49. Practice Guidelines for blood component therapy: a report by the American Society of Anesthesiologists Task Force on Blood Component Therapy. Anesthesiology 1996;84(3):732–47.
50. Segal JB, Dzik WH. Paucity of studies to support that abnormal coagulation test results predict bleeding in the setting of invasive procedures: an evidence-based review. Transfusion 2005;45(9):1413–25.
51. Kleinman S, Chan P, Robillard P. Risks associated with transfusion of cellular blood components in Canada. Transfus Med Rev 2003;17(2):120–62.
52. Stanworth SJ, Brunskill SJ, Hyde CJ, et al. Is fresh frozen plasma clinically effective? A systematic review of randomized controlled trials. Br J Haematol 2004; 126(1):139–52.
53. Iorio A, Basileo M, Marchesini E, et al. The good use of plasma. A critical analysis of five international guidelines. Blood Transfus 2008;6(1):18–24.
54. McVay PA, Toy PT. Lack of increased bleeding after liver biopsy in patients with mild hemostatic abnormalities. Am J Clin Pathol 1990;94(6):747–53.
55. McVay PA, Toy PT. Lack of increased bleeding after paracentesis and thoracentesis in patients with mild coagulation abnormalities. Transfusion 1991;31(2):164–71.

56. Leslie SD, Toy PT. Laboratory hemostatic abnormalities in massively transfused patients given red blood cells and crystalloid. Am J Clin Pathol 1991;96(6):770–3.

57. Holland LL, Brooks JP. Toward rational fresh frozen plasma transfusion: the effect of plasma transfusion on coagulation test results. Am J Clin Pathol 2006;126(1): 133–9.

58. Abdel-Wahab OI, Healy B, Dzik WH. Effect of fresh-frozen plasma transfusion on prothrombin time and bleeding in patients with mild coagulation abnormalities. Transfusion 2006;46(8):1279–85.

59. Finkbiner RB, Mc GJ, Goldstein R, et al. Coagulation defects in liver disease and response to transfusion during surgery. Am J Med 1959;26(2):199–213.

60. Spector I, Corn M, Ticktin HE. Effect of plasma transfusions on the prothrombin time and clotting factors in liver disease. N Engl J Med 1966;275(19):1032–7.

61. Youssef WI, Salazar F, Dasarathy S, et al. Role of fresh frozen plasma infusion in correction of coagulopathy of chronic liver disease: a dual phase study. Am J Gastroenterol 2003;98(6):1391–4.

62. Grant A, Neuberger J. Guidelines on the use of liver biopsy in clinical practice. British Society of Gastroenterology. Gut 1999;45(Suppl 4):IV1–IV11.

63. Gilmore IT, Burroughs A, Murray-Lyon IM, et al. Indications, methods, and outcomes of percutaneous liver biopsy in England and Wales: an audit by the British Society of Gastroenterology and the Royal College of Physicians of London. Gut 1995;36(3):437–41.

Anticoagulation Monitoring

Valerie L. Ng, MD, PhD

KEYWORDS

- Warfarin • Heparin • Low-molecular-weight heparin
- Direct thrombin inhibitors • Xa inhibitors
- Non-standardized coagulation testing • Reagent variability

Anticoagulation is prescribed to prevent thrombosis, treat existing thrombosis, or prevent future recurrence in someone who has had a thrombotic episode. Two major classes of anticoagulants have been used for almost a century with an accompanying wealth of evidence to guide therapy: vitamin K antagonists ([VKAs] ie, warfarin) and heparin.

Warfarin and heparin have narrow therapeutic indices and significant morbidity associated with long-term treatment. As a result, there has long been a desire for safer, oral anticoagulants with high bioavailability and predictable pharmacokinetics. Recent times have witnessed an explosion of the development and preliminary clinical trials of new potential anticoagulants with many benefits and advantages when compared with VKAs or heparin. Some are taken orally and most have predictable pharmacokinetics and require no laboratory testing to monitor effect.[1–3] These new agents target multiple points in the coagulation cascade, with those most advanced in clinical trials being direct anti-Xa agents or direct thrombin inhibitors (DTI). Some of these agents have already been approved by the Food and Drug Administration for use in specific clinical situations. The reader is encouraged to stay abreast of this rapidly evolving field.

DISCOVERY OF HEPARIN AND VITAMIN K ANTAGONISTS

The discoveries of heparin and VKAs are fascinating glimpses into the scientific practices and larger cultural backdrops of the associated historical times. The discovery of heparin was steeped in controversy, with multiple scientists claiming credit.[4,5] Furthermore, reading the original description of its early crude preparations, made from autolyzing bovine liver, evokes vivid pungent and visceral reactions even today.[5]

Department of Pathology and Laboratory Medicine, Clinical Laboratory Room 3408, Alameda County Medical Center/Highland General Hospital, 1411 East 31st Street, Oakland, CA 94602, USA
E-mail address: vang@acmedctr.org

Clin Lab Med 29 (2009) 283–304
doi:10.1016/j.cll.2009.05.003
0272-2712/09/$ – see front matter © 2009 Elsevier Inc. All rights reserved.

The discovery of warfarin reads like a Horatio Alger success story.[4–6] It begins with the juxtaposition of the great depression in North America (1920s) and the fiscal inability of farmers to purchase additional cattle feed when the usual sweet clover feed had become moldy. Cattle eating the spoiled sweet clover predictably began hemorrhaging 15 days later, with fatal hemorrhage within 30 to 50 days of ingestion. The disease was named "sweet clover disease." In February 1933, one distraught rancher who had lost many cattle and doubtful of his local veterinarian's "sweet clover disease" explanation was referred to the "local agricultural experimental station." He loaded his truck with a dead heifer, 100 pounds of spoiled sweet clover, a milk can of unclotted blood, and drove 190 miles in a blizzard to present the truckload to a scientist, Karl Link, and his senior student, Wilhelm Schoeffel. After the rancher left, the subsequent exchange between Dr. Link and the rather melodramatic Mr. Schoeffel remains as enthralling today as it must have been then, and as captivating as any Shakespearean or Wagnerian drama (**Box 1**).

Beginning the next day and from the delivered moldy hay, the active anticoagulant, dicumarol, was ultimately isolated and crystallized in 1939. Notably, the work was funded by the Wisconsin Alumni Research Foundation, to which the patent rights were assigned and from which the name of the now most commonly used derivative, "warfarin," was derived.

Dicumarol was first developed as a rat poison, but acted slower than desired because of the substantial vitamin K content in grains and vegetables naturally available to the free living rat. A more effective and faster acting derivative, warfarin, was subsequently developed and quickly became a subject of interest for human use when reversal of its effect was demonstrated in 1951; an army inductee attempted suicide by ingesting rat poison (warfarin) but survived with vitamin K supplementation.[6] Notably and early in its development before adequate clinical efficacy evidence, President Eisenhower was treated with warfarin following his acute myocardial infarction in 1955 and initial heparin anticoagulation.[6]

Box 1
Excerpt from Link and attributed to Schoeffel

After farmer Carlson left, Schoeffel stormed back and forth in the laboratory shouting, "Vat da Hell, a farmer shtruggles nearly 200 miles in dis Sau-wetter, driven by a shpectre and den has to go home vit promises dat might come true in five, ten, fifteen years, maybe never. Who knows? 'Get some good hay–transfuse.' Ach!! Gott, how can you do dat ven you haf no money?" he snarled.

He dipped his hands into the milk can repeatedly and while rubbing them muttered, " Dere's no clot in dat blook! BLUT, BLUT VERFLUCHTES BLUT. 'Die Menschen dauern mich in ihren Jammertagen.'" (Faust Prolog., line 297) and then, "Vat vill he find ven he gets home? Sicker crows. And ven he and his good voman go to church tomorrow and pray and pray and pray, vat vill dey haf on Monday? MORE DEAD COWS!! He has no udder hay to feed–he can't buy any. And if he loses de bull he loses his seed. Mein Gott!! Mein Gott!! Vy didn't ve anti-shi-pate dis? Ya, ve should haf anti-shi-pated dis."

We took the blood and hay played about with them until about 7:00 p.m. when I headed for home. As I left the laboratory, Schoeffel grabbed me by the shoulders, looked my squarely in the face and said, "Before you go let me tell you something. Der is a desh-tiny dat shapes out ends, it shapes our ends I tell you! I vill clean up and gif you a document on Monday morning."

From Link KP. The discovery of dicumarol and its sequels. Circulation 1959;19:97–107; with permission.

WARFARIN–VITAMIN K ANTAGONIST THERAPY: USE THE INTERNATIONAL NORMALIZED RATIO TO MONITOR

Warfarin's mechanism of anticoagulation action is by inhibiting gamma carboxylation of the vitamin K–dependent coagulation factors. This results in a decreased level of active coagulation factors and an excess of precursor coagulation factors, or proteins induced by VKAs.

The demonstration of warfarin's effectiveness early in its development was hampered by highly variable laboratory assays. The development of the international normalized ratio (INR) system in the mid-1980s helped reduce laboratory assay variability and introduced an internationally standardized method for monitoring warfarin's effect. One must remember that INRs are reproducible between laboratories for only those patients who are stably anticoagulated (ie, at least 6 weeks of VKA therapy). It is speculated that this unique interlaboratory reproducibility of INRs is related to the presence of proteins induced by VKAs (see the article on prothrombin time [PT] and partial thromboplastin time [PTT] assay considerations elsewhere in this issue).

VKA treatment guidelines are developed by an international committee and updated periodically. Current evidence-based guidelines recommend a target INR of 2.5 (range, 2–3) for most thrombotic situations, with a slightly higher INR target of 3 (range, 2.5–3.5) for various types of mechanical heart valves.[7–10] The reader is referred to these recent guidelines for a detailed discussion on the many nuances of dosing VKAs, bridging to VKA therapy from initial heparin therapy, and duration of VKA anticoagulation.[7–10]

One small cautionary note: because the INR is derived from the measured PT, one must know if the PT reagent is sensitive to the presence of heparin. Some PT reagents are sensitive to heparin and if both heparin and warfarin are simultaneously present, may yield disproportionately long PT INRs, thereby unnecessarily decreasing anticoagulant dosing, and increasing the risk of clotting.[11]

Biologic Variability of International Normalized Ratios

Warfarin has complex pharmacodynamics and pharmacokinetics, and coupled with its narrow therapeutic index, requires frequent monitoring (ie, INR). Although cytochrome P-450 (ie, CYP2C9) and VKORC1 variant alleles influence warfarin metabolism and effect, the action of these two gene products only accounts for a fraction of the observed biologic variability (ie, only 30%–50% of the observed biologic variability was attributed to variant alleles in one Swedish study[12]). Other factors, such as dietary vitamin K intake, alcohol use, liver disease, other drugs taken concomitantly, and infections, have been well known to affect INRs.

What is the minimum INR biologic variability? One study of serial INRs from 35 stably anticoagulated patients over a 6-month period demonstrated an overall approximate 10% INR coefficient of biologic variability (CV), with approximate 12% CV for a target INR of 2.5 and approximate 9% for a target INR of 3.5.[13] The reference laboratory INR method was in good control; only 3.5% total CV was observed for control specimens with assigned INR values of 2.5 and 4.1. The CV corresponding to biologic variability was then used to determine the threshold at which an INR difference was beyond that expected for statistical variation and the development of a useful nomogram is depicted to guide therapeutic decision making (**Fig. 1**).[13]

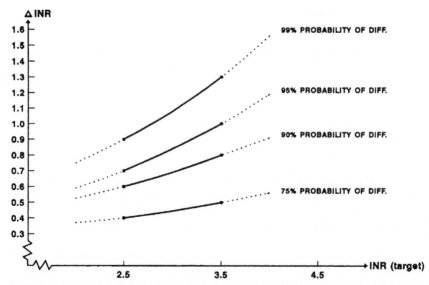

Fig. 1. Probability of significant difference between two consecutive INR measurements from patients on oral anticoagulant therapy. For example, a change in INR from 2.7 to 3.5 means a △INR of 0.8. From the nomogram, a △INR of 0.8 that results in an INR of 3.6 (x-axis) corresponds to a probability of biologic change of approximately 90%. (*From* Lassen JF, Brandslund I, Antonsen S. International normalized ratio for prothrombin times in patients taking oral anticoagulants: critical difference and probability of significant change in consecutive measurements. Clin Chem 1995;41:444–7; with permission.)

International Normalized Ratio Reproducibility for Vitamin K Antagonist–Treated Patients

Early studies relied on data from a limited number of coagulation laboratories to demonstrate the superior interlaboratory reproducibility of INRs when compared with prothrombin times. Subsequently, and with the widespread international adoption of the INR, real-life interlaboratory INR reproducibility and precision could be determined.

Interlaboratory Reproducibility of Clinical Laboratory–Derived International Normalized Ratios

The desired interlaboratory INR reproducibility is a CV less than or equal to 10% in the therapeutic range (INR 2–3 for routine VKA-based anticoagulation, INR 2.5–3.5 for mechanical heart valves).[14]

The actual observed interlaboratory INR reproducibility does not achieve this desired goal. There are relatively few recent publications on this subject because no major advances have been made since the flurry of publications in the 1990s describing significant INR variability caused by reagent or instrumentation effects (see the article on PT and PTT assay considerations elsewhere in this issue for more detail). The available published studies are not consistent in the type of specimens used. Some have used patient specimens, and others proficiency test materials, which may not have the same matrix as patient specimens.

Reproducibility studies with patient specimens

Arguably, these are the best type of specimens to use for interlaboratory reproducibility studies because they reflect real-world testing and are of the same matrix as patients who need testing. Earlier studies used rigorously controlled patient specimens: obtained fresh, platelet poor plasma separated within 2 hours of collection, aliquoted and stored at $-70°C$, transported between laboratories on dry ice, subjected to only one freeze-thaw before testing. Significant variability between laboratories was demonstrated such that 15% to 30% of paired INR values from the same specimen are categorized into different INR therapeutic ranges (with likely VKA dose adjustment) depending on which reagent-instrument combination was used and regardless of thromboplastin reagent sensitivity to coagulation factor deficiencies.[15,16] A more recent study by Testa and colleagues[17] reproduced the same proportion of INR discrepancies and demonstrated that even after optimizing the INR calibration process, 16% of patients with specimens tested by different thromboplastin reagents have VKA dosage adjustment solely dependent on which thromboplastin reagent had been used. Notably, portions of these studies have occurred within a single laboratory, demonstrating significant INR variability even while avoiding the known additional variability associated with testing by multiple laboratories.

Reproducibility studies using proficiency test specimens

Proficiency test specimens may be of a different composition than patient specimens, possibly introducing a "matrix" effect on proficiency test results and rendering conclusions not applicable to testing performed with fresh plasma specimens. Nonetheless, review of the most recent College of American Pathologists coagulation proficiency test participant summary reveals continued interlaboratory method (identified as reagent and instrument combination) INR discrepancies. The INR discrepancies increase proportionately with higher assigned INR values, often exceed the desired 10% interlaboratory variability within the same reagent-instrument category, and have even larger INR discrepancies when results are compared across different reagent-instrument combinations.[18]

POINT-OF-CARE TESTING INTERNATIONAL NORMALIZED RATIO ACCURACY AND REPRODUCIBILITY

Significant INR variability has been demonstrated within the controlled environment of a clinical laboratory. With point-of-care testing (POCT), additional test reliability concerns arose, most notably related to personnel competency and test environment (ie, temperature, humidity).[19,20] In recognition of these additional concerns associated with POCT, two key questions were posed when POCT INR test devices became commercially available: how do INRs generated from POCT devices compare with those generated by the laboratory; and what INR variability is introduced by non–health care personnel performing testing (ie, patient self-testing)?

Comparison of Point-of-care Testing versus Clinical Laboratory International Normalized Ratios

A number of studies have compared POCT-derived INRs with those generated in a central laboratory.[21] These studies varied in their design, but were similar in that patients had paired whole blood (obtained by fingerstick) INR testing and conventional plasma PT-INR testing within a short period of time (1–4 hours). Overall, the findings have been consistent: most paired values were in agreement. The caveat to these studies is INR agreement was defined as 80% concordance for paired INR values within 0.4 INR units and 90% concordance within 0.7 INR units.[22] These INR ranges were statistically defined based on studying INRs from 35 stably anticoagulated patients over 6 months to determine "critically significant differences."[13] If target INR values were 2.5 or 3, it is clear that some of the paired values deemed within acceptable agreement exceed the desired maximal INR variability of less than or equal to 10%.[14]

The intermethod INR variability (POCT versus clinical laboratory) is comparable with previously documented interlaboratory INR variability. POCT testing does not introduce additional variability for INR results.

International Normalized Ratios Derived from Different Point-of-care Testing have Comparable Variability as International Normalized Ratios from Different Laboratories

Most of these studies have been centered in the United Kingdom and led to the UK National External Quality Assessment Scheme (Coagulation). Some of these studies were performed using manipulated specimens (eg, lyophilized, artificially depleted of coagulation factors), so their conclusions may not be applicable to everyday POCT performance using fresh whole blood or plasma specimens.

Tripodi and colleagues[23] conducted a study in which patients brought in their own POCT coagulometers for testing of three quality assurance specimens by experienced laboratorians. The intent was to determine the value of periodic coagulometer checking to verify accuracy. The patients also had simultaneous comparison of their own INRs produced from self-testing with INRs determined by the laboratory using plasma collected at the time of the visit. The authors observed most quality assurance specimen values and paired self-testing versus plasma laboratory INR values were within ± 15% to 20% of the consensus values (note the observed variation was larger than the desirable ± 10% variation[14]).

Poller and coworkers[24] distributed 60 lyophilized artificially depleted and 60 lyophilized coumarin-treated plasmas to 10 centers for testing by experienced laboratorians on 10 POCT devices representing two models, each from a different manufacturer. A subset of three to five specimens from each group was selected as a quality assurance set to assess relative reliability of the different testing centers. Aberrant results were defined as those exceeding 15% deviation from the assigned INR. The authors observed significant aberrant INR results, varying by device, testing center, and type of specimen.

Meijer and associates[25] distributed a set of five "certified international normalized ratio plasmas" for testing on 539 POCT devices by experienced laboratory staff in nine Netherlands Thrombosis Centers. "Significant deviation" was defined as greater than or equal to 15% from the assigned INR value. They observed approximately 20% of participants had a significant deviation on at least one of the five certified plasmas, and significant differences related to test strip lots.

Finally, Kitchen and collaborators[26] reported on INR proficiency test results generated by experienced health care personnel using POCT INR devices over a 6-year period. Three different POCT devices were used by more than 10 participating centers. In general, POCT INR results differed by 11% to 14% between centers, comparable with the 12% variability for conventional hospital laboratory–based INR testing. Of note, 10% to 11% of centers generated POCT INRs exceeding the acceptable ± 15% deviation.

POCT INRs, when generated by experienced laboratory personnel, yield results comparable with laboratory generated INRs with no additional variation specifically attributable to the POCT device.

Know how Point-of-care Testing International Normalized Ratios Compares with Central Laboratory International Normalized Ratios

It is prudent (and required by regulation)[27–30] to determine how POCT INRs compare with central laboratory's INRs and from which to develop organizational policy and procedure.[31] There are publications demonstrating POCT INRs and central laboratory derived INR variability equivalent to interlaboratory INR variability.[22,32] There are other studies demonstrating a net positive systematic bias for POCT INRs when compared with paired clinical laboratory derived INRs.[33,34]

Regardless of what is published, the following is a real life example of why one needs to regularly monitor how POCT INR relates to clinical laboratory INRs. In 2005, a clinical pharmacist–managed anticoagulation clinic was initiated in my health care system. The laboratory assessed the INRs determined by the fingerstick POCT device chosen to best meet the needs of the clinical team and demonstrated reasonable INR correlation between methods for the target 2 to 3.5 therapeutic INR range. The POCT device was put into use and a single clinical pharmacist operated the clinic under a standardized protocol approved by the medical staff. The clinical pharmacist was supervised by the clinic's medical director. A subsequent comparison study of INR results between methods conducted in 2007 demonstrated acceptable POCT performance (**Fig. 2**).

One of the requirements of this anticoagulation clinic protocol was for the clinical pharmacist to refer any patient with a POCT outside the therapeutic range (ie, INR >4) to the clinical laboratory for a laboratory INR determination. In 2008, a scheduled 1-year audit of this POCT INR program revealed 45 (2.3%) of 1926 patients tested had INRs greater than 4, but only 19 (42%) of the 45 patients had a same-day laboratory INR determined. The primary reason for why patients did not present to the laboratory for a paired laboratory INR was inconvenience; patients did not want to wait for phlebotomy and did not want more blood drawn.

Fig. 3 demonstrates the paired INRs for these 19 patients. It is apparent that the POCT device had a systematic high bias present, which was not obvious in the initial or in the 2007 INR method comparison. This bias was apparent in the 2008 study because supratherapeutic POCT INR values were the focus; supratherapeutic INRs were uncommon and underrepresented in the earlier studies.

The clinical providers in anticoagulation clinic had been concerned about an increased risk of bleeding for patients who had a supratherapeutic POCT INR but

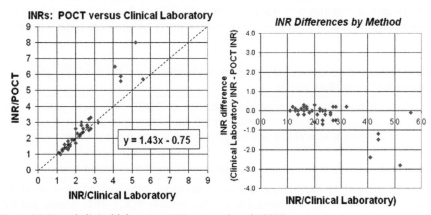

Fig. 2. POCT and clinical laboratory INR comparison in 2007.

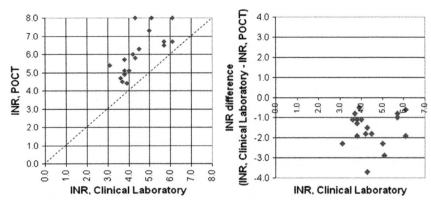

Fig. 3. POCT versus clinical laboratory INR comparison for the 19 patients whose POCT INR was supratherapeutic (INR ≥ 8).

did not present to the laboratory for a definitive laboratory INR determination. This concern was partially allayed by review of these comparative INR data with the providers. It was recognized that the actual risk of bleeding corresponds to the lower laboratory-derived INR and is less than initially considered based on only the elevated and systematically high-biased POCT result. Review of the POCT INRs for those patients who did not have a paired laboratory INR revealed all patients who had subsequent anticoagulation clinic visits had INRs in the therapeutic range. Furthermore, there were no untoward bleeding complications documented for these patients in the intervening period between clinic visits. These data ensured the providers that the VKA dosage adjustments taken based on only POCT INRs were appropriate.

The systematic high bias of the POCT INR device at supratherapeutic INRs coupled with the reality of patients not having a same-day laboratory INR determined has provided a rational basis for revising the anticoagulation clinic protocol. Because there were no bad outcomes, and because the POCT device reliably and predictably yielded a higher INR value than the laboratory for supratherapeutic POCT INRs, the POCT device was viewed to have a built-in "safety margin." Providers are alerted much earlier to possible supratherapeutic INRs with the POCT device than by laboratory INRs. Based on this information, laboratory INR testing for supratherapeutic POCT INRs is now recommended, instead of required. Providers are also asked to enact the same clinical changes on the supratherapeutic INRs as they did before this study, because their clinical actions at the time were correct and avoided patient adverse effects.

Patient Self-testing does not Introduce More Variability into Point-of-care Testing International Normalized Ratios

One study demonstrated comparable variability of POCT INRs from patient self-testing as INRs determined by experienced laboratory personnel using POCT devices.[22] Early concerns about test personnel training were not realized.

Clinical Outcomes for Point-of-care Testing International Normalized Ratios

Given the number of patients on chronic Coumadin treatment and the need for frequent INR monitoring, it is desirable to have reliable POCT INRs (ideally patient self-testing POCT INRs) to avoid the inconvenience of centralized INR monitoring.

Also, patient self-testing permits frequency of testing to be altered as necessary to maximize the time individualized INRs are in the therapeutic range.

Time in therapeutic range has been used as a surrogate measure of clinical outcome for patient INR self-testing studies. Although time in therapeutic range related to POCT INR testing has been variable between studies,[21] equivalent long-term clinical outcome for patient INR self-testing when compared with centralized laboratory INR testing has been demonstrated, with a few studies actually showing improved outcome for a select subset of patients (ie, fewer minor or major hemorrhages, thromboembolic events, or death).[35,36]

International Normalized Ratios Greater than 4.5 are not Reliable, so why Report?

The previous discussion demonstrates that INRs are generally reliable within the therapeutic range (ie, INR 2–4.5), regardless of who performs the testing, whether a POCT device or clinical laboratory instrument is used, and where the testing is performed. Even with this general statement, however, evidence has repeatedly demonstrated 15% to 20% of specimens yield INRs with greater than or equal to 15% CV when tested by different methods, a CV higher than the desired $\pm$ 10%.[14]

No one knows how reproducible INRs greater than 4.5 are between laboratories. There is no certified or calibrator material to determine the accuracy of INRs greater than 4.5. There are no studies on the variability of INRs greater than 4.5 related to use of different thromboplastin reagents or instruments. The limited study between a POCT and a clinical laboratory coagulometer suggests a high degree of variability (see **Fig. 3**).

The theoretical highest INR a laboratory could report is that linked to the upper limit of the PT measurable range. It is a simple mathematical exercise to determine this: simply convert the upper limit of the PT measurable range into an INR. For example, if the PT limit is 100 seconds, the geometric mean PT is 12.5 seconds and the reagent ISI is 1, the highest INR the laboratory could report is $(100/12.5)^{1.0} = 8$. If one used the same measured PT and geometric mean PT, but the reagent ISI is 1.3, the highest INR the laboratory could report is $(100/12.5)^{1.3} = 14.9$. Some laboratories have addressed this dilemma by simply capping their INR reporting at "INR greater than or equal to 10."

One should report INRs greater than 4.5 because international guidelines dictate different reversal VKA therapies to be undertaken when the INR is greater than 5 versus greater than 9.[21] These INR thresholds and ranges have different treatment recommendations. Even though the accuracy of INRs reported in this range is not known, one's clinical counterparts are relying on these numbers for treatment specific to the different ranges.

HEPARINS

Heparin is a negatively charged glycosaminoglycan comprised of repeating sulfated disaccharide units (**Fig. 4**) derived from animal or plant sources. Heparin has been used for treatment for almost a century; the reader is referred to the many excellent reviews on this subject for more detail.[37–40]

Unfractionated Heparin

Unfractionated heparin (UFH) is a mixture of glycosaminoglycans of varying molecular weights, ranging from the monomeric form to polymers as large as 30 kd. The large heterogeneous mixture of polysaccharide polymers in UFH accounts for its variable therapeutic action because there is polymer size-related variation in both metabolic clearance and inhibition of factors Xa and thrombin. After entering the intravascular

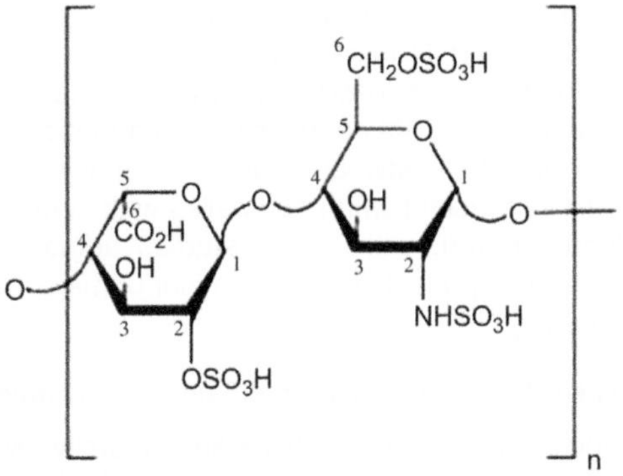

Fig. 4. Repeating disaccharide units of heparin.

space, heparin's anticoagulant activity is decreased because of binding to plasma proteins, endothelial cells, macrophages and von Willebrand factor. Sustained anticoagulant activity is dependent on the complex metabolic clearance of heparin, a saturable dose-dependent phase related to endothelial cell and macrophage binding and heparin depolymerization, and a nonsaturable phase related to renal clearance. Large-molecular-weight polymers are cleared more rapidly than low-molecular-weight species. The saturable phase results in an increased prolongation, increased intensity, and increased duration of the heparin effect disproportionate to the increased dosage.[37]

Low-molecular-weight Heparin

Low-molecular-weight heparins (LMWH) have come into widespread use and favor since their development in the late 1980s because of superior benefit/risk ratios relative to UFH. This type of heparin is also derived from animal or plant sources, but is size fractionated and restricted to polysaccharide polymers of less than or equal to 10,000 d. This relatively refined mixture results in a product with near 100% bioavailability at low doses. Dosing is based solely on body weight.

LWMH is administered typically by subcutaneous abdominal injections and has predictable pharmacokinetics. Peak effect is typically 3 to 5 hours after a subcutaneous injection, and metabolic clearance is primarily renal and not dose-dependent. LMWH is not recommended for patients with severe renal disease (defined as creatinine clearance <30 mL/min) caused by a prolonged effect related to decreased clearance. Finally, LMWH has a lower risk of osteoporosis and heparin-induced thrombocytopenia than UFH.[37–40]

No routine laboratory tests are needed to monitor LMWH dosing efficacy for most treated patients because of its predictable pharmacokinetics. The only exceptions are for pregnant patients (whose weight is constantly changing); those with renal failure; and neonates or other low-weight patients for whom weight-based dosing may not be accurate. For these exceptions, anti-Xa plasma levels are the preferred test for assessing and guiding accurate dosing.[41]

Synthetic Pentasaccharides and Meta-pentasaccharides

Fondaparinux is a chemically synthesized pentasaccharide containing the minimal heparin sequence necessary for antithrombin (AT) binding (**Fig. 5**).[2] The drug has complete bioavailability because its effect is not diminished by binding to plasma

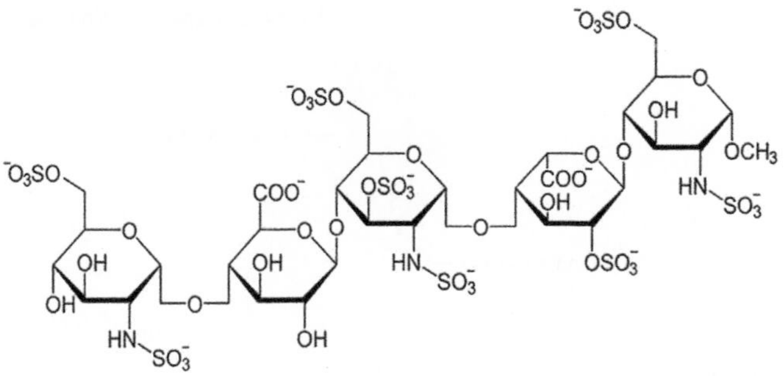

Fig. 5. Fondaparinux.

proteins or endothelial cells or macrophages. It is dosed once daily, administered as a subcutaneous injection, and has a plasma half-life of 17 hours. It is cleared by the kidneys, and accumulates in those with severe renal disease. Fondaparinux does not cross-react in vitro with antibodies associated with heparin-induced thrombocytopenia, raising a theoretical possibility of usefulness for patients with heparin-induced thrombocytopenia. This theoretical possibility is controversial, however, and awaits clinical trial evidence to support this specific use.[42–44]

Idraparinux (**Fig. 6**) is one of a family of meta-pentasaccharides.[2] This family is characterized by additional chemical modifications beyond that found in fondaparinux, resulting in enhanced affinity for AT and a much longer half-life.

Heparin (and Low-molecular-weight Heparin and Pentasaccharides): Mode of Action

Heparin has three major sites of action for clot inhibition (**Fig. 7**).[37–40] All heparins bind to AT through the unique pentasaccharide sequence. This binding dramatically accelerates the inhibitory activity of AT on thrombin.

For UFH, the large polymers bridge to and bind AT, FXa, and thrombin in a ternary complex. This ternary complex of protease (FXa, thrombin) and inhibitor (AT) is a stable complex, inhibiting the clot-initiating activities of FXa and thrombin. This ternary complex also inhibits FIXa, FXIa, and FXIIa. Inhibition of thrombin through the ternary complex in turn indirectly inhibits FV and FVIII activity.[37–40]

The ability of heparin to bridge and bind FXa and thrombin is directly related to the size of the heparin (see **Fig. 7**). Only heparin molecules with at least 18 polysaccharide units are large enough to bridge and bind heparin to FXa and thrombin. For UFH, it is

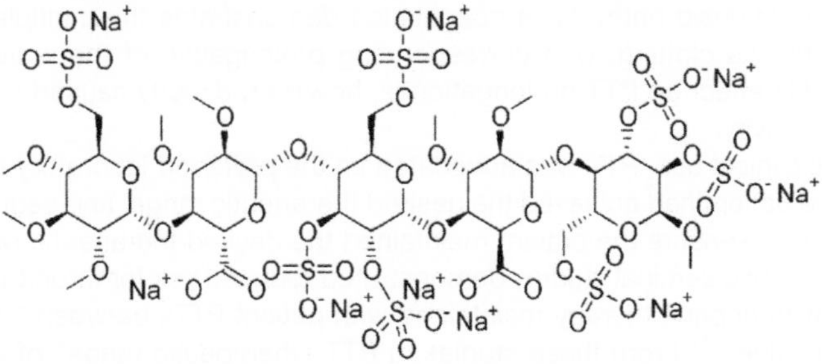

Fig. 6. Idraparinux.

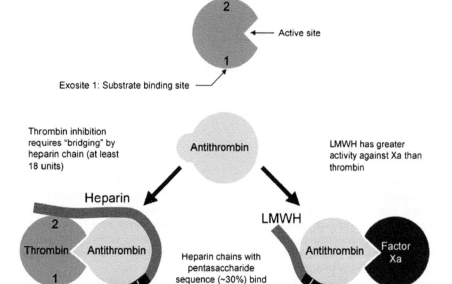

Fig. 7. Comparison of mechanisms of action of UFH, LMWH, and fondaparinux. Abbreviations: AT, antithrombin; Xa, activated factor X. (*From* Haines ST. US Pharm 2001;Suppl:3–11; with permission.)

estimated only one third of the administered dose binds all three factors to exert an anticoagulant effect.[37]

LMWH is shorter than UFH. It is large enough to bind both AT and FXa, but too short to bridge to and bind thrombin. Its activity is predominantly directed at FXa inhibition.[37]

Fondaparinux contains the unique pentasaccharide sequence capable of binding to AT only. Its activity is predominantly directed at FXa inhibition.[2]

LABORATORY TESTING TO MONITOR UNFRACTIONATED HEPARIN ANTICOAGULANT EFFECT

Review of the intrinsic pathway of coagulation demonstrates the multiple points at which UFH blocks clotting, with corresponding prolongation of the activated PTT. The major UFH effect on PTT prolongation is, however, directly caused by inhibition of thrombin activity.

Early in its clinical use, PTT was advocated as the preferred laboratory test for establishing the patient had achieved the desired therapeutic range, and sequential PTT determinations to ensure the patient maintained the desired therapeutic range.

In the 1970s, two seminal studies demonstrated reduced risk for thromboembolism associated with heparin therapy maintained with patient PTTs between 1.5 and 2.5x the "control value."[37] From these studies, a PTT "therapeutic range" of 1.5 to 2.5x was widely adopted.

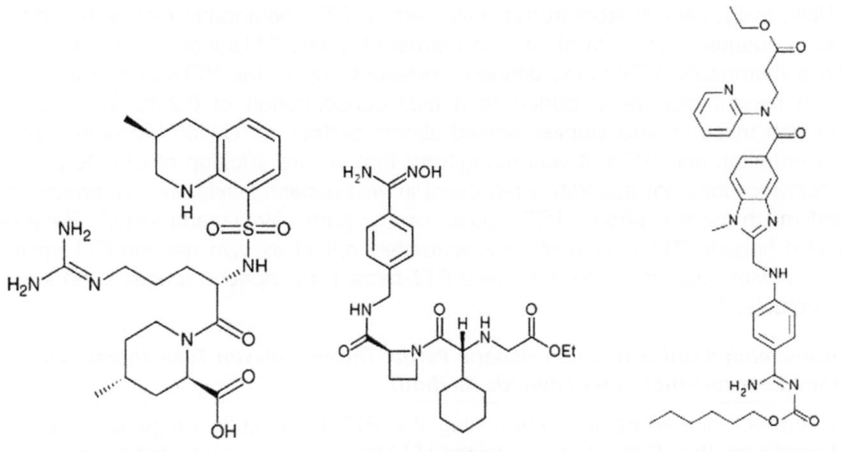

| Argatroban | Ximelagatran | Dabigatran etexilate |

Fig. 8. Univalent small molecule direct thrombin inhibitors. Ximelagatran has been withdrawn from use because of hepatotoxicity.

Unfortunately, the wide variability in different PTT reagents and test methods influencing actual PTT values was not recognized at the time of these studies. Subsequent exhortations for PTT reagent standardization[45–48] or consensus recommendations for PTT assay calibration and performance[49] have not materialized with standardized commercial PTT reagents.

Furthermore, changes in laboratory practice over the past few decades have substituted PTT reference ranges instead of the historical reporting of a "control" value in parallel with a patient sample. These changes have resulted in practitioners using the arithmetic mean of the PTT reference range as a substitute for the PTT "control" value. The "x" amount of PTT prolongation is usually calculated by dividing the patient's measured PTT by the arithmetic mean of the reference range.

Historically, UFH therapeutic ranges were defined as 0.2 to 0.4 U/mL determined by a protamine titration neutralization assay. This therapeutic range corresponds to the 0.3 to 0.7 anti-Xa units defined with an anti-Xa activity assay.[50]

Interlaboratory PTT variability is pronounced and directly related to PTT reagent sensitivity and coagulometer (see the article on PT and PTT assay considerations elsewhere in this issue for more detail). With current PTT assays, the interlaboratory PTT variability indicates widespread subtherapeutic anticoagulation. Specifically, for the typical 1.5 to 2.5x PTT prolongation range, the actual PTT ranges corresponding to therapeutic heparin ranges (determined by anti-Xa activity assay) actually range from 1.5 to 2.7x, to 3.7 to 6.2x. The wide variability in these PTT reagents is directly related to the specific PTT reagent-instrument combination.[37]

Unfractionated Heparin Partial Thromboplastin Time Therapeutic Ranges cannot be Determined with in Vitro Heparin Addition Studies

If offering PTT testing for heparin therapeutic monitoring, the first step is for a clinical laboratory to verify that the 1.5x to 2.5x PTT prolongation range specific to the laboratory's reagent-instrument combination does reflect the therapeutic heparin range in anti-Xa units.

Historically, clinical laboratories have verified PTT therapeutic ranges by adding known quantities (in vitro) of UFH to normal plasmas. PTTs were then determined and a therapeutic PTT range defined, corresponding to the PTTs of specimens to which heparin had been added to a final concentration of 0.2 to 0.4 mIU/mL. Although these in vitro studies yielded almost perfect correlation between heparin concentration and PTTs, it was recognized that in vitro addition of UFH to plasma specimens does not accurately represent in vivo heparin levels; ex vivo specimens yield much more scattered PTT values for any particular heparin level.[51] Because in vitro heparin PTT curves did not accurately reflect ex vivo heparin PTT values, using in vitro specimens to determine PTT-heparin therapeutic ranges is no longer acceptable.[51]

Recommended Unfractionated Heparin Partial Thromboplastin Time Therapeutic Range Determination (Brill-Edwards Method)

The correct procedure for determining the PTT therapeutic range is commonly referred to as the "Brill-Edwards" method.[51] This procedure uses plasma specimens obtained from patients receiving known doses of heparin (ex vivo specimens).[52] PTT values are compared with anti-Xa activity levels determined in parallel from the same specimens to determine the PTT therapeutic range (ie, corresponding to 0.3–0.7 anti-Xa units/mL).

Heparin Resistance: Usually a Partial Thromboplastin Time Artifact

Heparin resistance has been commonly considered when a heparinized patient's PTT does not prolong to the desired 1.5 to 2x range. Recent studies using anti-Xa activity assays to determine actual heparin activity, however, have demonstrated that most patients thought to be "heparin resistant" did have therapeutic heparin anti-Xa levels. The mistake in labeling these patients as "heparin resistant" was caused by inadequately prolonged PTTs. It has since been determined that the inadequately prolonged PTTs were caused by elevated FVIII levels and the known effect of FVIII elevation on PTT shortening (see the article on PT and PTT assay considerations elsewhere in this issue for more detail).[50,53–56] True heparin resistance does occur and is usually related to relative deficiencies of AT. The rare cases of true heparin resistance occur in patients with hereditary homozygous AT deficiency. Although acquired AT deficiency is common in the critically ill, AT levels are still detectable and do not typically decrease to the undetectable levels associated with hereditary homozygous AT deficiency to result in true heparin resistance.[57,58]

Low-molecular-weight Heparin: for the Rare Occasion when One Needs to Monitor Effect, use an Anti-Xa Activity Assay

The pharmacokinetic predictability of LMWH has obviated the need for laboratory testing to monitor therapeutic effect for most treated individuals. For the rare situations where it is desirable to measure the circulating level of LMWH, anti-Xa activity assays are recommended.[41] This is because LMWH, by virtue of binding only AT and FXa and inability to bridge or bind thrombin, has only minimal if any effect on the PTT. The PTT is not helpful.

Anti-Xa activity assays determine the amount of anti-Xa activity in a specimen. The anti-Xa activity can be presumed to be caused by any UFH, LMWH, or fondaparinux in the sample. Any of these heparins present in the specimen bind to AT and the complex inhibits FXa. FXa activity is measured using a chromogenic substrate resembling the natural FXa substrate. Factor Xa in the specimen cleaves the chromogenic substrate and releases a colored compound detected with a spectrophotometer. UFH, LMWH, or fondaparinux in the specimen prevents FXa cleavage of the colored substrate, resulting in proportionately decreased amounts of colored compound generated and extrapolation to the corresponding amount of anti-FXa activity. Conversely, absence of UFH, LMWH, or fondaparinux results in maximal colored substrate cleavage by FXa; high levels of colored compound generated; and extrapolation to low (or absent) anti-Xa activity. Excess AT is provided in the reaction to avoid artifactual results related to insufficient in vitro AT.

Unfortunately, anti-Xa activity assays are not standardized. There are many different commercially available anti-Xa activity assays reliant on two major methodologies: clot-based versus chromogenic substrate assays. Chromogenic anti-Xa activity assays are the preferred methodology and recommended for LMWH monitoring.[41]

Unfortunately, there is considerable interassay result variability between different commercial anti-Xa assays.[59–61] Furthermore, there is variability in LMWH results in a single anti-Xa assay, including significant variability from different LMWH lots from the same manufacturer.[62] Given the variable composition of the different commercial LMWHs and related variable performance in laboratory assays, one should calibrate the chromogenic anti-Xa assays using the LMWH dispensed by the pharmacy against an international standard.[41] There is limited evidence that a single LMWH calibration curve can be extrapolated for use with multiple different LMWHs.[63,64]

High-dose Unfractionated Heparin: Activated Clotting Time

This area is truly amazing because of the widespread use of the activated clotting time for monitoring high-dose UFH, although there is a sheer paucity of evidence demonstrating accuracy or effectiveness of activated clotting time for this indication. High-dose UFH is typically used for interventional cardiology procedures; cardiac surgery (especially those needing cardiac bypass); or extracorporeal membrane oxygenation. Although there is ample evidence that high-dose anticoagulation is necessary to prevent blood clotting on the external circuits or during procedures, there is no evidence demonstrating accuracy of the various activated clotting time devices used for measuring degree of anticoagulation. Review of College of American Pathologists activated clotting time proficiency test summary reports demonstrates values returned from a single proficiency test specimen tested by multiple laboratories exceed recommended target therapeutic ranges. "Matrix" effects may be responsible for this variability, because the proficiency test specimens may not be the same as fresh whole heparinized blood. Other studies, however, have demonstrated significant lack of agreement between various commercially available devices when the same specimen is tested on both in parallel. These differences are so significant that values from one device indicate a different therapeutic range than values obtained from another devide.[49,65,66]

Unfortunately, there is no alternative. But the high variability and imprecision of the activated clotting time has led one group to comment "…the target times employed stem more from historical clinician comfort than outcome studies."[66]

DIRECT FXA INHIBITORS (XABANS)

There is limited information on oral direct FXa inhibitors, because many are in the midst of clinical trials and no definitive statement can be made regarding their clinical applicability.[67]

Two xabans (rivaroxaban and apixaban) have received the most attention. Both have excellent bioavailability, predictable pharmacokinetics, are taken orally, bind reversibly to FXa, and have plasma half-lives of many hours. They differ in metabolism; rivaroxaban is excreted renally, whereas apixaban is excreted fecally.

Laboratory Testing is Less Predictable than the Xaban Effect

The predictable pharmacokinetics of the xabans has obviated laboratory testing for many of the published clinical trials. For those studies in which laboratory coagulation testing was done, a dose-dependent prolongation of the PT or increasing anti-Xa activity was demonstrated for both xabans.[68,69] Apixaban was additionally demonstrated to prolong PTTs in a dose-dependent manner, whereas having minimal effect on the thrombin time.[69]

A safe assumption is the dose-dependence observed with the xabans is likely reagent and methodology dependent. There have not been sufficient studies assessing interassay variability. Given that every other coagulation test application for anticoagulant monitoring (excepting the INR for chronic warfarin therapy) has demonstrated significant interassay and interlaboratory variability, however, there is every reason to believe such variability will similarly exist with whatever test is recommended for xaban monitoring. What this means is that the laboratory must know whether thromboplastin (for PT) or partial thromboplastins reagent (for PTT) is sensitive to the presence of a xaban. This is important to know, especially if any patients might be treated with more than one anticoagulant with a possible cumulative effect of unknown magnitude on either the PT or PTT.

Tobu and colleagues[70] assessed the effect of one synthetic factor Xa inhibitor (JTV-803) on a variety of coagulation tests. Studies were conducted with in vitro addition of JTV-803, and many of the assays were either developed within their own laboratory or used commercially available assays. The relevance of these results is unclear, given that no ex vivo specimens were tested for comparison. They observed the following:

- Dose-dependent effect, variable between reagents: prolonged celite activated clotting time; prolonged PT; prolonged INR; prolonged PTT; prolonged dilute Russell's viper venom test; increased percent inhibition in an amidolytic anti-Xa assay; decreased percent platelet aggregation by platelet aggregometry; increased percent serine protease inhibition (trypsin, tissue-type plasminogen activator); dose-dependent decrease in thrombin activatable fibrinolytic inhibitor levels; and reduced fibrinopeptide A generation
- Minimal effect: mild dose-dependent prolongation of the Heptest
- No effect: thrombin time, Ecarin clotting time, tissue factor pathway inhibitor levels, functional or immunologic assays, urokinase inhibition, chymotrypsin inhibition

DIRECT THROMBIN INHIBITORS

Thrombin plays a central role in hemostasis, acting at multiple points in the clotting cascade.[38–40] It has both prothrombotic (ie, cleavage of fibrinogen to fibrin to start clot formation, activation of FXIII, platelet activation, and inhibition of fibrinolysis by a thrombin-activatable fibrinolysis inhibitor) and anticoagulant (ie, protein C activation) effects, and effects on endothelium and vascular smooth muscle cells.[38–40] Thrombin itself is inhibited by AT and this interaction is the physiologic basis for the therapeutic actions of the heparins (UFH, LMWH, fondaparinux).[38–40]

DTI do exactly that, inhibit thrombin directly by inhibiting the enzymatic activation of thrombin without the need for AT or other cofactors. DTIs fall into two major classes: hirudin and its synthetic analogs, and chemical inhibitors.

Hirudin

Hirudin is the natural anticoagulant of the leech and was originally isolated from the salivary gland of the medicinal leech, *Hirudo medicinalis*.[71] It is a 65 amino acid polypeptide of approximately 7000 kd. It is a potent inhibitor of thrombin and binds in a 1:1 ratio with thrombin.[71] It has "bivalent" binding potential, blocking both the "substrate recognition" and "catalytic site" on thrombin responsible for fibrinogen cleavage.[71] This exquisite binding specificity limits hirudin's action to thrombin; no other components of the clotting cascade are affected.[71]

Hirudin Analogs

A variety of hirudin analogs have been created and undergone clinical trials, publications of which are only now appearing. The hirudin analogs can be divided roughly into two major categories depending on their ability to bind either both (bivalent) or only one (univalent) of the two key thrombin sites. This distinction is also conveniently linked to the broad categories: recombinantly derived modified hirudin analogs (eg, lepirudin and bivalirudin) are capable of bivalent binding, whereas synthetic small molecule hirudin analogs (eg, argatroban, melagatran, and dabigatran; **Fig. 8**) are capable of only univalent binding.[1,3,71,72]

Each of the different DTIs differs in potency; recommended clinical use; metabolism and excretion (liver versus renal); and adverse effects. This area is evolving rapidly and the reader is referred to existing reviews on the specific DTI for more detailed information and to stay current with published literature in this field.[3,71,72]

Laboratory Testing to Monitor Direct Thrombin Inhibitor Anticoagulant Effect

No coagulation test has emerged as the preferred test for monitoring DTI effect.[3,41] Cautionary notes abound in the literature about using the PT to monitor DTI effect because of variability related to PT reagent sensitivity (ISI). This should have been predicted based on the long history of coagulation test variability attributable to different PT reagent sensitivities. The PT variability is of such significance that published studies warn readers to avoid converting PTs to INRs, because the INRs in turn are quite variable and misleading.[68,70,73] There are additional effects on the PT when more than one anticoagulant is in use (eg, warfarin or DTI or heparin).[68,70,73]

Similar concerns have been raised for using the PTT to monitor DTI effects because of lack of PTT standardization.[48,74,75] The Ecarin clotting time has been proposed,[76] but to date has not been widely available or standardized.

One group examined the effect of hirudin, PEG-hirudin, argatroban, and efgatran on the PT and INR. They tested plasma specimens to which these drugs had been added in vitro and demonstrated a dose- and reagent-dependent prolongation of the PT and INR. The significant effect of DTIs alone on prolonging PTs and INRs led to a cautionary note against the use of PTs-INRs for monitoring patients treated with both warfarin and DTIs because the resultant PT-INR is disproportionately prolonged because of the added effects of both drugs.[73]

SUMMARY

This is a dissatisfying end to an exciting time in clinical anticoagulant therapy. With the exception of the INR for monitoring patients on chronic warfarin therapy, any other coagulation test used to monitor any other anticoagulant suffers from a lack of standardization and the presence of significant variability of results depending on which reagent or test method is used.

For the laboratorian, caveat emptor. It is absolutely critical to know how the assay performs with the target patient population, and to educate providers on how to use the coagulation test results generated. Laboratorians and patient care providers should demand assay standardization.

REFERENCES

1. Hirsh J, O'Donnell M, Eikelboom JW. Beyond unfractionated heparin and warfarin: current and future advances. Circulation 2007;116(5):552–60.
2. Gerotziafas GT, Samama MM. Heterogeneity of synthetic factor Xa inhibitors. Curr Pharm Des 2005;11(30):3855–76.
3. Di Nisio M, Middeldorp S, Buller HR. Direct thrombin inhibitors. N Engl J Med 2005;353(10):1028–40.
4. Duxbury BM, Poller L. The oral anticoagulant saga: past, present, and future. Clin Appl Thromb Hemost 2001;7(4):269–75.
5. Wardrop D, Keeling D. The story of the discovery of heparin and warfarin. Br J Haematol 2008;141(6):757–63.
6. Link KP. The discovery of dicumarol and its sequels. Circulation 1959;19(1): 97–107.
7. Hirsh J, Bauer KA, Donati MB, et al. Parenteral anticoagulants: American College of Chest Physicians Evidence-Based Clinical Practice Guidelines (8th edition). Chest 2008;133(6 Suppl):141S–59S.
8. Hirsh J, Guyatt G, Albers GW, et al. Executive summary: American College of Chest Physicians Evidence-Based Clinical Practice Guidelines (8th edition). Chest 2008;133(6 Suppl):71S–109S.
9. Kearon C, Kahn SR, Agnelli G, et al. Antithrombotic therapy for venous thromboembolic disease: American College of Chest Physicians Evidence-Based Clinical Practice Guidelines (8th edition). Chest 2008;133(6 Suppl):454S–545S.
10. Salem DN, O'Gara PT, Madias C, et al. Valvular and structural heart disease: American College of Chest Physicians Evidence-Based Clinical Practice Guidelines (8th edition). Chest 2008;133(6 Suppl):593S–629S.
11. Leech BF, Carter CJ. Falsely elevated INR results due to the sensitivity of a thromboplastin reagent to heparin. Am J Clin Pathol 1998;109(6):764–8.
12. Takeuchi F, McGinnis R, Bourgeois S, et al. A genome-wide association study confirms VKORC1, CYP2C9, and CYP4F2 as principal genetic determinants of warfarin dose. PLoS Genet 2009;5(3):e1000433. Available at: http://www.plosgenetics.org/article/info:doi/10.1371/journal.pgen.1000433. Accessed July 13, 2009.
13. Lassen JF, Brandslund I, Antonsen S. International normalized ratio for prothrombin times in patients taking oral anticoagulants: critical difference and probability of significant change in consecutive measurements. Clin Chem 1995;41(3):444–7.
14. Adcock D, Brien W, Duff S, et al. Procedures for validation of INR and local calibration of PT/INR systems; approved guideline. Wayne (PA): Clinical and Laboratory Standards Institute; 2005. H54-A.
15. Ng VL, Levin J, Corash L, et al. Failure of the international normalized ratio to generate consistent results within a local medical community. Am J Clin Pathol 1993;99(6):689–94.
16. Ng VL, Valdes-Camin R, Gottfried EL, et al. Highly sensitive thromboplastins do not improve INR precision. Am J Clin Pathol 1998;109(3):338–46.

17. Testa S, Morstabilini G, Fattorini A, et al. Discrepant sensitivity of thromboplastin reagents to clotting factor levels explored by the prothrombin time in patients on stable oral anticoagulant treatment: impact on the international normalized ratio system. Haematologica 2002;87(12):1265–73.
18. Coagulation Resource Committee C. CGL-A. Coagulation limited. Participant summary 2009. Northfield (IL): College of American Pathologists.
19. Ng VL. QC for the future: laboratory issues - POCT and POL concerns. Lab Med 2005;36(10):621–5.
20. Ng V. My three wishes for point-of-care testing. Journal of Point-of-Care Testing 2008;7:99–101.
21. Ansell J, Hirsh J, Hylek E, et al. Pharmacology and management of the vitamin K antagonists: American College of Chest Physicians Evidence-Based Clinical Practice Guidelines (8th Edition). Chest 2008;133(6 Suppl): 160S–98S.
22. Oral Anticoagulation Monitoring Study Group. Point-of-care prothrombin time measurement for professional and patient self-testing use. A multicenter clinical experience. Oral Anticoagulation Monitoring Study Group. Am J Clin Pathol 2001;115(2):288–96.
23. Tripodi A, Bressi C, Carpenedo M, et al. Quality assurance program for whole blood prothrombin time-international normalized ratio point-of-care monitors used for patient self-testing to control oral anticoagulation. Thromb Res 2004; 113(1):35–40.
24. Poller L, Keown M, Chauhan N, et al. European concerted action on anticoagulation: use of plasma samples to derive international sensitivity index for whole-blood prothrombin time monitors. Clin Chem 2002;48(2):255–60.
25. Meijer P, Kluft C, Poller L, et al. A national field study of quality assessment of CoaguChek point-of-care testing prothrombin time monitors. Am J Clin Pathol 2006;126(5):756–61.
26. Kitchen S, Kitchen DP, Jennings I, et al. Point-of-care international normalised ratios: UK NEQAS experience demonstrates necessity for proficiency testing of three different monitors. Thromb Haemost 2006;96(5):590–6.
27. The Joint Commission. Standard QC.1.80. Oakbrook Terrace (IL): Joint Commission Resources; 2008.
28. College of American Pathologists. Point of care testing inspection checklist item POC.07568. Northfield (IL): College of American Pathologists; 2007.
29. Centers for Medicare and Medicaid Services. Centers for Disease Control and Prevention. 493.1253 Standard; Establishment and verification of method performance specifications. Available at: http://wwwn.cdc.gov/clia/regs/subpart_k.aspx#493.1253. Accessed April 11, 2009.
30. ISO 15189. Medical laboratories: particular requirements for quality and competence: Standard 5.6.6; 2003. Switzerland: ISO (The International Organization for Standardization).
31. CLSI. C54-A. Verification of comparability of patient results within one health care system; approved guideline. Wayne (PA): CLSI; 2008.
32. Sunderji R, Gin K, Shalansky K, et al. Clinical impact of point-of-care vs laboratory measurement of anticoagulation. Am J Clin Pathol 2005;123(2):184–8.
33. Chapman DC, Stephens MA, Hamann GL, et al. Accuracy, clinical correlation, and patient acceptance of two handheld prothrombin time monitoring devices in the ambulatory setting. Ann Pharmacother 1999;33(7–8):775–80.
34. Shermock KM, Bragg L, Connor JT, et al. Differences in warfarin dosing decisions based on international normalized ratio measurements with two point-of-care

testing devices and a reference laboratory measurement. Pharmacotherapy 2002;22(11):1397–404.

35. Kortke H, Korfer R. International normalized ratio self-management after mechanical heart valve replacement: is an early start advantageous? Ann Thorac Surg 2001;72(1):44–8.

36. Menendez-Jandula B, Souto JC, Oliver A, et al. Comparing self-management of oral anticoagulant therapy with clinic management: a randomized trial. Ann Intern Med 2005;142(1):1–10.

37. Hirsh J, Raschke R. Heparin and low-molecular-weight heparin: the Seventh ACCP Conference on Antithrombotic and Thrombolytic Therapy. Chest 2004; 126(3 Suppl):188S–203S.

38. Weitz JI, et al. Chapter 130. Anticoagulant and fibrinolytic drugs. In: Hoffman M, Benz EJ Jr, Shattil SJ, et al, editors. Hematology: basic principles and practice. 4th edition. Philadlephia: Elsevier Churchill Livingstone; 2005. p. 2249–67.

39. Colman RW, Clowes AW, Marder VJ, et al, editors. Hemostasis and thrombosis: basic principles and clinical practice. 5th edition. Philadelphia: Lippincott Williams & Wilkins; 2005.

40. Greer JP, Arber DA, Rodgers GM, et al, editors. Wintrobe's clinical hematology. 12th edition. Philadelphia: Lippincott Williams & Wilkins; 2008.

41. Laposata M, Green D, Van Cott EM, et al. College of American Pathologists Conference XXXI on laboratory monitoring of anticoagulant therapy: the clinical use and laboratory monitoring of low-molecular-weight heparin, danaparoid, hirudin and related compounds, and argatroban. Arch Pathol Lab Med 1998;122(9): 799–807.

42. Papadopoulos S, Flynn JD, Lewis DA. Fondaparinux as a treatment option for heparin-induced thrombocytopenia. Pharmacotherapy 2007;27(6):921–6.

43. Lobo B, Finch C, Howard A, et al. Fondaparinux for the treatment of patients with acute heparin-induced thrombocytopenia. Thromb Haemost 2008;99(1): 208–14.

44. Efird LE, Kockler DR. Fondaparinux for thromboembolic treatment and prophylaxis of heparin-induced thrombocytopenia. Ann Pharmacother 2006;40(7–8): 1383–7.

45. Hales SC, Johnson GS, Wagner D. Comparison of six activated partial thromboplastin time reagents: intrinsic system factors' sensitivity and responsiveness. Clin Lab Sci 1990;3(3):194–6.

46. van den Besselaar AM, Neuteboom J, Meeuwisse-Braun J, et al. Preparation of lyophilized partial thromboplastin time reagent composed of synthetic phospholipids: usefulness for monitoring heparin therapy. Clin Chem 1997;43(7): 1215–22.

47. Kitchen S, Jennings I, Woods TA, et al. Wide variability in the sensitivity of APTT reagents for monitoring of heparin dosage. J Clin Pathol 1996;49(1):10–4.

48. Eby C. Standardization of APTT reagents for heparin therapy monitoring: urgent or fading priority? Clin Chem 1997;43(7):1105–7.

49. Olson JD, Arkin CF, Brandt JT, et al. College of American Pathologists Conference XXXI on laboratory monitoring of anticoagulant therapy: laboratory monitoring of unfractionated heparin therapy. Arch Pathol Lab Med 1998;122(9):782–98.

50. Levine MN, Hirsh J, Gent M, et al. A randomized trial comparing activated thromboplastin time with heparin assay in patients with acute venous thromboembolism requiring large daily doses of heparin. Arch Intern Med 1994;154(1):49–56.

51. Brill-Edwards P, Ginsberg JS, Johnston M, et al. Establishing a therapeutic range for heparin therapy. Ann Intern Med 1993;119(2):104–9.

52. CLSI. One-stage prothrombin time (PT) test and activated partial thromboplastin time (APTT) test. Approved guideline - second edition. Wayne (PA): Clinical and Laboratory Standards Institute; 2008.

53. Ten Boekel E, Bartels P. Abnormally short activated partial thromboplastin times are related to elevated plasma levels of TAT, F1+2, D-dimer and FVIII: C. Pathophysiol Haemost Thromb 2002;32(3):137–42.

54. Ten Boekel E, Bock M, Vrielink GJ, et al. Detection of shortened activated partial thromboplastin times: an evaluation of different commercial reagents. Thromb Res 2007;121(3):361–7.

55. Raschke RA, Guidry JR, Foley MR. Apparent heparin resistance from elevated factor VIII during pregnancy. Obstet Gynecol 2000;96(5 Pt 2):804–6.

56. Rosborough TK, Shepherd ME. Heparin resistance as detected with an antifactor Xa assay is not more common in venous thromboembolism than in other thromboembolic conditions. Pharmacotherapy 2003;23(2):142–6.

57. Lehman CM, Rettmann JA, Wilson LW, et al. Comparative performance of three anti-factor Xa heparin assays in patients in a medical intensive care unit receiving intravenous, unfractionated heparin. Am J Clin Pathol 2006;126(3):416–21.

58. Messori A, Vacca F, Vaiani M, et al. Antithrombin III in patients admitted to intensive care units: a multicenter observational study. Crit Care 2002;6(5):447–51.

59. Kitchen S, Iampietro R, Woolley AM, et al. Anti Xa monitoring during treatment with low molecular weight heparin or danaparoid: inter-assay variability. Thromb Haemost 1999;82(4):1289–93.

60. Kitchen S, Theaker J, Preston FE. Monitoring unfractionated heparin therapy: relationship between eight anti-Xa assays and a protamine titration assay. Blood Coagul Fibrinolysis 2000;11(2):137–44.

61. Kovacs MJ, Keeney M, MacKinnon K, et al. Three different chromogenic methods do not give equivalent anti-Xa levels for patients on therapeutic low molecular weight heparin (dalteparin) or unfractionated heparin. Clin Lab Haematol 1999; 21(1):55–60.

62. Gosselin RC, King JH, Janatpour KA, et al. Variability of plasma anti-Xa activities with different lots of enoxaparin. Ann Pharmacother 2004;38(4):563–8.

63. McGlasson DL. Using a single calibration curve with the anti-Xa chromogenic assay for monitoring heparin anticoagulation. Lab Med 2005;36(5):297–9.

64. Robertson JD, Brandao L, Williams S, et al. Use of a single anti-Xa calibration curve is adequate for monitoring enoxaparin and tinzaparin levels in children. Thromb Res 2008;122(6):867–9.

65. Spinler SA, Wittkowsky AK, Nutescu EA, et al. Anticoagulation monitoring part 2: unfractionated heparin and low-molecular-weight heparin. Ann Pharmacother 2005;39(7–8):1275–85.

66. Nichols JH, Christenson RH, Clarke W, et al. Executive summary. The National Academy of Clinical Biochemistry Laboratory Medicine Practice Guideline: evidence-based practice for point-of-care testing. Clin Chim Acta 2007; 379(1–2):14–28 [discussion: 29–30].

67. Francis CW. New issues in oral anticoagulants. Hematology Am Soc Hematol Educ Program 2008;2008:259–65.

68. Mueck W, Eriksson BI, Bauer KA, et al. Population pharmacokinetics and pharmacodynamics of rivaroxaban–an oral, direct factor Xa inhibitor–in patients undergoing major orthopaedic surgery. Clin Pharmacokinet 2008;47(3):203–16.

69. Kubitza D, Becka M, Voith B, et al. Safety, pharmacodynamics, and pharmacokinetics of single doses of BAY 59-7939, an oral, direct factor Xa inhibitor. Clin Pharmacol Ther 2005;78(4):412–21.

70. Tobu M, Iqbal O, Hoppensteadt DA, et al. Effects of a synthetic factor Xa inhibitor (JTV-803) on various laboratory tests. Clin Appl Thromb Hemost 2002;8(4): 325–36.
71. Greinacher A, Warkentin TE. The direct thrombin inhibitor hirudin. Thromb Haemost 2008;99(5):819–29.
72. Warkentin TE, Greinacher A, Koster A. Bivalirudin. Thromb Haemost 2008;99(5): 830–9.
73. Tobu M, Iqbal O, Hoppensteadt D, et al. Anti-Xa and anti-IIa drugs alter international normalized ratio measurements: potential problems in the monitoring of oral anticoagulants. Clin Appl Thromb Hemost 2004;10(4):301–9.
74. Tripodi A, Chantarangkul V, Arbini AA, et al. Effects of hirudin on activated partial thromboplastin time determined with ten different reagents. Thromb Haemost 1993;70(2):286–8.
75. Poller L. Standardization of the APTT test. Current status. Scand J Haematol Suppl 1980;37:49–63.
76. Nowak G. The ecarin clotting time, a universal method to quantify direct thrombin inhibitors. Pathophysiol Haemost Thromb 2003;33(4):173–83.

Antiphospholipid Syndrome Review

Charles Eby, MD

KEYWORDS

• Antiphospholipid syndrome • Lupus • Anticoagulant
• Anticardiolipin • β2 glycoprotein I

The antiphospholipid syndrome (APS) is an autoimmune disorder presenting with tissue injury in various organs attributed to large or small vessel thrombosis or, in some instances, possible nonthrombotic inflammatory mechanisms, associated with in vitro evidence of antibodies to certain proteins, or protein-phospholipid complexes. Clinicians in nearly every discipline encounter patients of all ages with presentations that lead to consideration of APS in the differential diagnosis, especially in obstetrics, rheumatology, hematology, neurology, cardiology, vascular medicine, and dermatology. Like a mirage, however, although the pathophysiology, diagnosis, and management of APS may seem clear and straightforward from a distance, closer inspection reveals a more complex, incomplete, and uncertain image. This article reviews the evolution of APS from the first description of lupus anticoagulant (LAC) to the current criteria used to guide clinical research, critiques laboratory methods used to identify autoantibodies, comments on prognosis and management, and summarizes insights into the pathophysiology of this elusive disorder.

EVOLUTION OF THE ANTIPHOSPHOLIPID SYNDROME

Three observations, over 28 years, provide examples of the gradual development of an association between circulating anticoagulants and adverse events. In 1952, Conley and Hartmann[1] coined the term "lupus anticoagulant" to describe prolonged whole blood clotting times in two women diagnosed with lupus erythematosus who did not manifest abnormal bleeding or bruising tendencies. Both women also had biologic false-positive tests for syphilis. In 1963, Bowie and colleagues[2] at the Mayo Clinic reported an association between circulating anticoagulants, based on incomplete correction of either a prolonged prothrombin time (PT) or recalcification time (equivalent to a partial thromboplastin time) on 50:50 mixing with normal plasma, and thrombotic complications in 11 systemic lupus erythematosus (SLE) patients. Six of the patients also had biologic false-positive tests for syphilis. In 1980, French investigators reported fetal loss and venous thrombosis associated with circulating

Department of Pathology and Immunology, Washington University School of Medicine, Campus box 8118, St. Louis, MO 63110, USA
E-mail address: eby@wustl.edu

Clin Lab Med 29 (2009) 305–319
doi:10.1016/j.cll.2009.06.001 labmed.theclinics.com

inhibitors in three women who did not have SLE.[3] The phospholipid-dependent behavior of LAC and the observation that many LAC-positive SLE patients also had biologically false-positive tests for syphilis led a group of rheumatologists at the Hammersmith Hospital in London to develop a sensitive radioimmunoassay for antibodies to cardiolipin, the negatively charged phospholipid antigen in the VDRL reagent.[4] Cohort studies confirmed associations between phospholipid antibodies (anticardiolipin [aCL] and LAC), and thrombosis, pregnancy loss, or thrombocytopenia in patients without[5] and with[6] SLE, leading to the designations of primary and secondary APS, respectively.

Conversion to an ELISA method[7] to detect aCL antibodies stimulated unbridled testing of patients with various vascular and autoimmune disorders without consistent guidelines for performing or interpreting aCL results. Investigators were also reporting positive aCL antibodies associated with acute infections and adverse drug reactions, indicating that aCL antibodies were not specific for APS. Recognizing the need for specific APS classification criteria to advance understanding of the underlying pathophysiology and to improve diagnosis and management of this complex disorder through recruitment of fairly homogeneous patient populations for future studies, experts developed initial clinical criteria and laboratory testing guidelines, which have been periodically revised based on expert consensus and clinical evidence of variable strength (**Table 1**). The first classification, proposed by the Hammersmith group, and widely adopted, included three clinical categories (arterial and venous thromboembolic events, pregnancy loss, and thrombocytopenia) and two laboratory criteria (LAC and cardiolipin antibodies), the latter restricted to IgG or IgM isotypes with titers greater than 20 affinity purified IgG or affinity purified IgM units, respectively.[8] The units were based on a calibrator derived from the sera of selected positive aCL patients. Patients who exhibited at least one clinical criteria and one repeatedly positive laboratory test, to exclude patients temporarily positive because of acute infections or possible drug reactions, were classified as having APS. Subdivision into primary and secondary APS was based on the absence or presence of SLE or other connective tissue disorders, respectively.

In 1995, recognizing the need for more consistent LAC test performance, the International Society of Thrombosis and Haemostasis Subcommittee on LAC/Phospholipid-Dependent Antibodies published general guidelines consisting of four steps (**Table 2**).[9] (1) Sensitivity is to enhance by using at least two different methods to activate clotting in the presence of a limited amount of phospholipid. (2) Specificity is improved by including a mixing step to rule out coagulopathies, and (3) a confirm step to demonstrate shortening of the clotting time, was dependent on addition of phospholipid. A plasma sample that fulfills the criteria for LAC based on steps 1 to 3 may still be a false-positive result if a high titer factor VIII inhibitor were present and an intrinsic pathway activator was used, or the plasma contained certain anticoagulants. (4) The final step requires ruling out the possibility of a false-positive LAC result by performing selected coagulation factor activities, or obtaining clinical information regarding the patient's medications and signs and symptoms of bleeding.

In 1998, an international multidisciplinary symposium workshop reviewed the growing body of evidence combined with expert experience and opinion and updated the classification criteria for APS (see **Table 1**).[10] Major changes included the removal of thrombocytopenia as a clinical criterion because of insufficient evidence of an independent association with antiphospholipid antibodies, addition of specific criteria for pregnancy complications attributed to phospholipid antibodies, inclusion of the International Society of Thrombosis and Haemostasis guidelines for LAC testing, and the requirement that aCL antibody testing methods include β_2 glycoprotein I (β2GPI).

Table 1 Evolving consensus criteria for classification of antiphospholipid syndrome[a]			
	Hammersmith Group 1987	**Sapporo Conference 1998**	**Sydney Conference 2006**
Clinical criteria	1. Venous or arterial thrombosis 2. Pregnancy loss 3. Thrombocytopenia	1. Thrombosis confirmed by imaging or histo pathology except superficial phlebitis 2a. ≥1 unexplained fetal death ≥10 wk gestation, normal morphology b. ≥1 birth ≤34 wk gestation due to preeclampsia, eclampsia, or placental insufficiency c. ≥3 consecutive spontaneous abortions <10 wk gestation, absent maternal anatomic, hormonal, chromosomal (paternal too) abnormalities	1. Superficial phlebitis no longer accepted 2. a, b, c, no changes
Laboratory criteria	1. Repeatedly positive LAC and/or 2. Repeatedly positive IgG or IgM ACA >20 GPL or MPL, respectively	1. Repeatedly positive LAC per International Society of Thrombosis and Haemostasis 1995 guidelines 2. Medium and high titer IgG/IgM ACA in presence of β2GPI	1. No changes 2. IgG/IgM ACA titers >40 GPL/MPL (requirement for β2GPI presence removed) 3. Repeatedly positive IgG/IgM β2GPI cut off >99th percentile
Minimal interval between positive tests	6 wk	6 wk	12 wk

Abbreviations: ACA, anticardiolipin antibody; β2GPI, beta-2 glycoprotein I; GPL, affinity purified IgG; LAC, lupus anticoagulant; MPL, affinity purified IgM.
[a] APS diagnosis requires at least one clinical and one laboratory criteria be met.

Earlier investigators noted improved precision of aCL antibody ELISA results when sera were diluted in bovine serum compared with saline. Subsequent studies confirmed that most phospholipid antibodies associated with APS recognized β2GPI bound to negatively charged cardiolipin, whereas antibodies that recognized cardiolipin in the absence of β2GPI were typically associated with infectious or inflammatory states and were often temporary.[11] The physiologic role of β2GPI is incompletely understood, but accumulating evidence supports direct pathologic consequences from some antibodies that recognize this protein.[12]

Table 2

International Society of Thrombosis and Haemostasis Scientific Subcommittee on LAC/Phospholipid-Dependent Antibodies 1995 guidelines for detection of lupus anticoagulants

Step 1	Prolonged phospholipid-dependent coagulation based on ≥2 different screening tests
Step 2	Failure to correct prolonged screening test by mixing patient plasma with normal platelet poor plasma
Step 3	Shortening or correction of prolonged screening test by addition of excess phospholipid
Step 4	Exclusion of other coagulopathies

In 2004, during a subsequent international antiphospholipid antibody symposium, another workshop was convened, and APS classification criteria were revised again (see **Table 1**).[13] Focusing on laboratory criteria, the requirement for β2GPI to be a component of aCL testing was removed, and antibodies recognizing purified β2GPI in an ELISA assay were added. To improve the specificity of the serologic tests, thresholds for aCL and β2GPI antibodies were included; however, the lack of method and calibrator standardization for the latter diminishes their usefulness.[12] The minimum time between repeatedly positive LAC or aCL/β2GPI serologies was empirically increased to 12 weeks. Based on systematic literature reviews that confirmed a consistent and strong association between positive LAC tests and thrombosis, supported a stronger thrombotic risk for combinations of positive APL tests compared with a single positive test, and noted weak or absent thrombotic risk for isolated aCL antibody positivity,[14,15] the committee recommended subclassification of patients enrolled in studies as follows: (1) more than one positive test, (2) LAC positive only, (3) aCL antibody positive only, and (4) β2GPI antibody positive only. Finally, the expert committee recommended abolishing primary and secondary APS categories noting an absence of data supporting differences in clinical outcomes based on this classification.[16]

The Sapporo and Sydney conferences established specific APS classification criteria to enhance the homogeneity of subjects enrolled in clinical studies. There are other clinical manifestations and laboratory features that may be associated with APS, but evidence and expert opinion did not support their inclusion in the criteria (**Table 3**). In diseases where the fundamental pathophysiology is understood, with

Table 3

Associated clinical and laboratory features of antiphospholipid syndrome

Clinical[a]	Laboratory
Cardiac valve thickening, nodules	IgA-aCL
Livedo reticularis[b]	IgA anti β2GPI
Renal thrombotic microangiopathy[c]	Antibodies to other phospholipids[e]
Thrombocytopenia[d]	Antibodies to prothrombin
Nonischemic neurologic deficits	

Abbreviations: aCL, anticardiolipin; β2GPI, beta-2 glycoprotein I.
  [a] Exclusion of patients who fulfill one or more of the definitive clinical criteria.
  [b] Persistent mottled pattern of the skin, not reversible with warming.
  [c] Histologic diagnosis, exclusion of other causes of microangiopathy.
  [d] Exclusion of other causes of thrombocytopenia.
  [e] Phosphatidylserine, phosphatidylethanolamine.

discrete signs and symptoms supported by accurate and precise diagnostic tests, high rates of diagnostic sensitivity and specificity can be achieved. Unfortunately, APS fails on all these counts. Is this autoimmune entity a thrombotic disorder, a complex inflammatory disorder, or sometimes both? How does a clinician decide if a patient with some findings associated with APS, but not meeting the more stringent clinical or laboratory classification criteria, should be given the diagnosis of APS? If the latter is done, what therapy, if any, should be recommended? What test menu should a clinical laboratory director recommend to clinicians who suspect APS, and more importantly, how should the laboratory director interpret the results? Unfortunately, there are currently no definitive answers to these questions.

Furthermore, clinicians recognize additional subsets of APS not dependent on unique laboratory findings. A growing body of case reports, having in common the sudden onset of multiorgan failure caused by microvascular thrombi, typically occurring in patients previously diagnosed with APS and often associated with a triggering event (infection, trauma), has given rise to the diagnosis of catastrophic APS.[17] Evidence for a unique pathophysiology is lacking, prognosis is very poor, and therapy typically includes aggressive immune suppression therapy, intravenous immunoglobulin, plasma exchange, and anticoagulation. Finally, some clinicians consider the clinical evidence supporting a diagnosis of APS so compelling, they conclude that the pathogenesis must be mediated by phospholipid antibodies, even when the results of standard antiphospholipid tests are negative, and thereby applying a diagnosis of seronegative APS.[18,19]

LABORATORY COMPONENTS OF ANTIPHOSPHOLIPID SYNDROME DIAGNOSIS

Antiphospholipid antibodies are polyclonal and heterogeneous in terms of their clinical associations and in vitro behaviors. Two different approaches are used to detect them: serologic (aCL and anti-β2GPI antibodies) and clot-based (LAC) methods. There are many unresolved analytical and standardization problems with both types of tests, and disappointing results from external quality assurance surveys highlighting poor agreement between laboratories give one pause,[20–23] knowing that clinicians often make long-term management decisions based on the results of these assays. Preanalytical variables can also affect the accuracy of LAC testing, and determination of reference intervals for LAC and serologic results, and the accompanying interpretations, or lack thereof, are crucial factors that affect patient care.[24]

LUPUS ANTICOAGULANT TESTING

LAC antibodies interfere with phospholipid-dependent activation of coagulation factors in vitro. LAC tests indirectly detect the presence of antiphospholipid antibodies, primarily targeting epitopes on β2GPI and prothrombin. Given the many ways to initiate coagulation, investigators developed multiple assays for LAC detection, and given the heterogeneity of LAC antibodies, no method is consistently the most sensitive, and no gold standard exists. Manufactures have taken a handful of LAC methods and produced a supermarket of kits and reagents that laboratories use on many different coagulation instrument makes and models. The two most popular LAC screening strategies in the United States are the dilute Russell viper venom time,[25] which activates factor X (common pathway), and the activated partial thromboplastin time (aPTT) (intrinsic pathway) performed with reagents containing reduced phospholipid and designed to be "LAC sensitive." Other methods include dilute thromboplastin time (extrinsic pathway) and kaolin or silica clotting times (intrinsic pathway, but with no phospholipid in the reagent). Two negative screening tests are considered sufficiently sensitive to exclude LAC.[26] Test specificity is enhanced by repeating the positive screening test method on a 1:1 mixture of patient and normal pooled plasma (NPP) to correct for coagulopathies. A 1:1 mix clotting time within the reference interval established by each laboratory is considered a negative LAC result, although weak LAC may be missed because of dilution. If the 1:1 mix clotting time is prolonged, a confirmation step is performed with the same activation method used for screening plus additional negatively charged phospholipid (which may be "in house" prepared lysed platelet membranes, or commercial bilayer or hexagonal phase phospholipids). Phospholipid-dependent shortening of a clotting time indicates the presence of a LAC.

Many analytical variables impact on LAC testing. First, there is no LAC-positive standard available to use for method comparisons and quality control. Pools of monoclonal β2GPI and prothrombin antibodies derived from human B cells of LAC-positive patients could potentially meet this need,[27] and may soon be available. Plasma used in mixing steps should be from a normal pool rather than an individual, and must be free of platelet contamination. Each decision step (screen, mix, and confirm) requires determination of cut-offs points. Using two standard deviations above the mean from a small group of healthy controls for cut-offs labels 2.5% of the population as positive. Investigators using a three standard deviation or 99th percentile cut-off have reported improved specificity without missing "clinically relevant" positive LACs.[28] To reduce the impact of between-day imprecision, some commercial and in-house laboratory LAC methods perform each step in parallel on patient and NPP, calculate the ratios of patient/control NPP, and compare them with cut-offs derived from a control population using the same ratio technique.[29]

Another strategy for interpreting mixing study results is Rosner's index of circulating anticoagulant.[30] Integrated test systems can be used to complete analysis of patient plasmas with positive screen results. Patient plasma is mixed 1:1 with NPP and clotting times (aPTT, PT, Russell viper venom time, silica activated) are performed with low and high phospholipid concentrations.[28] The results are analyzed based on the difference (delta) between the clotting times, or normalized ratios are calculated using NPP tested in parallel.[31] Interlaboratory comparisons of LAC results from external quality assurance surveys are generally good for LAC negative and strongly positive plasmas, but disappointing for specimens with weak LAC activity, anticoagulants, and factor deficiencies,[20,21,32] highlighting the need for standardized calibrators, revised guidelines, and improved commercial tests.[24]

Accurate LAC testing also depends on careful attention to the quality of the test specimen. Serum is unacceptable. Citrated plasma (0.105–0.109 M) depleted of platelets ($<10 \times 10^9/L$) by centrifugation before freezing is required to prevent false-negative errors caused by absorption of APL antibodies to platelet fragments. Filtration of thawed plasmas can remove vWF and factor VIII in addition to residual platelet membranes,[33] possibly producing false-positive screen results with aPTT-dependent methods because of depletion of factor VIII. Ideally, LAC testing should not be performed on patients with severe coagulopathies, or receiving concurrent anticoagulation therapy. Plasma samples from patients anticoagulated with the pentasaccharide fondaparinux, intravenous direct thrombin inhibitors, and very likely in the near future, oral direct factor Xa and IIa inhibitors, should not be tested because of drug interferences that cannot be reversed. Complex screening algorithms using PT, aPTT, thrombin time, repeat thrombin time after heparin neutralization, and anti-FXa tests can detect the presence of anticoagulants, but they increase costs and are difficult to automate. There are also concerns regarding the accuracy of LAC results for patients anticoagulated with heparin or warfarin.[34] Heparin can be neutralized before testing, and most commercial LAC reagents have a finite capacity to neutralize heparin, which exceeds typical therapeutic levels. Although there is evidence supporting the accuracy of LAC testing of plasmas containing heparin following neutralization with polybrene using in-house methods and reagents,[35] similar validation studies are required with other LAC methods. Plasmas from patients taking warfarin and other coumarins can produce false-positive LAC screening and confirm tests; however, specificity should be achieved with a mixing step to replace vitamin K–dependent coagulation factor deficiencies in patients with international normalized ratios (INRs) in the therapeutic range. An integrated test approach performed on a 1:1 mix of patient and NPP seems to be sensitive and specific for LAC detection in patients taking warfarin.[36]

There are also postanalytical issues to address. Laboratories report LAC results in many different formats. For instance, some provide semiquantitative categories for positive results, without data to support clinical relevance.[24,31] International guidelines for reporting and interpreting LAC results could improve the clinical management of patients suspected of APS.

DETECTION OF ANTIPHOSPHOLIPID ANTIBODIES BY ELISA

For over 20 years, output from aCL ELISA testing has been quantified in arbitrary units where 1 unit equals 1 μg of affinity purified IgG or IgM from the serum of aCL antibody–positive patients. There was a period when most laboratories prepared their own reagents and plates and used a single source of positive human serum for calibration, resulting in good interlaboratory agreement.[37] The optical density of the calibration curve is relatively flat below 10 and above 90 affinity purified IgG,[38] however, making results in these ranges imprecise. Correlation of clinical events with aCL antibody isotypes (IgG, IgM, or IgA) and strength of positive serologic results produced semiquantitative cut-offs to improve specificity. For example, even though the cut-off between negative and positive IgG aCL antibody results is typically between 10 and 20 affinity purified IgG, levels greater than 40 affinity purified IgG (moderate or high) are recommended to support a diagnosis of APS.[13]

Commercial aCL kits have replaced "in-house" prepared assays and manufacturers do not adhere to uniform reagent and plate specifications, test procedures, or use a common calibration standard. As a result, interlaboratory agreement for quantitative results is often poor,[22] especially for proficiency testing samples with low aCL antibody concentrations. Similar problems with discordant interlaboratory quantitative results apply to commercial β2GPI ELISA assays.[23] Problems with standardization extend beyond manufacturer reagent and calibrator differences and include variations among laboratories regarding cut-off determinations, test performance, and data interpretation. In a recent Italian study, 35 clinical laboratories performed aCL ELISA assays on blinded samples consisting of normal plasmas or plasmas spiked with purified IgG from an APS patient to produce strongly positive results.[39] Although sensitivity and specificity based on positive and negative determinations were 94% and 96%, respectively, the variable strength of positive results was substantial, even between laboratories using the same commercial kit. An analysis of β2GPI ELISA results identified similar degrees of imprecision. Calls for improved standardization by hemostasis experts and organizations seem insufficient to motivate manufacturers to cooperate, citing regulatory hurdles to modification of currently licensed kits as a major disincentive.[24]

Although there is unanimity among experts regarding the disappointing lack of standardization of phospholipid antibody serologic testing, controversy exists when selecting combinations of phospholipid antibody serologic targets, immunoglobulin isotypes, and thresholds for positivity from the perspectives of enhancing sensitivity or specificity for diagnosing APS and predicting thrombotic or pregnancy-related complications. Detection of all aCL antibody isotypes (IgG, IgA, and IgM) in the presence of β2GPI provides the greatest sensitivity and least specificity. Isolated IgA aCL is uncommon, and considered by most, but not all, experts not to warrant inclusion in the APS consensus criteria.[13] A minority of investigators dispute the specificity of IgM aCL[40,41] or the use of testing for aCL antibodies at all with the current assay problems, recommending instead anti-IgG β2GPI alone to maximize specificity.[41]

MANAGEMENT

Identifying LAC in an asymptomatic patient with a prolonged aPTT, or antiphospholipid antibodies when screening patients with SLE, raises the issue of primary prophylaxis. Currently, there is no evidence to recommend thromboprophylaxis in patients with incidentally discovered LAC or aCL antibodies in whom the risk of thrombosis is likely to be less than 1% per year.[42] SLE patients are at increased risk for thrombotic complications, and the risk seems higher when combined with antiphospholipid antibodies, leading to a consensus recommendation for low-dose aspirin (81 mg/d)[43]; however, this strategy has not been validated in prospective, randomized studies. A label of APS for a patient with arterial or venous thrombosis, or a woman with pregnancy-related complications, has definite implications for treatment. The best quality evidence is for venous thromboembolic events, which account for approximately 32% of APS-associated clinical events.[44] Two prospective, randomized trials comparing standard intensity oral anticoagulation (INR 2–3) with a higher intensity regimen (INR target >3) in venous thromboembolic events patients diagnosed with APS showed no significant difference in recurrent thrombosis incidents[45,46] for high-intensity versus moderate anticoagulation arms, respectively. Therefore, the recommended INR target is 2 to 3. Expert consensus supports indefinite anticoagulation for secondary prevention of venous thromboembolic events in APS patients, based primarily on one prospective study,[47] and expert consensus.[48] Subjects with spontaneous deep venous thromboses were randomized to 6 months or prolonged oral anticoagulation. When therapy was stopped at 6 months, subjects with a single positive test for IgG aCL antibodies had a recurrence rate of 23 of 105 compared with 3 of 106 for aCL antibody–positive patients on indefinite anticoagulation.[47]

Another challenging management issue is secondary prevention in patients with arterial thromboembolic events, particularly strokes and transient ischemic attacks, who have antiphospholipid antibodies. The prospective Warfarin Aspirin Recurrent Stroke Study included a subset of LAC or aCL antibody–positive stroke patients (N = 1770) who were randomized to aspirin, 325 mg/d, or moderate-intensity warfarin therapy. There was no significant difference for the risk of recurrent thrombotic events between LAC-aCL antibody–positive and –negative patients, or between treatment options among LAC-aCL antibody–positive patients.[49] Based on the results of the Warfarin Aspirin Recurrent Stroke Study, aspirin is recommended for secondary prevention of strokes in APS patients by some expert groups.[50] Other experts do not endorse this practice, however, because of concerns regarding the test methodology and criteria used to define antiphospholipid (aPL)-positive status.[51]

Strategies for secondary prevention of pregnancy loss in women with APS are also controversial. Recurrent pregnancy loss may occur in up to 5% of couples, and aPL antibodies have been reported in 20% to 31%[52,53] of affected women. A generally accepted approach, based on small randomized trials, is to begin treatment with low-dose aspirin before conception, and add prophylactic doses of unfractionated heparin or low-molecular-weight heparin once a viable pregnancy is confirmed.[54] A meta-analysis of early and subsequent small randomized controlled trials concluded,[55] however, that there was insufficient evidence to support a specific approach to thromboprophylaxis of recurrent pregnancy loss in women with APS.

Monitoring acute and chronic phases of anticoagulation therapy can be difficult in LAC-positive patients. If a patient's baseline aPTT is prolonged, dosing unfractionated heparin using nomograms based on aPTT prolongation may lead to excessive or inadequate antithrombotic therapy. Alternatives include using a chromogenic anti-Xa heparin activity assay that does not rely on clotting, or therapeutic doses of low-molecular-weight heparins, which do not require monitoring. An unlikely combination is a LAC-positive patient with a prolonged aPTT suspected of having heparin-induced thrombocytopenia, and requiring immediate anticoagulation. Direct thrombin inhibitor dosing is typically determined by aPTT prolongation, and alternative monitoring methods (Ecarin venom activates prothrombin and is not phospholipid dependent[34]) or alternative immediate acting anticoagulants that do not require monitoring (fondaparinux or, if eventually approved by the Food and Drug Administration, oral factor Xa or thrombin inhibitors) could be used.

In the presence of LACs, mildly prolonged baseline PTs and exaggerated INR responses to warfarin therapy may occur with certain commercial thromboplastins.[56–58] The consequence could be inadequate antithrombotic therapy despite an INR within the therapeutic target range of 2 to 3. This artifact is not unique to one type or brand of thromboplastin, and may occur despite a normal baseline PT-INR.[56] To identify this potential analytical INR inaccuracy in LAC patients anticoagulated with warfarin, one can concurrently measure a chromogenic factor X (therapeutic range 20%–40%), which is unaffected by LAC, and contrast that value with the INR.[56,58] If both tests provide results within the therapeutic target range, then INRs derived with the current thromboplastin are valid. If not, then either another thromboplastin should be evaluated, or warfarin monitoring can be done solely with the chromogenic factor X assay.

Rarely, a patient presents with sudden onset of excessive bleeding, and screening laboratory testing detects markedly prolonged aPTT and PT. The aPTT does not correct on mixing, but the PT does, LAC testing is positive, and performance of PT-based factor activities uncovers an acquired prothrombin deficiency without an inhibitor pattern on dilution. Circulating prothrombin antibodies are common in APS patients,[59] and they are one of the associated serologic findings (see **Table 3**). Antibodies typically have a low affinity for prothrombin, however, and rarely cause a clinically evident coagulopathy. Based on published case series, LAC-associated hypoprothrombinemia usually occurs in children and young adults and is linked to rheumatic disorders, particularly SLE.[60,61] Although management of these patients is challenging, most patients respond to corticosteroid therapy.

PATHOPHYSIOLOGY

Heterogeneity, a defining clinical quality of APS, can also be applied to its incompletely understood pathophysiology. Thrombotic complications correlate more strongly with the presence of LAC than positive serologic tests,[14] analogous to in vitro heparin-dependent platelet activation assays versus serologic detection of anti-PF4 antibodies for confirmation of heparin-induced thrombocytopenia. In vitro prolongation of clotting, however, does not provide an explanation for an increased in vivo risk for thrombosis. Initial attention focusing on deregulation of the protein C pathway by phospholipid antibodies as a likely prothrombotic mechanism has not yielded promising results. A more exciting area of research, initiated by de Groot and colleagues in the Netherlands, involves the consequences of β2GPI cross-linking by autoantibodies. Experimental evidence supports the following model (**Fig. 1**): auto-antibodies linking two molecules of β2GPI by domain 1 increase β2GPI affinity for negatively charged phospholipid surfaces and bring β2GPI domain 5 in contact with putative receptors including apoER2', a member of the LDL receptor super family, capable of activation and subsequent signal transduction. Downstream conse-quences also include weak platelet activation.[62,63] Using a mouse model to investi-gate phospholipid antibody–induced fetal loss, Salmon and colleagues results support an intriguing interaction between antibody-mediated complement activation, complement C5a–dependent induction of tissue factor expression, and subsequent neutrophil oxidative burst and trophoblast injury (**Fig. 2**).[64] In addition, heparin and low-molecular-weight heparin, but not hirudin, a direct thrombin inhibitor, inhibit complement activation and prevent fetal loss in the same mouse model,[65] suggesting

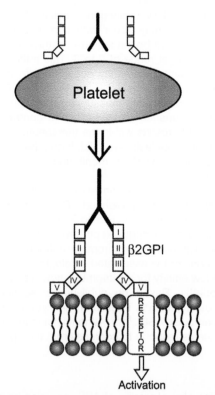

Fig. 1. Model of β2GPI antibody-mediated platelet activation. Autoantibodies to epitopes in domain I form β2GPI dimers with increased affinity for negatively charged phospholipid membranes. β2GPI domain V binds to transmembrane receptors including lipoprotein receptor family-8 (alias ApoER2) and platelet glycoprotein Ibα, activating signaling path-ways and contributing to platelet activation.

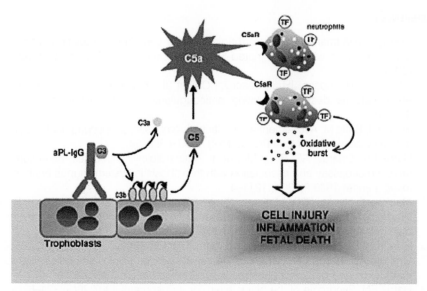

Fig. 2. Mechanism of APL-induced tissue factor (TF) increase and fetal death. APL antibodies are preferentially targeted to the placenta where they activate complement leading to the generation of the potent anaphylatoxin C5a. C5a attracts and activates neutrophils. As a result of C5a-C5a receptor interaction, neutrophils express TF. TF on neutrophils contribute to oxidative burst and subsequent trophoblast injury and ultimately fetal death. (*From* Redecha P, Tilley R, Tencati M, et al. Tissue factor: a link between C5a and neutrophil activation in antiphospholipid antibody-induced fetal injury. Blood 2007;110:2423–31; with permission.)

that treating women with APS and recurrent fetal loss with heparin may improve future pregnancy outcomes by an anti-inflammatory rather than an antithrombotic mechanism. Based on these promising findings, future basic research discoveries may translate into more specific diagnostic tests capable of detecting subsets of "phospholipid antibodies" with thrombotic and inflammatory consequences and novel therapeutic approaches to abrogate them.

SUMMARY

Given the inherent uncertainties surrounding the reliability of the laboratory tests that must be "positive" to apply a label of APS syndrome to patients with common vascular and obstetric disorders, it is indeed challenging for clinicians and laboratory scientists to balance the ill-defined trade-offs between sensitivity and specificity when evaluating different assays, determining cut-offs, and making management decisions. Fortunately, there are ongoing efforts to improve understanding of APS through basic research, clinical trials, and diagnostic testing refinements. In 2010, another consensus conference will update APS classification criteria, and revised guidelines for LAC testing are forthcoming from the International Society of Thrombosis and Haemostasis. It is hoped that one of the consequences of these efforts is better standardization of LAC and serologic antiphospholipid antibody tests, and some substance will be added to the mirage termed "antiphospholipid syndrome."

REFERENCES

1. Conley C, Hartmann R. A hemorrhagic disorder caused by circulating anticoagulant in patients with disseminated lupus erythematosus. J Clin Invest 1952;31: 621–2.
2. Bowie EJ, Thompson JH Jr, Pascuzzi CA, et al. Thrombosis in systemic lupus erythematosus despite circulating anticoagulants. J Lab Clin Med 1963;62: 416–30.
3. Soulier J, Boffa M. Avortement a repetition, thromboses, et anticoagulant circulant anti-thromboplastine. Nouv Presse Med 1980;9:859–64.
4. Harris EN, Gharavi AE, Boey ML, et al. Anticardiolipin antibodies: detection by radioimmunoassay and association with thrombosis in systemic lupus erythematosus. Lancet 1983;2(8361):1211–4.
5. Mackworth-Young CG, Loizou S, Walport MJ. Primary antiphospholipid syndrome: features of patients with raised anticardiolipin antibodies and no other disorder. Ann Rheum Dis 1989;48(5):362–7.
6. Hughes GR. The anticardiolipin syndrome. Clin Exp Rheumatol 1985;3(4):285–6.
7. Gharavi AE, Harris EN, Asherson RA, et al. Anticardiolipin antibodies: isotype distribution and phospholipid specificity. Ann Rheum Dis 1987;46(1):1–6.
8. Harris EN. Syndrome of the black swan. Br J Rheumatol 1987;26(5):324–6.
9. Brandt JT, Triplett DA, Alving B, et al. Criteria for the diagnosis of lupus anticoagulants: an update. On behalf of the subcommittee on lupus anticoagulant/antiphospholipid antibody of the scientific and standardization committee of the ISTH. Thromb Haemost 1995;74(4):1185–90.
10. Wilson WA, Gharavi AE, Koike T, et al. International consensus statement on preliminary classification criteria for definite antiphospholipid syndrome: report of an international workshop. Arthritis Rheum 1999;42(7):1309–11.
11. McNeil HP, Simpson RJ, Chesterman CN, et al. Anti-phospholipid antibodies are directed against a complex antigen that includes a lipid-binding inhibitor of coagulation: beta 2-glycoprotein I (apolipoprotein H). Proc Natl Acad Sci U S A 1990; 87(11):4120–4.
12. Giannakopoulos B, Passam F, Ioannou Y, et al. How we diagnose the antiphospholipid syndrome. Blood 2009;113(5):985–94.
13. Miyakis S, Lockshin MD, Atsumi T, et al. International consensus statement on an update of the classification criteria for definite antiphospholipid syndrome (APS). J Thromb Haemost 2006;4(2):295–306.
14. Galli M, Luciani D, Bertolini G, et al. Lupus anticoagulants are stronger risk factors for thrombosis than anticardiolipin antibodies in the antiphospholipid syndrome: a systematic review of the literature. Blood 2003;101(5):1827–32.
15. Galli M, Luciani D, Bertolini G, et al. Anti-beta 2-glycoprotein I, antiprothrombin antibodies, and the risk of thrombosis in the antiphospholipid syndrome. Blood 2003;102(8):2717–23.
16. Levine JS, Branch DW, Rauch J. The antiphospholipid syndrome. N Engl J Med 2002;346(10):752–63.
17. Merrill JT, Asherson RA. Catastrophic antiphospholipid syndrome. Nat Clin Pract Rheumatol 2006;2(2):81–9.
18. Asherson RA. The primary, secondary, catastrophic, and seronegative variants of the antiphospholipid syndrome: a personal history long in the making. Semin Thromb Hemost 2008;34(3):227–35.
19. Wong RC, Favaloro EJ. Clinical features, diagnosis, and management of the antiphospholipid syndrome. Semin Thromb Hemost 2008;34(3):295–304.

20. Jennings I, Kitchen S, Woods TA, et al. Potentially clinically important inaccuracies in testing for the lupus anticoagulant: an analysis of results from three surveys of the UK National External Quality Assessment Scheme (NEQAS) for blood coagulation. Thromb Haemost 1997;77(5):934–7.
21. Arnout J, Meijer P, Vermylen J. Lupus anticoagulant testing in Europe: an analysis of results from the first European Concerted Action on Thrombophilia (ECAT) survey using plasmas spiked with monoclonal antibodies against human beta2-glycoprotein I. Thromb Haemost 1999;81(6):929–34.
22. Favaloro EJ, Silvestrini R. Assessing the usefulness of anticardiolipin antibody assays: a cautious approach is suggested by high variation and limited consensus in multilaboratory testing. Am J Clin Pathol 2002;118(4):548–57.
23. Favaloro EJ, Wong RC, Jovanovich S, et al. A review of beta2 -glycoprotein-I antibody testing results from a peer-driven multilaboratory quality assurance program. Am J Clin Pathol 2007;127(3):441–8.
24. Favaloro EJ, Wong RC. Laboratory testing and identification of antiphospholipid antibodies and the antiphospholipid syndrome: a potpourri of problems, a compilation of possible solutions. Semin Thromb Hemost 2008;34(4):389–410.
25. Thiagarajan P, Pengo V, Shapiro SS. The use of the dilute Russell viper venom time for the diagnosis of lupus anticoagulants. Blood 1986;68(4):869–74.
26. Tripodi A. Laboratory testing for lupus anticoagulants: diagnostic criteria and use of screening, mixing, and confirmatory studies. Semin Thromb Hemost 2008; 34(4):373–9.
27. Le Querrec A, Arnout J, Arnoux D, et al. Quantification of lupus anticoagulants in clinical samples using anti-beta2GPI and anti-prothrombin monoclonal antibodies. Thromb Haemost 2001;86(2):584–9.
28. Devreese K, Hoylaerts M. Laboratory diagnosis of the antiphospholipid syndrome: a plethora of obstacles to overcome. Eur J Haematol 2009;83:1–16.
29. Gardiner C, MacKie IJ, Malia RG, et al. The importance of locally derived reference ranges and standardized calculation of dilute Russell's viper venom time results in screening for lupus anticoagulant. Br J Haematol 2000;111(4):1230–5.
30. Rosner E, Pauzner R, Lusky A, et al. Detection and quantitative evaluation of lupus circulating anticoagulant activity. Thromb Haemost 1987;57(2):144–7.
31. Jacobsen EM, Barna-Cler L, Taylor JM, et al. The lupus ratio test: an interlaboratory study on the detection of lupus anticoagulants by an APTT-based, integrated, and semi-quantitative test. Fifth International Survey of Lupus Anticoagulants–ISLA 5. Thromb Haemost 2000;83(5):704–8.
32. Tripodi A, Biasiolo A, Chantarangkul V, et al. Lupus anticoagulant (LA) testing: performance of clinical laboratories assessed by a national survey using lyophilized affinity-purified immunoglobulin with LA activity. Clin Chem 2003;49(10): 1608–14.
33. Favaloro EJ. Preanalytical variables in coagulation testing. Blood Coagul Fibrinolysis 2007;18(1):86–9.
34. Greaves M, Cohen H, Machin SJ, et al. Guidelines on the investigation and management of the antiphospholipid syndrome. Br J Haematol 2000;109(4):704–15.
35. Jacobsen EM, Trettenes E, Wisloff F, et al. Detection and quantification of lupus anticoagulants in plasma from heparin treated patients, using addition of polybrene. Thromb J. Available at: http://www.thrombosisjournal.com/content/pdf/ 1477-9560-4-3.pdf. Accessed May 26, 2009.
36. Aboud MR, Roddie C, Ward CM, et al. The laboratory diagnosis of lupus anticoagulant in patients on oral anticoagulation. Clin Lab Haematol 2006;28(2):105–10.

37. Harris EN, Gharavi AE, Patel SP, et al. Evaluation of the anti-cardiolipin antibody test: report of an international workshop held 4 April 1986. Clin Exp Immunol 1987;68(1):215–22.

38. Passam F, Krilis S. Laboratory tests for the antiphospholipid syndrome: current concepts. Pathology 2004;36(2):129–38.

39. Pengo V, Biasiolo A, Bison E, et al. Antiphospholipid antibody ELISAs: survey on the performance of clinical laboratories assessed by using lyophilized affinity-purified IgG with anticardiolipin and anti-beta2-glycoprotein I activity. Thromb Res 2007;120(1):127–33.

40. Pengo V. A contribution to the debate on the laboratory criteria that define the antiphospholipid syndrome. J Thromb Haemost 2008;6(6):1048–9.

41. Galli M, Reber G, de Moerloose P, et al. Invitation to a debate on the serological criteria that define the antiphospholipid syndrome. J Thromb Haemost 2008;6(2):399–401.

42. Vila P, Hernandez MC, Lopez-Fernandez MF, et al. Prevalence, follow-up and clinical significance of the anticardiolipin antibodies in normal subjects. Thromb Haemost 1994;72(2):209–13.

43. Alarcon-Segovia D, Boffa MC, Branch W, et al. Prophylaxis of the antiphospholipid syndrome: a consensus report. Lupus 2003;12(7):499–503.

44. Cervera R, Piette JC, Font J, et al. Antiphospholipid syndrome: clinical and immunologic manifestations and patterns of disease expression in a cohort of 1,000 patients. Arthritis Rheum 2002;46(4):1019–27.

45. Crowther MA, Ginsberg JS, Julian J, et al. A comparison of two intensities of warfarin for the prevention of recurrent thrombosis in patients with the antiphospholipid antibody syndrome. N Engl J Med 2003;349(12):1133–8.

46. Finazzi G, Marchioli R, Brancaccio V, et al. A randomized clinical trial of high-intensity warfarin vs. conventional antithrombotic therapy for the prevention of recurrent thrombosis in patients with the antiphospholipid syndrome (WAPS). J Thromb Haemost 2005;3(5):848–53.

47. Schulman S, Svenungsson E, Granqvist S. Anticardiolipin antibodies predict early recurrence of thromboembolism and death among patients with venous thromboembolism following anticoagulant therapy. Duration of Anticoagulation Study Group. Am J Med 1998;104(4):332–8.

48. Kearon C, Kahn SR, Agnelli G, et al. Antithrombotic therapy for venous thromboembolic disease: American College of Chest Physicians Evidence-Based Clinical Practice Guidelines (8th edition). Chest 2008;133(6 Suppl):454S–545S.

49. Mohr JP, Thompson JL, Lazar RM, et al. A comparison of warfarin and aspirin for the prevention of recurrent ischemic stroke. N Engl J Med 2001;345(20):1444–51.

50. Brey RL, Chapman J, Levine SR, et al. Stroke and the antiphospholipid syndrome: consensus meeting Taormina 2002. Lupus 2003;12(7):508–13.

51. Ruiz-Irastorza G, Hunt BJ, Khamashta MA. A systematic review of secondary thromboprophylaxis in patients with antiphospholipid antibodies. Arthritis Rheum 2007;57(8):1487–95.

52. Erkan D, Merrill JT, Yazici Y, et al. High thrombosis rate after fetal loss in antiphospholipid syndrome: effective prophylaxis with aspirin. Arthritis Rheum 2001;44(6):1466–7.

53. Laskin CA, Spitzer KA, Clark CA, et al. Low molecular weight heparin and aspirin for recurrent pregnancy loss: results from the randomized, controlled HepASA Trial. J Rheumatol 2009;36(2):279–87.

54. Tincani A, Branch W, Levy RA, et al. Treatment of pregnant patients with antiphospholipid syndrome. Lupus 2003;12(7):524–9.

55. Gates S, Brocklehurst P, Davis L. Prophylaxis for venous thromboembolic disease in pregnancy and the early postnatal period. Cochrane Database Syst Rev 2002(2):CD14001689.

56. Moll S, Ortel TL. Monitoring warfarin therapy in patients with lupus anticoagulants. Ann Intern Med 1997;127(3):177–85.

57. Tripodi A, Chantarangkul V, Clerici M, et al. Laboratory control of oral anticoagulant treatment by the INR system in patients with the antiphospholipid syndrome and lupus anticoagulant. Results of a collaborative study involving nine commercial thromboplastins. Br J Haematol 2001;115(3):672–8.

58. Rosborough TK, Shepherd MF. Unreliability of international normalized ratio for monitoring warfarin therapy in patients with lupus anticoagulant. Pharmacotherapy 2004;24(7):838–42.

59. Fleck RA, Rapaport SI, Rao LV. Anti-prothrombin antibodies and the lupus anticoagulant. Blood 1988;72(2):512–9.

60. Baca V, Montiel G, Meillon L, et al. Diagnosis of lupus anticoagulant in the lupus anticoagulant-hypoprothrombinemia syndrome: report of two cases and review of the literature. Am J Hematol 2002;71(3):200–7.

61. Erkan D, Bateman H, Lockshin MD. Lupus anticoagulant-hypoprothrombinemia syndrome associated with systemic lupus erythematosus: report of 2 cases and review of literature. Lupus 1999;8(7):560–4.

62. Urbanus RT, Derksen RH, de Groot PG. Platelets and the antiphospholipid syndrome. Lupus 2008;17(10):888–94.

63. de Groot PG, Derksen RH. Pathophysiology of the antiphospholipid syndrome. J Thromb Haemost 2005;3(8):1854–60.

64. Redecha P, Tilley R, Tencati M, et al. Tissue factor: a link between C5a and neutrophil activation in antiphospholipid antibody induced fetal injury. Blood 2007;110(7):2423–31.

65. Girardi G, Redecha P, Salmon JE. Heparin prevents antiphospholipid antibody-induced fetal loss by inhibiting complement activation. Nat Med 2004;10(11):1222–6.

Thrombotic Thrombocytopenic Purpura and Heparin-Induced Thrombocytopenia: Two Unique Causes of Life-Threatening Thrombocytopenia

Marisa B. Marques, MD

KEYWORDS

• TTP • HIT • Thrombocytopenia • Heparin • Plasma exchange

Physicians of all specialties encounter patients with coagulation disorders, owing to the wide range of presentations of hemostasis disarray, from mild bleeding to overt thrombosis. Thrombocytopenia is among the top reasons for hematology consultation because it arises from a myriad of pathogenic mechanisms. Although bone marrow failure syndromes, primary or secondary, probably account for most thrombocytopenia cases and patients with these conditions tend to bleed, patients with thrombotic thrombocytopenic purpura (TTP) and heparin-induced thrombocytopenia (HIT) rarely bleed. Notwithstanding the fact that these entities cause significant morbidity and mortality, and their appropriate diagnosis and management are crucial to avoid complications, their clinical and laboratory features overlap often with a number of totally distinct conditions. This review will summarize the practical and essential aspects of these syndromes, namely how they can be diagnosed and their impact on patient care.

THROMBOTIC THROMBOCYTOPENIC PURPURA
Historical Perspective

The first case of TTP was described by Moschkowitz[1] in 1924 after he conducted an autopsy of a young woman who died suddenly and was found to have disseminated

Division of Laboratory Medicine, Department of Pathology, University of Alabama at Birmingham, 619 19th Street South, West Pavilion–P230G, Birmingham, AL 35249, USA
E-mail address: mmarques@uab.edu

Clin Lab Med 29 (2009) 321–338
doi:10.1016/j.cll.2009.03.003   labmed.theclinics.com
0272-2712/09/$ – see front matter © 2009 Elsevier Inc. All rights reserved.

platelet thrombi in arterioles and capillaries. For much of the last century, TTP remained a mystery and most patients succumbed to the disease. In 1977, Bukowski and colleagues[2] reported success with plasma exchange. Insights into the pathogenesis of TTP expanded in 1982 with Moake and colleagues'[3] observation that plasma from patients with chronic relapsing TTP had ultra-large von Willebrand factor (vWF) multimers. This observation directly led to many studies published in the 1990s describing a plasma enzyme responsible for the cleavage of vWF after its release from endothelial cells and platelets (vWF-cleaving protease or vWF-CP). Furthermore, it was discovered that many patients with TTP had an acquired deficiency of vWF-CP, which led to the accumulation of ultra-large vWF multimers and, consequently, massive platelet clumping and severe thrombocytopenia.[4,5] Before these discoveries, a hallmark prospective randomized clinical trial from Canada conclusively demonstrated that therapeutic plasma exchange (TPE) was superior to plasma infusion and significantly improved survival of patients with TTP.[6] Although TTP is still somewhat of a mystery, these studies have clearly expanded our understanding of its pathogenesis and had a major impact on the long-term prognosis of affected patients.

Pathogenesis of Thrombotic Thrombocytopenic Purpura

The normal vWF-CP turns ultra-large vWF multimers into smaller fragments that circulate in plasma. In its absence, as seen in patients with familial or acquired TTP, such large vWF multimers accumulate and, owing to their high affinity for the glycoprotein Ib/V/IX on the platelet membrane, cause spontaneous agglutination and thrombocytopenia under conditions of increased fluid shear stress.[7] vWF-CP, a 190- kDa protein primarily synthesized in the liver, is a member of the ADAMTS family and is designated ADAMTS-13.[8] Severe deficiency of ADAMTS-13 is most commonly defined as activity of less than 5% to 10% and is caused by an autoantibody detectable in most patients with acquired TTP.[4,5,9] Systemic occlusive vWF-platelet-rich thrombi are the hallmark pathologic feature of TTP, causing widespread organ ischemia, especially in the brain, heart, and kidneys (**Fig. 1**). Consequently, microangiopathic hemolytic anemia (MAHA) ensues as the red blood cells pass through the affected vessels and break into fragments called schistocytes (**Fig. 2**).

Diagnosis of Thrombotic Thrombocytopenic Purpura

TTP does not present with a specific set of symptoms. Most patients have common and vague complaints such as weakness, nonlocalized abdominal pain, nausea, and vomiting. In others, neurologic symptoms are prominent and dominant even as the initial manifestation, and range from headache and mild confusion to generalized seizures and coma. Some patients complain of recent onset of increased tendency to bleed from mucosal surfaces, including menorrhagia, or the sudden appearance of purpura in the lower extremities. Thus, TTP may be missed unless the patient has a complete blood cell count (CBC) and the physician recognizes the possibility of TTP because of profound thrombocytopenia and MAHA. Because these findings are not rare or specific, awareness plays an important role in the prompt recognition of TTP and referral for TPE.

The classic pentad of thrombocytopenia, hemolytic anemia, fever, renal dysfunction, and neurologic symptoms is present in only a minority of TTP patients. Our current approach to clinical suspicion of the disease requires only thrombocytopenia and MAHA without an alternative explanation.[10] The difficulty in making the diagnosis of TTP lies in the fact that several other conditions also present with a low platelet count and MAHA. This group of disorders is called thrombotic microangiopathies or TMAs. First and foremost, atypical hemolytic uremic syndrome (HUS not associated

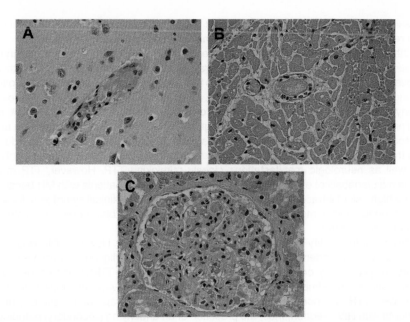

Fig. 1. Photomicrograph of the classical platelet-rich thrombi from a patient with fatal thrombotic thrombocytopenic purpura (TTP). (*A*) Brain; (*B*) Heart; (*C*) Kidney. The involved vessels are at the center of the field, except in 1C, where several capillary loops are occluded by the hyaline thrombi (hematoxilyn and eosin [H&E], ×40 magnification).

with infection with *Escherichia coli* O157H7) in adults has all the features of TTP with prominent acute renal failure and often anuria. However, because the renal involvement in TTP may be of multiple forms, uremia does not exclude the diagnosis of TTP. On the other hand, neurologic compromise increases the likelihood of TTP. Thus, it is currently common practice to use the term TTP-HUS to encompass both

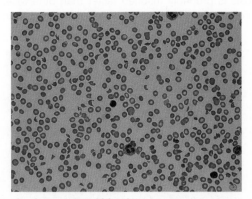

Fig. 2. Photomicrograph of a peripheral blood smear containing numerous fragmented red blood cells (schistocytes), the hallmark of microangiopathic hemolytic anemias (MAHA). In addition, the smear contains reticulocytes, which are released as a consequence of the brisk hemolysis, and platelets are absent, all consistent with a diagnosis of TTP (Wright stain, ×20 magnification).

possibilities.[11] This approach ensures that if the actual diagnosis is TTP, the patient will receive emergent TPE to circumvent the 90% risk of mortality without TPE.

Other TMAs that must be in the differential diagnosis of TTP include malignant hypertension (MH) and disseminated intravascular coagulation (DIC). All of them present with systemic signs and symptoms that arise from ischemia of multiple organs owing to small and medium vessel disease. Although MH is a purely clinical diagnosis, many physicians underestimate its ability to cause thrombocytopenia and MAHA. By definition, the diagnosis of MH requires high blood pressure and papilledema on fundoscopic examination. Because the organs most affected in hypertensive individuals are the same involved in TTP (**Fig. 3**), individuals with MH have impaired renal function as well as neurologic manifestations closely mimicking TTP. However, TTP must remain a diagnosis of exclusion and TPE is not indicated in patients with MH because of the high risk of intracerebral bleed during the procedure. Clinical symptoms, thrombocytopenia, and hemolysis in MH tend to improve as the blood pressure is slowly brought into control.

DIC is another entity that can be easily confused with TTP. However, DIC is always secondary to an underlying condition such as infection, malignancy, massive tissue injury, or pregnancy complication among others, whereas TTP is often a de novo phenomenon superimposed on someone who was otherwise previously healthy. However, TTP can occur as a complication of chemotherapy or pregnancy, or in patients with HIV infection; thus, the presence of an underlying (secondary) pathology cannot exclude TTP. Histologically, the thrombi in DIC are mainly composed of fibrin, whereas in TTP they are mostly rich in platelets (**Fig. 4**). The distinction between DIC and TTP is significantly improved by routine laboratory studies discussed later in this article.

Classification of Thrombotic Thrombocytopenic Purpura

The two main types of TTP are *acquired*, resulting from an autoantibody directed against ADAMTS-13 and *familial* TTP, where the enzyme is missing. The latter is rare and is usually diagnosed in childhood or early adulthood. In many patients, renal insufficiency is the dominant manifestation of familial TTP, which typically occurs acutely after an upper respiratory tract infection. If there is already a family history of TTP, the diagnosis is probably reached faster than otherwise. Other conditions under the umbrella of "TTP syndromes" include transplant-associated

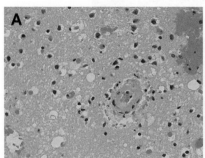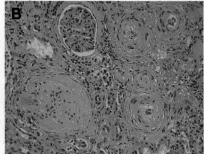

Fig. 3. Photomicrograph of the vascular lesions identified at autopsy of a patient with malignant hypertension (MH). (*A*) Brain; (*B*) Kidney. In contrast with TTP, where the vessels appear normal, these vessels in malignant hypertension depict both chronic and irreversible changes (H&E, ×40 magnification).

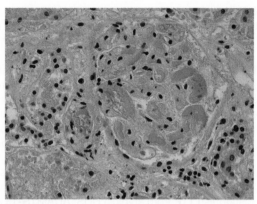

Fig. 4. Photomicrograph of a glomerulus involved by fibrin thrombi in a patient with disseminated intravascular coagulation (DIC). Many capillary loops contain a deep pink deposit consistent with organized fibrin (H&E, ×40 magnification).

microangiopathy, catastrophic antiphospholipid antibody syndrome, and pregnancy-associated microangiopathic hemolytic anemia.[12] As the names imply, their pathogenesis differs from acquired de novo TTP, they require unique management, and their discussion goes beyond the scope of this review.

Epidemiology and Risk Factors of Thrombotic Thrombocytopenic Purpura

Because TTP is a rare condition that affects only approximately 1000 persons per year in the United States, many patients are not promptly diagnosed because of lack of familiarity with the condition. TTP is much more prevalent among women, and the incidence among African Americans is nine times higher than that among persons of other races.[12] In a TTP cohort from our institution, we found that smoking was more prevalent among patients than in the general population, although a correlation has not been confirmed.[13]

The Role of the Clinical Laboratory in Thrombotic Thrombocytopenic Purpura

The clinical laboratory is essential to suspect the diagnosis of TTP and to differentiate it from other TMAs. Routinely available tests such as the CBC, lactate dehydrogenase (LDH), blood urea nitrogen (BUN), creatinine, prothrombin time (PT), partial thromboplastin time (PTT), D-Dimer, and fibrinogen will show the characteristic features of TTP or suggest an alternative etiology such as DIC. In a recent study of patients with severe ADAMTS-13 deficiency between our institution and the Massachusetts General Hospital, we calculated the 99% confidence interval for the presenting platelet count as between 13 and 22 × 10^9 per L and for maximum creatinine as between 1.14 and 2.04 mg per dL.[14] Typically, LDH is several-fold increased because of both massive hemolysis and ischemic changes of LDH-rich organs such as heart, brain, and kidney. Because TTP is characterized by platelet thrombi (see **Fig. 1**), routine assays that detect coagulation factor deficiencies secondary to the activation of secondary hemostasis, such as PT and PTT, are rarely abnormal.[15] Fibrinogen, on the other hand, being an acute phase reactant, is expected to be increased. Because the D-Dimer level is a very sensitive marker of fibrin generation, a quantitative assay could potentially show a result in TTP above the reference range but not as high as that seen in severe DIC (40- to 50-fold increases in the latter). However, when we compared the D-Dimer level of patients with TTP versus those with DIC, we did not find a statistically significant difference, whereas platelet count and PT results were more discriminatory.[15] In a recently published report of cardiac involvement by TTP, mortality and acute morbidity of TTP were associated with higher troponin T levels at admission to the hospital.[16]

ADAMTS-13 deficiency and the presence of its inhibitor can be of value to confirm the clinical diagnosis of TTP, as an activity of less than 10% strongly supports the diagnosis (highly specific for TTP) over other TMAs. However, a patient without ADAMTS-13 deficiency may still have TTP and will respond to TPE, and milder enzyme deficiencies are common in conditions such as systemic inflammatory states and decompensated liver cirrhosis, potentially causing diagnostic confusion.[12] According to a recent summary report, various published series of TTP suggest that ADAMTS-13 activity assays have sensitivities ranging from 89% to 100% and specificity greater than 91%.[17] Thus, despite the initial enthusiasm for the discovery of ADAMTS-13 and its potential to distinguish TTP from atypical HUS, ADAMTS-13 activity continues to be neither as sensitive nor specific for TTP as hoped, and thus, its role in patient management remains unclear. Furthermore, several different assays whose results are not always in agreement are currently being used. At present, there is no indication that should a rapid ADAMTS-13 test become available that it would be clinically useful in deciding which patients to refer to TPE. The standard of care mandates that we initiate TPE in all patients with the *clinical diagnosis of TTP* to circumvent the high risk of mortality. Furthermore, the significance of persistent, severe ADAMTS-13 deficiency during recovery, when the patient is asymptomatic, is also unknown. Thus, it is likely that the initial ADAMTS-13 deficiency facilitates the development of TTP, but it is also possible that the full clinical syndrome requires another, as-yet-unidentified, factor consistent with a two-hit phenomenon.

Additional unanswered questions regarding TTP and ADAMTS-13 include discerning the triggers of the autoantibody and if the actual inhibitor titer plays a role in either the clinical course of TTP and/or its response to TPE. An older study suggested that a higher inhibitor titer predicts increased mortality, refractoriness to TPE, and a more severe presentation,[18] although others have not confirmed this association.[19,20] In a United Kingdom TTP cohort, there was not a correlation between titer and clinical severity, and the absolute antibody level was not associated with mortality.[17]

Treatment of Thrombotic Thrombocytopenic Purpura

The American Society for Apheresis (ASFA) classifies TTP as a category I indication for TPE.[21] After emergent initiation of TPE with normal plasma as replacement fluid, mortality in acquired TTP decreases to less than 10% during the acute episode.[6,11] TPE's benefits stem from several ostensible reasons: removal of the ultra large-vWf multimers and the ADAMTS-13 IgG inhibitor, as well as infusion of normal enzyme with vWF-CP activity. Daily TPE replacing at least one plasma-volume with plasma or cryo-poor plasma[12] must be continued until the platelet count is 150×10^9 per L or higher and hemolysis has ceased (stable hemoglobin and normal LDH). There is much less agreement regarding the role of additional TPEs (tapering) after these laboratory parameters are achieved, based on a lack of evidence for or against its continuation. Major factors that influence the decision to continue plasma exchange include the patient's tolerance to plasma (based on the potential to cause severe hypocalcemia and/or allergic reactions), the available vascular access, and patient and/or clinician preferences.

Response to TPE is usually defined as maintenance of normal platelet count and lack of hemolysis for at least 2 days after discontinuation of TPE.[13] In our retrospective study of factors influencing response and relapse rates, obesity and more profound anemia at presentation were predictors of response to TPE.[13] Other investigators had previously reported similar findings.[22] Age also appeared to affect response to TPE, according to our data and that of Dervenoulas and colleagues,[23] which suggested that younger patients tend to have a better outcome.[13] As described earlier in this article, ADAMTS-13 inhibitor titer has been studied as a potential indicator of treatment response.[18–20] However, our investigation into the possibility of a correlation between inhibitor level and the number of TPEs required to achieve response failed to show an association.[24]

Clinical or laboratory parameters that predict mortality from TTP have also been examined. Although it appears that older patients have an increased risk of death from TTP,[23] data on race are controversial. An analysis of national mortality data from TTP found that African Americans were more likely to succumb from the disease,[25] whereas our results, by contrast, suggested a survival advantage for patients from this ethnic group.[13] It is important to note, however, that the older study[25] evaluated outcomes of TTP before TPE becoming the standard of care and possibly reflecting disparate TPE rates. For patients with familial TTP, chronic plasma transfusion to replace ADAMTS-13 is the treatment of choice.

Glucocorticoids, cyclosporine, vincristine, splenectomy, and, more recently, rituximab (monoclonal antibody to CD20) have all been used in combination with TPE to treat TTP, although randomized clinical trial data are lacking. The National Institutes of Health has funded a prospective multicenter study to determine the role of rituximab, and patient enrollment is imminent.[26] Until these results become available, despite a number of anecdotal reports about the experience with this immunosuppressive agent, its role in TTP is unknown. Another unanswered question is that of the risk of platelet transfusion during an acute episode of TTP. The previous standard of care has held that platelet transfusion is contraindicated in TTP, but a recently published review concluded that it is still uncertain if this practice is harmful or not.[27] On the other hand, experts in TTP suggest a role for the therapeutic use of antiplatelet agents in conjunction with TPE despite significant thrombocytopenia.[12]

Follow-up and Prognosis of Thrombotic Thrombocytopenic Purpura

TTP *remission* has been defined as persistence of the initial favorable response to TPE, whereas *relapse* refers to another episode of TTP occurring at least 4 weeks after discontinuation of TPE.[11] The need to restart apheresis within 1 month of the last TPE is considered an *exacerbation* of the same recent episode. It is unfortunate that published reports have used various definitions and made it difficult to interpret the available data regarding the rate and predictors of relapse. However, it is generally accepted that relapse occurs in approximately 30% of patients who achieve true remission, generally months to years since the initial episode. Prediction of who may relapse and how to prevent or manage relapse continues to be the subject of much debate. We found that male gender and more severe thrombocytopenia ($13 \pm 8 \times 10^9$ per L) at initial diagnosis, as well as a higher pre-/post-TPE LDH ratio were predictors of relapse in our patient population.[13] However, these findings have not been corroborated by a prospective analysis of other TTP patients, and there are no data to currently guide or justify preventive interventions to avoid acute relapsing episodes of TTP. This is an area of major interest to clinical laboratories for the future of TTP management.

HEPARIN-INDUCED THROMBOCYTOPENIA
Historical Perspective

The first cases of HIT were probably described in 1957 and consisted of 10 postoperative patients who developed arterial thrombosis while receiving heparin.[28] Five years later, 11 more surgical patients with unexplained arterial embolization despite having been receiving heparin for 10 days or more were reported.[29] In both publications, the authors did not mention platelet counts because routine CBCs were not common practice until the 1970s.[30] The term "heparin-induced thrombocytopenia" was first coined in 1969,[31] and the central features of HIT as we know them today were described subsequently by Rhodes and colleagues.[32,33] The immune basis of HIT was initially doubted because of its distinct differences with other immune thrombocytopenias (less severe thrombocytopenia and lack of bleeding), as well as the other unique features (thrombosis) of the disease,[30] but HIT was eventually accepted into a platelet immunobiology workshop in 1989.[34] At the time, "HIT Type 2" referred to what we now call HIT, whereas "HIT Type 1" defines the transient, clinically insignificant decrease in platelet count that occurs very early after the onset of heparin use and is not immunologically mediated.

Pathogenesis of Heparin-induced Thrombocytopenia

HIT is caused by platelet-activating antibodies that recognize a complex of platelet factor 4 (PF4; an alpha granule component) and heparin.[35] During normal platelet activation and degranulation, tetramers of PF4 attach to glycosaminoglycans on the platelet membrane. In patients receiving heparin, the drug forms complexes with free and bound PF4. In a minority of patients, an immune response to these complexes develops (see Epidemiology and Risk Factors for Heparin-induced Thrombocytopenia).[30] Although IgG, IgM, and IgA may be formed against PF4-heparin complexes, it appears that IgG is essential to mediate thrombocytopenia through strong platelet activation and aggregation that results from Fcγlla receptor cross-linking (**Fig. 5**).[36,37] Several other reasons have been described to explain the risk of arterial and venous thrombosis in patients with HIT. Visentin and colleagues[38] demonstrated that HIT antibodies could also bind to endothelial cells and activate secondary hemostasis with the generation of fibrin. Another mechanism of thrombosis in HIT involves the release of procoagulant platelet microparticles in the presence of HIT antibodies, which can be detected by electron microscopy (see **Fig. 5**).[30,39] Furthermore, in 2001, two independent groups reported that antibodies to PF4-heparin complexes can induce monocytes to express tissue factor.[40,41]

Diagnosis of Heparin-induced Thrombocytopenia

HIT is perhaps one of the most paradoxically difficult diagnoses to make because, on the one hand, thrombocytopenia is easily identified in the CBC but, on the other, hospitalized patients at risk for HIT often have many other possible reasons for their thrombocytopenia. In addition, missing the diagnosis of HIT may be disastrous owing to life-threatening thrombosis, whereas overdiagnosing HIT carries an increased bleeding risk because of introducing the anticoagulants that must be used for its treatment. With this in mind, the discussion that follows will contain several unanswered questions and many controversial issues.

To diagnose HIT, one must monitor platelet counts of patients receiving heparin according to the American College of Chest Physicians recommendations (Appendix 1).[42] A platelet count that has fallen by at least 50% from the baseline (before initiation of heparin) should be considered suspicious for HIT even if the platelet count is still

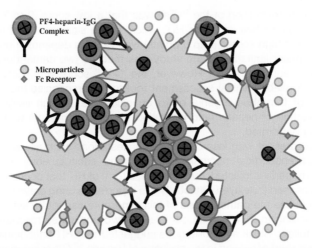

PF4-heparin-IgG
Complex

○ Microparticles
◆ Fc Receptor

Fig. 5. Schematic representation of the pathogenesis of heparin-induced thrombocytopenia (HIT) based on Kelton and Warkentin.[30] Immune complexes of PF4-heparin-IgG form large aggregates in the circulation of patients with HIT. The aggregates cause platelet activation via their Fcγlla receptors, which bind IgG. During activation, platelets release procoagulant microparticles that activate secondary hemostasis and lead to thrombin formation.

within the "normal" reference range.[43] Unless the patient has another reason for thrombocytopenia, the median platelet count at diagnosis of HIT is approximately 55×10^9 per L with very few patients having counts below 20×10^9 per L.[44] Thus, the degree of thrombocytopenia and its relationship to the patient's baseline platelet count are useful indicators of the possibility of HIT. Because profound thrombocytopenia is rare and HIT is a hypercoagulable state, patients are not expected to show symptoms and signs of bleeding. In the setting of unexplained thrombocytopenia accompanied by bleeding, HIT becomes less likely than other processes such as DIC or another drug-induced immune phenomenon. Timing of the thrombocytopenia is also helpful, because patients who have not received heparin in the previous 100 days will develop thrombocytopenia and detectable HIT antibodies only after about day 4 of heparin exposure, at a median time of 6.5 or 7.0 days ("Typical-Onset HIT").[45] Those patients with a history of heparin exposure within the previous 100 days are expected to develop thrombocytopenia much earlier, at a median of 10.5 hours after the initiation of heparin therapy ("Rapid-Onset HIT").[45] Although most patients with HIT present with isolated thrombocytopenia, the diagnosis must always be considered if arterial or venous thrombosis develop during therapy with heparin. Venous thromboembolism (VTE) is four times more common than arterial thrombosis[46,47] and the involved vessel is affected by patient-specific risk factors, such as recent arterial surgery predisposing to arterial thrombosis and central venous catheters predisposing to VTE.[48,49] As a "clinical rule," symptomatic VTE noted at least 5 days into prophylaxis with heparin or low molecular weight heparin, where day 0 is the first day of drug exposure, should remind physicians to consider the diagnosis of HIT.[50]

Based on these three parameters (degree of thrombocytopenia, timing, and thrombosis), the "4Ts" clinical score was developed and studied in two academic medical centers.[51] The fourth T comes from the possibility of "oTher" explanations for thrombocytopenia. To calculate the 4Ts score, each patient may be assigned 0, 1, or 2 points per parameter, depending on the set criteria, for a maximum of 8 points.[51]

The study's main conclusion of the "4Ts" was that a low score (0 to 3 points) has a high negative predictive value for HIT, whereas the significance of intermediate (4 to 5 points) and high scores (6 to 8 points) was variable depending on the clinical setting.[51] One major limitation of the study was that the two centers used different criteria for the diagnosis of HIT. However, the "4Ts" score was shown to be the best currently available clinical assessment tool to help recognize the possibility of other causes of thrombocytopenia or to conclude that a high likelihood of HIT demands cessation of heparin (and institution of specific therapy) while laboratory tests are being performed.

HIT can also present with less common manifestations such as cavernous sinus thrombosis, adrenocortical necrosis, and necrotic subcutaneous lesions where subcutaneous heparin is injected. Furthermore, a form of HIT that occurs after heparin exposure has ceased ("Delayed-Onset HIT") is reported to bring grave clinical consequences.[44] Because the pathogenesis of this syndrome cannot be simply explained by antibody binding to PF4-heparin complexes, two postulated mechanisms for its development follow. Blank and colleagues suggested that HIT antibodies can cause endothelial injury and activation in the absence of heparin.[52] Other independent investigators suggested that HIT antibodies can perhaps cause platelet activation by binding to noncomplexed PF4 or PF4-chondroitin sulfate complexes attached to the platelet membrane.[53–55]

The laboratory diagnosis of HIT is still a matter of much debate and is based on assays of two main types: solid-phase enzyme immunoassay (EIA) to simply detect the presence of a reactive antibody and functional assays to detect platelet activation upon incubation with the patient's antibody-containing serum. Several commercial EIAs that test for antibodies to PF4-heparin or PF4-polyvinyl sulfonate complexes are available and widely used in the United States. EIAs produce results in just a few hours and can be used in real-time for patient management. Unfortunately, a positive result does not mean that the patient truly has HIT because only a fraction of patients who form an immune response to the PF4-heparin complexes actually develop thrombocytopenia and/or thrombosis. Thus, EIAs are very sensitive but much less specific for the diagnosis of HIT.[38,50]

In the so-called "Iceberg Model" of HIT, the bottom of the iceberg corresponds to all patients exposed to heparin, including those who do and do not mount an immune response to PF4-heparin complexes (the latter is the majority). The next level up corresponds to those who develop an HIT antibody, but most of these are asymptomatic, followed by those with isolated thrombocytopenia (approximately 30% to 50% of those who seroconverted), and finally, at the tip of the iceberg, the 10% to 30% of thrombocytopenic patients with thrombosis.[50] Based on this model, it is strongly recommended that an EIA not be performed in patients routinely exposed to heparin unless there is a strong clinical suspicion of HIT based on the preceding definitions of thrombocytopenia, the rate of fall in platelet count, and/or the presence of thrombosis. That is because a positive EIA result, even in the absence of obvious clinical findings, would preclude the continuation of heparin and cause institution of alternative anticoagulants, which have several pitfalls. Furthermore, even in the event of thrombocytopenia, a low "4Ts" score can be used to justify not testing patients for HIT antibodies because of the likely scenario that the test may be positive but the thrombocytopenia is not truly the result of HIT.[51] Another downfall of the EIA is that it detects IgG, IgM, and IgA immunoglobulins. Because our understanding of the pathogenesis of HIT involves only IgG binding to platelet Fc receptors, it is clear that a positive EIA may not be clinically significant for all patients. Indeed, Lo and colleagues[56] calculated that there is a 100% chance of HIT overdiagnosis if any positive EIA result is used in isolation, ie, irrespective of the clinical scenario. Interestingly, a recently published study of the immune response in HIT found IgG antibodies on the first day of a positive EIA, sometimes with concomitant IgA and IgM in patients with HIT, as well as those with asymptomatic seroconversion, with the caveat that the former have higher IgG levels.[57] In the past 2 years, an IgG-specific EIA has become commercially available but its usefulness in patient management has not been clearly established.[58] One possibility that has been discussed to increase the specificity of the HIT EIA might be to increase the cutoff OD value to consider a sample as positive. Although there are published studies suggesting a correlation between higher OD and likelihood of HIT,[59–62] one must be cautious because ODs are relative readings that vary significantly with the operating characteristics of the assay itself and with that of the spectrophotometer. The utility of the specific OD value, thus, remains to be determined.

On the other hand, we, as well as other laboratories, have frequently noted patients with thrombocytopenia suspected to be HIT and an initially negative EIA who subsequently develop a clearly positive result, including patients who have died and/or developed thrombosis.[63,64] Thus, although a negative EIA result in the setting of HIT is rare, it is imperative to consider that EIAs, despite being the most sensitive method for HIT antibodies, may yield false negative results. To avoid missing the diagnosis of HIT, the patient's unique clinical features, such as those used to calculate the "4Ts" score, plus the type of heparin exposure and clinical situation must be taken into account in addition to the laboratory data.

The second type of assay for HIT is based on platelet activation. Although platelet aggregation is now rarely used for the purpose of diagnosing HIT because of a very low sensitivity (around 50%), the serotonin release assay (SRA) is considered the "gold standard" for the identification of clinically significant antibodies.[43,44] Unfortunately, the SRA is technically demanding, more time-consuming than the EIA, uses radiolabeled serotonin, and requires fresh platelets from previously identified donors whose platelets are known to aggregate in the presence of HIT antibodies. For all these reasons, the SRA is not widely available, and most of the studies that describe its usefulness have been performed by a group of experts at McMaster University.[30] Although a positive SRA is certainly very specific for HIT, the test is usually positive only when the EIA demonstrates a high concentration of antibody (OD value often > 2.0). Thus, patients with a high clinical suspicion of HIT, positive EIA, but a negative SRA must be carefully evaluated for the risks and benefits of continuing heparin exposure. We, and others, have seen patients with strong clinical features of HIT, including thrombosis, who have had a negative SRA.[43]

Although much less common and less studied, HIT can occur in children and neonates. A particular high-risk group of pediatric patients include those with congenital heart disease who are exposed to large doses of heparin during cardiopulmonary bypass.[65]

Epidemiology and Risk Factors for Heparin-induced Thrombocytopenia

The current literature suggests that a minority, between 5% and 30%, of patients who develop IgG anti-PF4-heparin complexes develop clinical HIT and that likelihood is strongly linked to the type of patient population.[30,67] Indeed, in a study of hundreds of patients undergoing cardiac or orthopedic surgery, the authors found that the former were much more likely to form HIT IgG, but those undergoing orthopedic procedures who did mount an immune response were more likely to develop clinical signs of HIT.[67] Among nonsurgical patients exposed to heparin, it is likely that 10% develop an immune response, but only a minority develop HIT. On the other hand, HIT in medical patients can complicate the use of prophylactic subcutaneous heparin and the use of heparin-coated catheters.[43] Overall, it is expected that 3% to 5% of all patients exposed to unfractionated heparin for at least 5 days and no more than 1% of those receiving low molecular weight heparin will develop HIT during or after discontinuation of the drug.[43] The difference in immunogenicity between unfractionated heparin and the low molecular weight heparins is probably based on the chain length and the amount of sulfation per saccharide unit of the two preparations.[66] Among the different sources of unfractionated heparin, drug purified from bovine lung is more immunogenic than heparin derived from porcine intestinal mucosa.[68]

The Role of the Clinical Laboratory in Heparin-induced Thrombocytopenia

The reporting of absolute thrombocytopenia or a significant fall in the platelet count in patients exposed to heparin marks the beginning of the essential role that the clinical laboratory plays in HIT. In an ideal scenario, the clinical pathologist would help calculate the "4Ts" score and decide for or against ordering an EIA and/or the SRA based on the unique features and pitfalls of the tests as discussed above. If one or both tests are performed, their interpretation should always involve the clinical pathologist who may be more familiar with HIT and its diagnosis than the patient's physician. If the diagnosis of HIT is confirmed, the need for anticoagulation once more involves the clinical laboratory because the only direct thrombin inhibitors (DTIs) approved by the Food and Drug Administration for HIT (lepirudin and argatroban) require monitoring by the partial thromboplastin time (PTT). Subsequently, the platelet count response during lepirudin or argatroban use must also be monitored with the CBC. Last, after platelet count recovery and initiation of warfarin to replace the parenteral drugs, the clinical laboratory will monitor the patient's International Normalized Ratio (INR). The laboratory medicine consultation does not end here; because both DTIs can prolong the PT/INR in addition to their therapeutic effect on the PTT, balancing the DTI tapering concurrent with addition of warfarin can be complicated.

Treatment of Heparin-induced Thrombocytopenia

The proper management of patients with HIT starts with discontinuing all heparin exposure, including that from heparin-coated catheters and line flushes. Second, because patients with HIT and isolated thrombocytopenia have been shown to have a 30-day risk of thrombosis greater than 50%, an alternative anticoagulant must be initiated promptly.[42,46] Since the American College of Chest Physicians has recently published "Treatment and prevention of heparin induced thrombocytopenia: ACCP evidence-based clinical practice guidelines" the readers are referred to the complete document for details and Appendix 1 at the end of this review, which contains the strongest recommendations (Grades 1B and 1C).[42]

Follow-up and Prognosis of Heparin-induced Thrombocytopenia

Although HIT can cause fatal thrombosis, most patients recover. However, HIT's long-term prognosis is unique among other drug-induced immune thrombocytopenias. HIT antibodies are transient and expected to disappear in a median of 50 days as assessed by the SRA and 85 days by the EIA.[45] In addition, although not suggested without caveats, when patients with previously detected antibodies to the PF4-heparin complexes (including clinical signs of HIT) have been re-challenged transiently with heparin at a time when antibody is no longer detectable, they do not develop thrombocytopenia or thrombosis.[45,69] Despite this observation, the current guidelines suggest that patients with a history of HIT antibodies should not be reexposed to heparin, unless they must undergo cardiac surgery, for which heparin remains the first choice for anticoagulation (see Appendix 1).[42]

SUMMARY

TTP and HIT are two perfect examples of diagnoses that must be made expeditiously to avoid bad outcomes, but that diagnosis can be very difficult and is often confusing. Patients with both conditions are best served by a multidisciplinary approach, including experts in laboratory medicine, transfusion medicine, hematology, and hematopathology, and pharmacists as well. For TTP, apheresis medicine physicians, often within laboratory medicine, usually have more experience with such patients than their internal medicine counterparts, and their input is critical. With respect to HIT, the difficulties in first establishing the diagnosis, and subsequently monitoring the efficacy and risks of DTI anticoagulants, mandates close collaboration between the patient's physicians, laboratory medicine consultants, and hospital-based pharmacists.

ACKNOWLEDGMENT

I am indebted to Dr. Vishnu V. B. Reddy for the photomicrographs used throughout this review. His collaboration has markedly enhanced the educational value of the concepts described here.

APPENDIX 1

Excerpt from the recommendations of the 8th edition of the American College of Chest Physicians consensus conference regarding "Treatment and prevention of heparin induced thrombocytopenia: ACCP evidence-based clinical practice guidelines". (*Adapted from* Warkentin TE, Greinacher A, Koster A, et al. Treatment and prevention of heparin induced thrombocytopenia: ACCP evidence-based clinical practice guidelines. Chest 2008;133(Suppl):340S–80S; with permission from the American College of Chest Physicians.):

Grade 1B (unless otherwise specified):

2.1.1. For patients with strongly suspected (or confirmed) HIT, whether or not complicated by thrombosis, we recommend use of an alternative, non-heparin anticoagulant (danaparoid, lepirudin [Grade 1C], argatroban [Grade 1C], fondaparinux [Grade 2C], bivalirudin [Grade 2C] over the further use of UFH or LMWH therapy or initiation/continuation of a VKA.

2.2.1. For patients with strongly suspected or confirmed HIT, we recommend against the use of VKA (coumarin) therapy until after the platelet count has substantially recovered (ie, usually to at least $150 \times 10^9/L$) over starting VKA therapy at a lower platelet count; that VKA therapy be started only with low, maintenance doses (maximum, 5 mg of warfarin or 6 mg of phenprocoumon) rather than with higher initial doses; and the non-heparin anticoagulant (eg, lepirudin, argatroban, danaparoid) be continued until the platelet count has reached a stable plateau, the INR has reached the intended target range, and after a minimum overlap of at least 5 days between non-heparin anticoagulation and VKA therapy rather than a shorter overlap.

2.3.1. For patients with strongly suspected HIT, whether or not complicated by thrombosis, we recommend against use of LMWH.

3.1.1. For patients with a history of HIT who are HIT antibody negative and require cardiac surgery, we recommend the use of UFH over a non-heparin anticoagulant.

3.2.1. For patients with acute HIT (thrombocytopenic, HIT antibody positive) who require cardiac surgery, we recommend one of the following alternative anticoagulant approaches (in descending order): delaying surgery (if possible) until HIT has resolved and antibodies are negative (see 3.1.1.) or weakly positive (see 3.1.2.); using bivalirudin for intraoperative anticoagulation during cardiopulmonary bypass (if techniques of cardiac surgery and anesthesiology have been adapted to the unique features of bivalirudin pharmacology) or during "off-pump" cardiac surgery.

3.3.1. For patients with strongly suspected (or confirmed) acute HIT who require cardiac catheterization or PCI, we recommend a non-heparin anticoagulant (bivalirudin, argatroban [Grade 1C], lepirudin [Grade 1C], or danaparoid [Grade 1C]) over UFH or LMWH.

Grade 1C (unless otherwise specified):

1.1. For patients receiving heparin in whom the clinician considers the risk of heparin-induced thrombocytopenia (HIT) to be >1.0%, we recommend platelet count monitoring over no platelet count monitoring.

1.1.1. For patients who are starting UFH or LMWH treatment and who have received UFH within the past 100 days, or those patients in whom exposure history is uncertain, we recommend obtaining a baseline platelet count and then a repeat platelet count within 24 h of starting heparin over not obtaining a repeat platelet count.

1.1.2. For patients in whom acute inflammatory, cardiorespiratory, neurologic, or other unusual symptoms and signs develop within 30 min following an IV UFH bolus, we recommend performing an immediate platelet count measurement, and comparing this value to recent prior platelet counts, over not performing a platelet count.

1.1.7. For patients who are receiving fondaparinux thromboprophylaxis or treatment, we recommend that clinicians do not use routine platelet count monitoring.

1.1.9. In patients who receive heparin, or in whom heparin treatment is planned (eg, for cardiac or vascular surgery), we recommend against routine HIT antibody testing in the absence of thrombocytopenia, thrombosis, heparin-induced skin lesions, or other signs pointing to a potential diagnosis of HIT.

1.1.10. For patients who are receiving heparin or have received heparin within the previous 2 weeks, we recommend investigating for a diagnosis of HIT if the platelet count falls by ≥ 50%, and/or a thrombotic event occurs, between days 5 and 14 (inclusive) following initiation of heparin, even if the patient is no longer receiving heparin therapy when thrombosis or thrombocytopenia has occurred.

1.2. For postoperative cardiac surgery patients, we recommend investigating for HIT antibodies if the platelet count falls by ≥ 50%, and/or a thrombotic event occurs, between postoperative days 5 and 14 (inclusive, day of cardiac surgery = day 0).

2.1.5. For patients with strongly suspected or confirmed HIT, whether or not there is clinical evidence of lower-limb deep vein thrombosis (DVT), we recommend routine ultrasonography of the lower-limb veins for investigation of DVT over not performing routine ultrasonography.

2.2.2. For patients receiving a VKA at the time of diagnosis of HIT, we recommend use of vitamin K (10 mg PO or 5 to 10 mg IV).

3.2.2. For patients with subacute HIT (platelet count recovery, but continuing HIT antibody positive), we recommend delaying surgery (if possible) until HIT antibodies (washed platelet activation assay) are negative, then using heparin (see Recommendation 3.1.1.) over using a non-heparin anticoagulant.

REFERENCES

1. Moschcowitz E. Hyaline thrombosis of the terminal arterioles and capillaries: a hitherto undescribed disease. Proc NY Pathol Soc 1924;24:21–4.
2. Bukowski RM, King JW, Hewlett JS. Plasmapheresis in the treatment of thrombotic thrombocytopenic purpura. Blood 1977;50:413–7.
3. Moake JL, Rudy CK, Troll JH, et al. Unusually large plasma factor VIII: von Willebrand factor multimers in chronic relapsing thrombotic thrombocytopenic purpura. N Engl J Med 1982;307:1432–5.
4. Furlan M, Robles R, Galbusera M, et al. Von Willebrand factor-cleaving protease in thrombotic thrombocytopenic purpura and the hemolytic-uremic syndrome. N Engl J Med 1998;339:1578–84.
5. Tsai HM, Lian EC. Antibodies to von Willebrand factor cleaving protease in acute thrombotic thrombocytopenic purpura. N Engl J Med 1998;339:1585–94.
6. Rock G, Shumak KH, Buskard NA, et al. Comparison of plasma exchange with plasma infusion in the treatment of thrombotic thrombocytopenic purpura. Canadian Apheresis Study Group. N Engl J Med 1991;325:393–7.
7. Arya M, Anvari B, Romo GM, et al. Ultralarge multimers of von Willebrand factor form spontaneous high-strength bonds with the platelet glycoprotein Ib-IX complex: studies using optical tweezers. Blood 2002;99:3971–7.
8. Zheng X, Chung C, Takayama TK, et al. Structure of von Willebrand factor-cleaving protease (ADAMTS13), a metalloprotease involved in thrombotic thrombocytopenic purpura. J Biol Chem 2001;276:41059–63.
9. Veyradier A, Obert B, Houllier A, et al. Specific von Willebrand factor-cleaving protease in thrombotic microangiopathies: a study of 111 cases. Blood 2002; 98:1765–72.
10. Sadler JE, Moake JL, Myata T, et al. Recent advances in thrombotic thrombocytopenic purpura. Hematology Am Soc Hematol Educ Program 2004;407–23.
11. George JN. How I treat patients with thrombotic thrombocytopenic purpura-hemolytic uremic syndrome. Blood 2000;96:1223–9.
12. Crowther MA, George JN. Thrombotic thrombocytopenic purpura: 2008 update. Cleve Clin J Med 2008;75:369–75.
13. Tuncer HH, Oster RA, Huang ST, et al. Predictors of response and relapse in a cohort of adults with thrombotic thrombocytopenic purpura-hemolytic uremic syndrome: a single-institution experience. Transfusion 2007;47:107–14.
14. Staropoli JF, Stowell CP, Tuncer HH, et al. An inquiry into the relationship between ABO blood group and thrombotic thrombocytopenic purpura. Vox Sang 2009;96: 344–8.
15. Park YA, Waldrum MR, Marques MB. Common assays distinguish thrombotic thrombocytopenic purpura-hemolytic uremic syndrome and disseminated intravascular coagulation. Transfusion 2006;46(Suppl):4A.
16. Hughes C, McEwan JR, Longair I, et al. Cardiac involvement in acute thrombotic thrombocytopenic purpura: association with troponin T and IgG antibodies to ADAMTS 13. J Thromb Haemost 2009;7:529–36.
17. Scully M, Yarranton R, Liesner R, et al. Regional UK TTP Registry: correlation with laboratory ADAMTS 13 analysis and clinical features. Br J Haematol 2008;142: 819–26.

18. Tsai HM. High titers of inhibitors of von Willebrand factor cleaving metalloprotei-nase in a fatal case of acute thrombotic thrombocytopenic purpura. Am J Hematol 2000;65:251–5.
19. Vesely SK, George JN, Lammle B, et al. ADAMTS13 activity in thrombotic thrombocytopenic purpura-hemolytic uremic syndrome: relation to presenting features and clinical outcomes in a prospective cohort of 142 patients. Blood 2003;102:60–8.
20. Bohm M, Betz C, Miesbach W, et al. The course of ADAMTS-13 activity and inhibitor titre in the treatment of thrombotic thrombocytopenic purpura with plasma exchange and vincristine. Br J Haematol 2005;129:644–52.
21. Szczepiorkowski ZM, Bandarenko N, Kim HC, et al. Guidelines on the use of therapeutic apheresis in clinical practice-evidence-based approach from the apheresis applications committee of the American Society for Apheresis. J Clin Apher 2007;22:106–75.
22. Nicol KK, Shelton BJ, Knovich MA, et al. Overweight individuals are at increased risk for thrombotic thrombocytopenic purpura. Am J Hematol 2003;74:170–4.
23. Dervenoulas J, Tsirigotis P, Bollas G, et al. Thrombotic thrombocytopenic purpura/hemolytic uremic syndrome (TTP/HUS): treatment outcome, relapses, prognostic factors. A single-center experience of 48 cases. Ann Hematol 2000;79:66–72.
24. Lakey MA, Boctor FN, Knight CS, et al. VWF-cleaving protease activity and inhibitor levels do not predict duration of treatment in TTP and HUS. J Clin Apher 2005;20:7.
25. Torok TJ, Holman RC, Chorba TL. Increasing mortality from thrombotic thrombocytopenic purpura in the United States—analysis of national mortality data, 1968–1991. Am J Hematol 1995;50:84–90.
26. George JN, Woodson RD, Kiss JE, et al. Rituximab therapy for thrombotic thrombocytopenic purpura: a proposed study of the Transfusion Medicine/Hemostasis Clinical Trials Network with a systematic review of rituximab therapy for immune-mediated disorders. J Clin Apher 2006;21:49–56.
27. Swisher KK, Terrell DR, Vesely SK, et al. Clinical outcomes after platelet transfusions in patients with thrombotic thrombocytopenic purpura. Transfusion 2009; in press.
28. Weismann RE, Tobin RW. Arterial embolism occurring during systemic heparin therapy. Arch Surg 1958;76:219–25.
29. Roberts B, Rosato FE, Rosato EF. Heparin: a cause of arterial emboli? Surgery 1963;55:803–8.
30. Kelton JG, Warkentin TE. Heparin-induced thrombocytopenia: a historical perspective. Blood 2008;112:2607–15.
31. Natelson EA, Lynch EC, Alfrey CP Jr, et al. Heparin-induced thrombocytopenia. An unexpected response to treatment of consumption coagulopathy. Ann Intern Med 1969;71:1121–5.
32. Rhodes GR, Dixon RH, Silver D. Heparin induced thrombocytopenia with thrombotic and hemorrhagic manifestations. Surg Gynecol Obstet 1973;136:409–16.
33. Rhodes GR, Dixon RH, Silver D. Heparin induced thrombocytopenia: eight cases with thrombotic-hemorrhagic complications. Ann Surg 1977;186:752–8.
34. Chong BH, Berndt MC. Heparin-induced thrombocytopenia. Blut 1989;58:53–7.
35. Amiral J, Bridey F, Dreyfus M, et al. Platelet factor 4 complexed to heparin is the target for antibodies generated in heparin-induced thrombocytopenia. Thromb Haemost 1992;68:95–6.
36. Kelton JG, Sheridan D, Santos A, et al. Heparin-induced thrombocytopenia: laboratory studies. Blood 1988;72:925–30.

37. Newman PM, Chong BH. Heparin-induced thrombocytopenia: new evidence for the dynamic binding of purified anti-PF4-heparin antibodies to platelets and the resultant platelet activation. Blood 2000;96:182–7.
38. Visentin GP, Ford SE, Scott JP, et al. Antibodies from patients with heparin-induced thrombocytopenia/thrombosis are specific for platelet factor 4 complexed with heparin or bound to endothelial cells. J Clin Invest 1994;93:81–8.
39. Warkentin TE, Hayward CP, Boshkov LK, et al. Sera from patients with heparin-induced thrombocytopenia generate platelet-derived microparticles with procoagulant activity: an explanation for the thrombotic complications of heparin-induced thrombocytopenia. Blood 1994;84:3691–9.
40. Pouplard C, Iochmann S, Renard B, et al. Induction of monocyte tissue factor expression by antibodies to heparin-platelet factor 4 complexes developed in heparin-induced thrombocytopenia. Blood 2001;97:3300–2.
41. Arepally GM, Mayer IM. Antibodies from patients with heparin-induced thrombocytopenia stimulate monocytic cells to express tissue factor and secrete interleukin-8. Blood 2001;98:1252–4.
42. Warkentin TE, Greinacher A, Koster A, et al. Treatment and prevention of heparin induced thrombocytopenia: ACCP evidence-based clinical practice guidelines. Chest 2008;133(Suppl):340S–80S.
43. Davoren A, Aster RH. Heparin-induced thrombocytopenia and thrombosis. Am J Hematol 2006;81:36–44.
44. Warkentin TE. Heparin-induced thrombocytopenia: pathogenesis and management. Br J Haematol 2003;121:535–55.
45. Warkentin TE, Kelton JG. Temporal aspects of heparin-induced thrombocytopenia. N Engl J Med 2001;344:1286–92.
46. Warkentin TE, Kelton JG. A 14-year study of heparin-induced thrombocytopenia. Am J Med 1996;101:502–7.
47. Greinacher A, Farner B, Kroll H, et al. Clinical features of heparin-induced thrombocytopenia including risk factors for thrombosis. A retrospective analysis of 408 patients. Thromb Haemost 2005;94:132–5.
48. Boshkov LK, Warkentin TE, Hayward CPM, et al. Heparin-induced thrombocytopenia and thrombosis: clinical and laboratory studies. Br J Haematol 1993;84:322–8.
49. Hong AP, Cook DJ, Sigouin CS, et al. Central venous catheters and upper-extremity deep-vein thrombosis complicating immune heparin-induced thrombocytopenia. Blood 2003;101:3049–51.
50. Linkins LA, Warkentin TE. The approach to heparin-induced thrombocytopenia. Semin Respir Crit Care Med 2008;29:66–74.
51. Lo GK, Juhl D, Warkentin TE, et al. Evaluation of pretest clinical score (4 T's) for the diagnosis of heparin-induced thrombocytopenia in two clinical settings. J Thromb Haemost 2006;4:759–65.
52. Blank M, Shoenfeld Y, Tavor S, et al. Anti-platelet factor 4/heparin antibodies from patients with heparin-induced thrombocytopenia provoke direct activation of microvascular endothelial cells. Int Immunol 2002;14:121–9.
53. Warkentin TE, Kelton JG. Delayed-onset heparin-induced thrombocytopenia and thrombosis. Ann Intern Med 2001;135:502–6.
54. Prechel MM, McDonald MK, Jeske WP, et al. Activation of platelets by heparin-induced thrombocytopenia antibodies in the serotonin release assay is not dependent on the presence of heparin. J Thromb Haemost 2005;3:2168–75.
55. Rauova L, Zhai L, Kowalska MA, et al. Role of platelet surface PF4 antigenic complexes in heparin-induced thrombocytopenia pathogenesis: diagnostic and therapeutic implications. Blood 2006;107:2346–53.

56. Lo GK, Sigouin CS, Warkentin TE. What is the potential for overdiagnosis of heparin-induced thrombocytopenia? Am J Hematol 2007;82:1037–43.

57. Warkentin TE, Sheppard JA, Moore JC, et al. Studies of the immune response in heparin-induced thrombocytopenia. Blood 2009; in press.

58. Sanders RD, Carroll SH, Jones TA, et al. Is the new IgG enzyme-immunoassay for HIT a solution for our diagnostic dilemma? Am J Clin Pathol 2008;130:491.

59. Pouplard C, Amiral J, Borg JY, et al. Decision analysis for use of platelet aggregation test, carbon 14-serotonin release assay, and heparin-platelet factor 4 enzyme-linked immunosorbent assay for diagnosis of heparin-induced thrombocytopenia. Am J Clin Pathol 1999;111:700–6.

60. Zwicker JI, Uhl L, Huang WY, et al. Thrombosis and ELISA optical density values in hospitalized patients with heparin-induced thrombocytopenia. J Thromb Haemost 2004;2:2133–7.

61. Warkentin TE, Sheppard JI, Moore JC, et al. Laboratory testing for the antibodies that cause heparin-induced thrombocytopenia: how much class do we need? J Lab Clin Med 2005;146:341–6.

62. Warkentin TE, Sheppard JI, Moore JC, et al. Quantitative interpretation of optical density measurements using PF4-dependent enzyme-immunoassays. J Thromb Haemost 2008;6:1304–12.

63. Refaai MA, Laposata M, Van Cott EM. Clinical significance of a borderline titer in a negative ELISA test for heparin-induced thrombocytopenia. Am J Clin Pathol 2003;119:61–5.

64. Chan M, Malynn E, Shaz B, et al. Utility of consecutive repeat HIT ELISA testing for heparin-induced thrombocytopenia. Am J Hematol 2008;83:212–7.

65. Boshkov LK, Kirby A, Shen I, et al. Recognition and management of heparin-induced thrombocytopenia in pediatric cardiopulmonary bypass patients. Ann Thorac Surg 2006;81:S2355–9.

66. Warkentin TE, Levine MN, Hirsh J, et al. Heparin-induced thrombocytopenia in patients treated with low-molecular-weight heparin or unfractionated heparin. N Engl J Med 1995;332:1330–5.

67. Warkentin TE, Sheppard JA, Horsewood P, et al. Impact of the patient population on the risk for heparin-induced thrombocytopenia. Blood 2000;96:1703–8.

68. Francis JL, Palmer GJ III, Moroose R, et al. Comparison of bovine and porcine heparin in heparin antibody formation after cardiac surgery. Ann Thorac Surg 2003;75:17–22.

69. Pötzsch B, Klövekorn W-P, Madlener K. Use of heparin during cardiopulmonary bypass in patients with a history of heparin-induced thrombocytopenia. N Engl J Med 2000;343:515.

Laboratory Evaluation of Hypercoagulability

Bernard Khor, MD, PhD, Elizabeth M. Van Cott, MD*

KEYWORDS

- Protein C • Protein S • Antithrombin III
- Activated protein C resistance • Factor V Leiden
- Prothrombin G20210A • Antiphospholipid antibodies

Venous thromboembolism affects 0.1% of the general population in the United States every year, resulting in over 50,000 deaths annually. Common predisposing conditions include the postoperative state, trauma, pregnancy, estrogen or progesterone use (including oral contraceptives), obesity, prolonged travel, smoking, dehydration, infection, prolonged bed rest, and immobility. In addition, several important medical conditions are associated with thrombosis, including chronic disseminated intravascular coagulation (DIC), malignancy, nephrotic syndrome, heparin-induced thrombocytopenia, paroxysmal nocturnal hemoglobinuria (PNH), systemic lupus erythematosis (SLE), polycythemia vera, essential thrombocythemia, ulcerative colitis, Crohn's disease, and Behcet's syndrome. These conditions can pose an even greater threat of thrombosis when superimposed on one of a number of well-characterized hereditary and acquired hypercoagulable conditions. A hypercoagulable condition is now identifiable by the laboratory in the majority of cases, particularly in young individuals or those with a positive family history and/or recurrent thrombosis. This discussion considers several important hypercoagulable states that predispose patients to venous, and in some instances, arterial thrombosis, focusing on activated protein C resistance/factor V Leiden, prothrombin G20210A, deficiencies of protein C, protein S or antithrombin, and antiphospholipid antibodies. The discussion includes the incidence of each hypercoagulable condition, the magnitude of the thrombotic risk it poses and synergistic interactions amongst the various hypercoagulable conditions. Salient advances in understanding the molecular pathogenesis of each condition are presented and discussed in the context of the interpretation and clinical utility of current laboratory testing and identifying potential targets of future testing. Finally, recommendations for laboratory testing are summarized.

ACTIVATED PROTEIN C RESISTANCE

The powerful prothrombotic potential of thrombin is tightly regulated. Endothelial cells express thrombomodulin and endothelial protein C receptor (EPCR) on their surface.[1]

Department of Pathology, Massachusetts General Hospital, Harvard Medical School, Jackson 235, 55 Fruit Street, Boston, MA 02114, USA
* Corresponding author.

Clin Lab Med 29 (2009) 339–366
doi:10.1016/j.cll.2009.03.002
0272-2712/09/$ – see front matter © 2009 Elsevier Inc. All rights reserved.

Thrombomodulin binds thrombin and inactivates thrombin's procoagulant activity. The thrombomodulin-thrombin complex then proteolytically activates EPCR-bound protein C (**Fig. 1**).[1] The activation of protein C by the thrombin-thrombomodulin complex is a key event in the protein C anticoagulant pathway. Activated protein C (APC), with its cofactor protein S, inactivates factors Va and VIIIa to help maintain hemostatic balance (see **Fig. 1**). Activated protein C also indirectly promotes fibrinolysis.[2] APC resistance was first reported in 1993 by Dählback and colleagues[3,4] and currently represents the most common known hereditary predisposition to venous thrombosis. APC resistance accounts for 20% of unselected patients with first-episode thrombosis, 50% of familial thrombosis, and 60% of thrombotic patients known to have normal levels of protein S, protein C, antithrombin, and antiphospholipid antibodies.[5-7] Several groups subsequently showed that the APC resistance observed by Dählback and colleagues was caused by a mutation in its substrate, Factor V (FV), termed FV_{Leiden}.[8-10]

Protein C cleaves FV at three arginine sites (R306, R506, and less importantly, R679), and the FV_{Leiden} mutation is a DNA substitution (G1691A) that changes the amino acid encoded at one of these sites (R506Q). This is thought to arise from a founder mutation that occurred more than 21,000 years ago.[11] Some studies attribute more than 95% of cases of APC resistance to the FV_{Leiden} mutation.[4,9,12] FV_{Leiden} is present in heterozygous form in 5% of the general Caucasian population and is less common or rare in other ethnic groups.[13-18] Homozygosity for FV_{Leiden} occurs at a frequency of about 1 in 5000. The risk of venous thrombosis is increased 3- to 7-fold in individuals heterozygous for FV_{Leiden}, and 80-fold in homozygotes.[19,20] This thrombotic risk is further increased in the presence of a second risk factor, such as oral contraceptive use (combined relative risk increased up to 48-fold),[21] pregnancy,[22] protein S deficiency,[23] hyperhomocysteinemia,[24] or advanced age.[18]

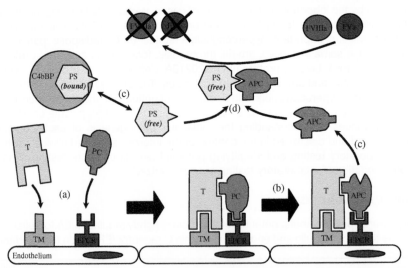

Fig. 1. Schematic of the protein C/protein S pathway. (a) Endothelial surface thrombomodulin (TM) and protein C receptor (EPCR) bind to plasma thrombin (T) and protein C (PC) respectively. (b) Thrombomodulin-bound thrombin generates activated protein C (APC). (c) APC and protein S (PS) can dissociate from their respective binding proteins, EPCR and C4b-binding protein (C4bBP). (d) APC and PS form a complex that proteolytically inactivates factors Va and VIIIa.

Some evidence suggests that the risk of PE is not as great as the risk of DVT in FV_{Leiden} individuals.[25] Studies have not consistently shown an increased risk for arterial thrombosis such as myocardial infarction or stroke, although FV_{Leiden} may be more common in affected patients who are young and who have other risk factors such as smoking.[26-30]

The study of the APC-factor V interaction has yielded valuable insights into how perturbations in this association lead to thrombophilia. It is now clear that APC exerts anticoagulant effects beyond inactivating factor Va by cleaving at R306 and R506, generating inactive FV (FV_{ai}). In addition, APC also generates an anticoagulant molecule (FV_{ac}) by cleaving full-length factor V at R506; this FV_{ac} acts as a cofactor with APC to degrade factor VIIIa.[29] Although the R506Q mutation in FV_{Leiden} abrogates both these effects, the major cause of APC resistance and thrombophilia in these patients is believed to be the decreased generation of the FV_{ac} anticoagulant.[29] This idea is further supported by the very high thrombotic risk observed in patients who are compound heterozygotes for factor V–deficient and FV_{Leiden} alleles (pseudo-homozygotes). Despite bearing only one FV_{Leiden} allele, the thrombotic risk in these patients is similar to that of FV_{Leiden} homozygotes, consistent with the notion that the predominant thrombophilic effect of FV_{Leiden} is related to the inability to generate the anticoagulant molecule FV_{ac}.[29]

Other, less common factor V mutations also affect APC resistance, with differing prothrombotic risks. Of these, one of the more significant is FV_{R2} (H1299R) which is tightly linked to several other mutations and collectively named the R2 haplotype.[29] FV_{R2} exhibits APC resistance entirely because of reduced APC cofactor activity and leads to an increased thrombotic risk when present in compound heterozygotes with FV_{Leiden}.[29,31] In the absence of FV_{Leiden}, mild APC resistance has been found to be present[32,33] or absent[33,34] with homozygous or heterozygous FV_{R2}; these studies used assays either with[32] or without[33,34] dilution into FV–deficient plasma. Factor V levels can either be reduced[34] or normal.[32] A link between heterozygous or homozygous FV_{R2} alone and thrombosis has not yet been clearly demonstrated. $FV_{Liverpool}$ (I359T) has been reported in a family in which $FV_{Liverpool}$ (I359T) alone was asymptomatic, but $FV_{Liverpool}$ (I359T) with a mutation on the other FV allele (a premature stop codon) was associated with low factor V levels, APC resistance, and increased thrombotic risk.[35] $FV_{Cambridge}$ (R306T) and $FV_{Hong Kong}$ (R306G) are rare mutations that both exhibit only mild APC resistance when studied in a recombinant, in vitro system (APC resistance was intermediate between that seen in normal individuals and that seen in FV_{Leiden}) and mildly reduced APC cofactor activity in vitro. These mutations have not been associated with increased risk of thrombosis.[36,37] Despite these in vitro results, patients with $FV_{Hong Kong}$ have not exhibited APC resistance.[37] $FV_{Hong Kong}$ was present in 4.7% of Hong Kong patients with thrombosis.[38] In contrast, $FV_{Cambridge}$ and $FV_{Hong Kong}$ were each found in only 0.4% of healthy Caucasians and in none of the other ethnic groups studied.[36]

Conversely, APC resistance can be a result of reasons other than hereditary factor V defects, especially when using an assay that does not include dilution of the patient plasma into factor V–deficient plasma. One study found APC resistance to be an independent risk factor for thrombosis even in the absence of FV_{Leiden}, using the original assay. However, the overlapping APC resistance results between controls and patients makes it difficult to apply this concept to individual patient care.[39] Patients have been reported to develop autoantibodies against factor V after exposure to bovine thrombin leading to APC resistance, with subsequent thrombosis of unclear etiology.[40-42] One study has also observed APC resistance (as measured by endogenous thrombin potential without dilution into factor V–deficient plasma) in unselected patients with untreated hematological malignancies, which may contribute to the increased risk of venous thrombosis observed in these patients.[43] Treatment of the malignancy ameliorated this APC resistance.[43] Lupus anticoagulants sometimes cause APC resistance. Mutations in the factor VIII gene causing resistance to activated protein C are theoretically possible but have not yet been described. Although one group reported that 6/32 (18.8%) of thrombosis patients with normal factor VIII had "factor VIII APC resistance" versus 1/38 (2.6%) of controls, the phenotype was not associated with any described genetic defect.[44]

Excitingly, APC has been shown in recent years to exhibit a diverse array of cytoprotective effects independent of its role in hemostasis. In this regard, APC has been shown to induce changes in gene expression profiles, anti-inflammatory activities, and anti-apoptotic activity, as well as protect the endothelial barrier.[45] Mutation studies have begun to dissect the distinct mechanisms by which APC exerts its anticoagulant effects and its cytoprotective effects. For example, whereas the anticoagulant activity of APC requires binding of its Gla-domain to phospholipid, its cytoprotective activity relies instead upon binding of APC to the EPCR.[45] As our understanding of how APC acts in this role, bringing about diverse changes ranging from interleukin (IL)-10 and tissue factor expression in sepsis to matrix metalloproteinase expression in rheumatoid arthritis, the way in which we define APC activity and thus APC resistance may evolve accordingly.[1,45–50]

The original assay for APC resistance is based on the prolongation of an activated partial thromboplastin time (PTT) in the presence or absence of exogenously supplied APC.[4,7] The exogenous APC degrades the patient's factors Va and VIIIa, thereby prolonging the PTT. The ratio of the PTT before and after adding APC is calculated, with a value of 2.0 or higher being typical of normal individuals, whereas individuals with FV_{Leiden} have a ratio less than 2.0 (each laboratory establishes its own cut-off). However, using a cut-off ratio of 2.0 achieves a sensitivity of only 50% to 86% and a specificity of 75% to 98% in adults.[51–54] There is considerable overlap between normals and heterozygotes in the 2.0 to 3.0 range of assay values, and raising the cut-off increases sensitivity but decreases specificity.[54] This original assay exhibits APC resistance from a range of causes other than FV_{Leiden}, including low protein S (<20%) or elevated factor VIII, and is inaccurate in individuals with an abnormal baseline PTT.[51,55] Therefore, it is not reliable in the context of warfarin, heparin, liver dysfunction, lupus anticoagulants, or low factor levels. Platelet contamination of plasma specimens can also lead to altered results with subsequent freezing and thawing.[3,56]

The "modified", second-generation assay for activated protein C resistance greatly improves the ability to distinguish between APC-resistant and healthy individuals (eg, Coatest APC resistance V, Chromogenix AB, Sweden), with sensitivity and specificity approaching 100%.[57,58] This is achieved by diluting the patient plasma 1:5 into factor V–deficient plasma before performing the PTT reactions, thus minimizing the effect of factor deficiencies and elevations that alter the baseline PTT. The dilution step allows the assay to be used in patients on oral anticoagulation, who have liver disease, those with low protein S, and those with an elevated factor VIII arising from acute phase reaction or pregnancy. Additionally, the addition of Polybrene neutralizes up to 1 IU/mL of unfractionated or low molecular weight heparin in the specimen. Heparin levels over 1 IU/mL can lead to a falsely elevated result (E.M. Van Cott, unpublished observations, 2009). The effects of specimen freezing and platelet contamination (<20,000 per μL) on the assay are also decreased.[59] Despite these improvements, some caveats remain. For example, direct thrombin inhibitors such as argatroban, hirudin, and bivalirudin can give falsely elevated APC resistance results.[60] In our experience, 20% of patients with lupus anticoagulants exhibit APC resistance with this assay.[61]

Suggestions proposed to deal with lupus anticoagulant interference include using higher plasma dilutions such as 1:10 or 1:20 or 1:40[62,63] and adding excess phospholipid to neutralize the lupus anticoagulant.[64] One theoretical disadvantage of using factor V–deficient plasma is the inability to detect any rare patient with APC resistance owing to mutations in factor VIII as postulated above.

Use of the normalized ratio appears to reduce intra- and interassay variability. This ratio is obtained by dividing the result of the patient's APC resistance assay by that of normal pooled plasma. However, some studies report that the use of the normalized ratio has not improved the ability of the assay to distinguish APC resistance from normal.[65–67]

More recently, Russell viper venom (RVV) assays from the snake *Daboia russelli russelli* have been developed. For example, the Siemens assay involves a dilute RVV time performed with and without activated protein C (generated by treating the specimen with a snake venom from *Agkistrodon contortrix* that activates endogenous protein C). The assay includes a phospholipid reagent intended to remove lupus anticoagulant interference. Specimens are not diluted into factor V–deficient plasma. Life Diagnostics offers a similar RVV-based assay. Both assays are affected by low protein C.

Other assays have been developed using a factor V activator from Russell viper venom (RVV-V, not to be confused with the well known factor X activator from RVV used in the two assays mentioned in the previous paragraph and in dilute RVV lupus anticoagulant assays). In the Pefakit system (Centerchem Inc, Norwalk, Connecticut or Acticlot from American Diagnostica, Stamford, Connecticut), specimens are diluted into factor V–deficient plasma. APC is then exogenously added to an aliquot of RVV-V–activated patient plasma. Wild-type FV, but not FV_{Leiden}, is degraded by APC. Subsequently, prothrombin is activated using venom from the Australian tiger snake (Noscarin, from *Notechis scutatus scutatus*) and the clotting time is measured, assessing for the presence of APC-resistant FV_{Leiden}, which would increase the velocity of thrombin activation.[68] The manufacturer reports that lupus anticoagulants do not interfere, because phospholipid is not present in the reagent.[67] Low factor V levels can interfere with this assay. An assay based on a factor IXa clotting time is also available (Aniara, Hyphen BioMed, Mason, Ohio). Another variation of the APC resistance assay uses a prothrombin time (PT)-based factor V assay (instead of a PTT-based assay) in factor V–deficient plasma.[69] This factor V assay involves plasma dilutions of up to 1:80. Therefore, lupus anticoagulants have not interfered with this assay. A chromogenic factor Va assay may also be suitable for patients with lupus anticoagulants.[59,70] Interestingly, APC resistance caused by lupus anticoagulants might have clinical significance, as studied by both the "modified" aPTT-based assay[61] and the original PTT-based assay.[71]

FV_{Leiden} testing can also be accomplished directly by DNA analysis. The FV_{Leiden} mutation is a point mutation (G1691A) that incidentally eliminates an MnlI restriction enzyme site. Various methods based on polymerase chain reaction (PCR) have been developed to detect this mutation.[8,67] Initial assays amplified DNA around the mutation site and assayed for the presence or absence of this MnlI site, with absence of this site correlating with presence of the FV_{Leiden} mutation.[8] Heterozygotes and homozygotes can be specifically identified by this method. Numerous modifications of PCR-based DNA testing have since been developed.[72] Automated PCR systems are commercially available. Several assays have been developed that do not require template amplification. The Invader assay (Third Wave Technologies Inc, Madison, Wisconsin) does not rely upon amplification of template DNA/RNA, but rather upon amplification of a signal generated by a cleavase DNA endonuclease upon recognition of a tertiary structure formed by selected fluorescein-labeled probes binding at the mutation site. By using differently labeled probes to the wild-type and FV_{Leiden} alleles, this method allows simultaneous detection of both alleles, enabling discrimination between heterozygous and homozygous samples. The Verigene system (Nanosphere Inc, Northbrook, Illinois) uses a solid array with capture oligonucleotides to bind DNA fragments of interest, followed by exposure to sequence-specific gold nanoparticle-bound probes. Silver is then catalytically coated onto the gold particles and read by light scattering. The silver signal amplification allows for extremely high sensitivity, and again template amplification is not required. Of note, the use of DNA testing without the concomitant use of an APC resistance assay will not identify the rare patient who has APC resistance caused by a mutation other than FV_{Leiden}. Conversely, there is at least one case report of a "molecular false positive," in which a DNA mutation was present that eliminated the MnlI site but did not cause APC resistance.[73]

Special Considerations for Activated Protein C Resistance Testing in Pediatrics

The normal range of the original assay for activated protein C resistance is higher in newborns than in older children and adults. The range decreases to the adult level by age 6 months.[74] As with adults, the assay has been greatly improved by diluting the patient plasma 1:5 in factor V–deficient plasma. In newborns, a 1:11 dilution performed better than a 1:5 dilution. Furthermore, the 1:11 dilution results correlate with DNA analysis, whereas the 1:5 dilution results did not.[75] Therefore, optimum assessment of activated protein C resistance in newborns may require a 1:11 dilution in factor V–deficient plasma. In children age 3 months to 16 years, the 1:5 dilution in factor V–deficient plasma correlated well with DNA analysis, but the nondiluted (original) method did not, even when the normalized ratio was used.[65] A 1:11 dilution in these children was not investigated. Clinically, infection-associated purpura fulminans has been reported in a neonate heterozygous for FV_{Leiden} and in two unrelated children doubly heterozygous for FV_{Leiden} and protein S deficiency.[76,77]

Recommendations for Activated Protein C Resistance Testing

A functional assay for APC resistance is advantageous, as it is automated, cost-effective, and detects causes of APC resistance other than FV_{Leiden}. The "modified" (second-generation) APC resistance assay, in which patient plasma is diluted 1:5 into factor V–deficient plasma, is recommended. Each laboratory should determine its own cut-off for an abnormal result, and all abnormal results should ideally be confirmed by DNA analysis for presence of the FV_{Leiden} mutation. Although concordance of the modified assay with DNA analysis is extremely high, it is reasonable to also perform DNA analysis on patients with a result that is at the very end of normal. If DNA analysis is not available, any patient with an abnormal result should be tested for a lupus anticoagulant. The College of American Pathologists Consensus Conference on Diagnostic Issues in Thrombophilia recommends that patients be tested for FV_{Leiden} either by the second-generation ("modified") functional APC resistance assay or by direct DNA detection methods.[78] The relatively low prevalence of the FV_{Leiden} mutation makes use of the functional APC resistance assay as a screening test cost-effective.[79]

PROTEIN C DEFICIENCY

Protein C is synthesized as a circulating, inactive glycoprotein whose activity is vitamin-K dependent.[80] Protein C deficiency occurs in 0.14% to 0.50% of the general population, and is inherited in an autosomal dominant fashion with variable penetrance.[81,82] It accounts for 3% of unselected patients with a first venous thrombosis and no known malignancy,[83] and up to 9% of patients younger than 70 years with venous thrombosis.[84] In the heterozygous state, it increases the risk for venous thrombosis sevenfold.[83] In symptomatic families, protein C deficiency is associated with an increased risk of venous thrombosis in patients younger than 55 (adjusted relative risk 11.3).[85] A recent study suggests that protein C–deficient subjects are also at a sevenfold increased risk of arterial thrombosis at an early age, compared with nondeficient family members.[86] A few prospective studies have been completed that suggest an association between low protein C and ischemic stroke.[28] Protein C levels in heterozygous individuals usually range between 35% and 65% of normal, although levels of up to 68% in heterozygotes have been reported.[87] The first thrombotic event usually presents between the ages of 10 and 50 years. Protein C–deficient individuals are also at increased risk for warfarin-induced skin necrosis. Homozygous deficient patients with severely decreased protein C levels present as newborns with purpura fulminans and DIC. This condition is incompatible with life unless anticoagulation and replacement therapy with fresh frozen plasma or protein C concentrates (Baxter Health Care Corporation, Glendale, California) are instituted. Like other hereditary hypercoagulable conditions, the presence of a second risk factor further increases thrombotic risk.

Protein C deficiencies can be categorized as being either quantitative (type I) or qualitative (type II) (**Table 1**), with the former being more common. In type I deficiencies, normally functioning protein C molecules are made in reduced quantity. Type II deficiencies are qualitative deficiencies, in which normal amounts of dysfunctional protein C are synthesized. The human protein C gene (*PROC*) comprises 9 exons and protein C deficiency has been linked to over 160 mutations to date (see **Table 1**).[88,89] Therefore, DNA testing of protein C deficiency is generally not available outside of specialized research laboratories. Instead, the laboratory assessment of protein C relies on assays of protein C function and antigen levels. Importantly, antigenic assays are immunoassays designed to measure the quantity of protein C regardless of its function. Thus, type I deficiencies are characterized by a decrease in both functional and antigenic protein C. In contrast, type II deficiencies exhibit normal protein C antigen levels with decreased functional levels. As a result, if only

Table 1
Classification and molecular basis of protein C deficiencies

Type	Functional Protein C	Protein C Antigen	Molecular Basis
I	Low	Low	Mostly missense mutations that tend to destabilize the protein; insertions, deletions, nonsense, promoter, and mRNA splicing mutations have also been described
II	Low	Normal	All described type II mutations are missense mutations, and tend to occur in polar surface residues that impact protein function, rather than stability • The N-terminal region contains glutamine residues that require vitamin-K dependant carboxylation for function. • Arg-1 mutations perturb interactions with the important cofactors calcium and phospholipids. These mutations have decreased protein C function in clotting-based assays; however, chromogenic assays may yield normal values • Arg 169 is cleaved by thrombin during protein C activation. Mutation at this residue generally leads to type II deficiency • His 211 is in the active site of protein C

antigenic assays are performed, type II deficiencies will not be detected. Accordingly, a functional assay should be used as the initial screening assay. If this result is decreased, an antigenic assay should then be performed to determine if the deficiency is type I or type II.

Commercially available functional assays use either clotting time–based or chromogenic methods. In both assays, protein C in patient plasma is activated, typically with the venom of a specific snake, and its activity is measured. The clotting time–based assay relies on the patient's activated protein C to degrade factors Va and VIIIa, thereby prolonging a PTT-based clotting time. A RVV-based assay is also available. The chromogenic assays measure the ability of the activated protein C to cleave a synthetic substrate (resembling its natural substrate) and liberate a chromogenic compound that is spectrophotometrically detected. Both clotting and chromogenic assays that tolerate up to 1 IU/mL heparin are available. Clotting-based assays can exhibit interferences from several sources. For instance, artifactually increased levels of protein C can be caused by lupus anticoagulants, whereas artifactually decreased levels of protein C can be caused by elevated factor VIII (above 200%, as can occur in patients with an acute phase reaction). In addition, falsely low values of protein C function have also been reported in patients with the FV_{Leiden} mutation, using a clotting-based assay.[90] With chromogenic assays, it is important to note that a type II protein C variant has been reported that is not detected in the chromogenic functional assay but is detected in the clot-based assay.[91,92] A study by the ECAT foundation shows significantly lower interlaboratory and intralaboratory variation using chromogenic, as opposed to clotting-based, assays of protein C function.[93]

Several conditions are known to cause acquired protein C deficiency, and these should be excluded before making a diagnosis of hereditary protein C deficiency. Protein C activity is vitamin K dependent. Therefore, oral anticoagulants or vitamin K deficiency cause decreases in protein C. In fact, protein C measurements cannot be reliably interpreted during oral anticoagulant therapy, even with the use of formulas comparing the ratio of other vitamin K–dependent factors to protein C. Patients should not have received oral anticoagulants for at least 10 days before testing. Liver disease may also lead to decreased protein C levels because of decreased hepatic synthesis. Protein C has a relatively short half-life of 6 to 8 hours, and is therefore one of the first of the hepatically synthesized coagulation proteins to decrease with liver disease, warfarin initiation, or the onset of vitamin K deficiency. Recent or active thrombosis, surgical procedures, or DIC consume protein C and thus lower protein C levels. L-asparaginase therapy decreases protein C by decreasing hepatic synthesis. A case of an acquired inhibitor (autoantibody) of protein C has been reported.[94] If an inhibitor is suspected, a protein C mixing study can be performed. Protein C has been reported to increase with oral contraceptives and pregnancy.[95] In nephrotic syndrome, protein C may increase, decrease, or remain normal. Women may have slightly decreased protein C levels in comparison with men, and premenopausal women may have slightly lower levels than postmenopausal women.[96]

Special Considerations for Protein C Testing in Pediatrics

At birth, protein C levels are decreased to 35% (range 17% to 53%) of normal adult values.[97] Levels rise to above 50% of adult values by age 6 months. However, protein C may remain below adult normal values until age 16 years or beyond.[98,99]

Recommendations for Testing for Protein C Deficiency

A functional assay should be performed as the screening assay. If a PTT-based clotting time assay is used and the result is decreased, a factor VIII assay should be performed. Factor VIII elevations may artifactually decrease protein C in PTT-based clotting time assays, but have no effect in chromogenic assays. Factor VIII elevations commonly occur during acute phase reactions. If the protein C functional assay is decreased, an antigenic assay should be performed to distinguish between type I and type II deficiencies.

If decreased protein C is established, acquired causes of decreased protein C must be excluded and testing should be repeated after any such conditions have resolved. Patients should not have received warfarin within 10 days before testing. Laboratory tests that can identify some acquired causes of decreased protein C include liver function tests and a DIC screen (D-dimer, PT, PTT, fibrinogen, platelet count, and if available, PTT waveform).[100] Because no confirmatory DNA test is readily available, definitive confirmation of a hereditary deficiency often requires additional approaches such as demonstrating protein C deficiency in a relative with a history of thrombosis.

PROTEIN S DEFICIENCY

Protein S is a 75-kDa glycoprotein, and, like protein C, its activity is vitamin K dependent.[101] It contains an N-terminal γ-carboxyglutamic (Gla) domain, a thrombin-sensitive region (TSR), four epidermal growth factor-like repeats, and a C-terminal sex hormone-binding globulin-like domain.[102] Protein S binds with high affinity to the β-chain of C4b binding protein (C4bBP) in plasma, with the excess circulating as free protein S.[101] In adults, 60% of plasma protein S is bound to C4bBP. The remainder, called free protein S, is the predominantly active form. Protein S is a required cofactor for activated protein C (APC)-mediated degradation of coagulation factors Va and VIIIa, increasing APC activity by approximately 20-fold. This cofactor activity appears to depend on the TSR and first EGF module of free protein S and is abrogated upon cleavage by thrombin.[102,103] Interestingly, protein S has also recently been shown to have anticoagulant activity independent of its APC cofactor function. For example, protein S interacts with factors Va and Xa, inhibiting prothrombin activation.[101] Also, protein S appears to act as a cofactor for tissue factor pathway inhibitor (TFPI), enhancing TFPI:factor Xa complex formation and thus inhibiting tissue factor–mediated factor X activation.[101,104] The pertinence of these novel functions of protein S remain to be clearly delineated, and assays of APC-cofactor–independent functions of protein S are not yet available for commercial use. Finally, the recent discovery that C4bBP-bound protein S also has anticoagulant activity, albeit less than and qualitatively different from that of free protein S, may add yet another dimension to how we assess protein S activity.[101,104,105]

Protein S deficiency is inherited in an autosomal dominant fashion with variable clinical expression. Its prevalence in the general population ranges from 0.03% to 0.13%.[106] By comparison, it is found in 1% to 13% of thrombophilic patients with venous thrombosis.[107] Within symptomatic families, a large multicenter prospective study found protein S deficiency to be associated with a significantly increased lifetime risk of venous thrombosis (adjusted relative risk 32.4).[85] However, these results cannot be generalized to unselected protein S–deficient persons, in whom this risk is lower and not well defined. As with protein C deficiency, the first thrombotic event tends to present between the ages of 10 to 50 years. Protein S deficiency is also associated with a 4.6-fold increased risk of arterial thrombosis in patients younger than 55,[86] although a prospective study did not find an association between low protein S and recurrent ischemic stroke.[108] Warfarin-induced skin necrosis has also been reported in the context of protein S deficiency. Functional protein S levels in heterozygous individuals have ranged from at least 20% to 64%.[87,109] Homozygous patients typically present as newborns with purpura fulminans and DIC, and require replacement therapy with fresh frozen plasma as well as anticoagulation for survival.[110] However, case reports have identified patients with untreated severe protein S deficiency but a relatively mild clinical phenotype.[111,112] As with the other hereditary hypercoagulable conditions, the presence of additional risk factors further increases the risk for thrombosis.

The gene encoding protein S (*PROS1*) comprises 15 exons spanning 80 kb on chromosome 3. Over 200 *PROS1* mutations have been identified in protein S–deficient patients, a different mutation segregating in almost every family (http://www.med.unc.edu/isth/ssc/communications/plasma_coagulation/proteins.htm).[105] While this diversity of mutations has led to valuable insights into the molecular bases of protein S deficiency, DNA testing is accordingly complicated, and generally not available outside of specialized research laboratories.[103]

Protein S deficiency is defined by its decreased APC-cofactor activity, and can be divided into three types (**Table 2**). Type I and type III deficiencies are quantitative defects with both low free protein S antigen levels and low protein S activity, and account for 95% of cases.[105] However, type I deficiency is associated with low total protein S antigen levels and can be attributed to monogenic *PROS1* defects, whereas type III deficiency is associated with normal total protein S antigen levels and most likely involves other genetic and/or environmental factors.[107] Although pure type III deficiency often cosegregates with the protein S Heerlen (S460P) allele, type I and type III protein S deficiencies cosegregate in many families, and these may represent phenotypic variants of the same disease.[105,113] Protein S type II deficiency accounts for about 5% of cases, representing a qualitative defect where levels of both total and free protein S antigen are normal, but protein S activity is diminished.[105] Type II deficiencies are associated with missense mutations in *PROS1*.[103] Notably, type II deficiencies will be missed if protein S is solely assessed by free and total antigenic assays. Thus, we suggest that a functional protein S assay should be used as the initial screening assay. If the result is abnormal, a free protein S antigen assay should be performed. If the free protein S antigen level is also decreased, a total protein S antigen assay can be performed to help distinguish between type I and type III deficiency, but total protein S antigen assays are not routinely required.[114]

Commercially available functional assays measure the ability of protein S to serve as a cofactor to APC, enhancing its degradation of factors Va and VIIIa and thereby prolonging the clotting time of the sample. APC is either added exogenously, or generated from endogenous protein C in the sample with specific snake venom (eg, Protac from *Agkistrodon contortrix*). Methods have been developed using PTT-, PT-, or factor

Table 2
Classification and molecular basis of protein S deficiencies

Type	Functional Protein S	Free Protein S	Total Protein S	Molecular Basis
I	Low	Low	Low	About 130 known candidate mutations throughout the protein S gene. Mostly missense mutations; frameshift, nonsense, and splice site mutations have also been described
II	Low	Normal	Normal	7 known mutations, including 5 missense and 2 splice site mutations
III	Low	Low	Normal	About 9 mutations thought to cosegregate with both type I and type III protein S deficiency

Xa-based clotting times. Assays that tolerate up to 1 to 2 IU/mL heparin are available. The factor Xa-based methods were designed to bypass factors above the common pathway, and factor Xa is either added exogenously (American Diagnostica, Stamford, Connecticut and Trinity Biotech, Berkeley Heights, New Jersey) or generated from factor X in the sample by adding RVV (Precision Biologic, Dartmouth, Nova Scotia). Chromogenic assays of protein S function have been developed, but are not commercially available. Lupus anticoagulants can interfere with factor Xa, PTT-based, or PT-based assays. With PTT-based protein S assays, as with PTT-based protein C assays, artifactually increased levels of protein S can be caused by lupus anticoagulants, whereas artifactually decreased levels of protein S can be caused by elevated factor VIII. Factor VIIa therapy can interfere in PT-based assays. Acute phase reactions might decrease protein S, regardless of the assay used. As previously discussed, C4bBP binds protein S and decreases free protein S antigen as well as protein S functional levels. C4bBP is commonly elevated during acute phase reactions; because a commercial assay for C4bBP may not be available, surrogate markers (such as factor VIII and fibrinogen) can help assess for an acute phase response. In PTT-based clotting assays, factor VIII elevations (>200%) artifactually reduce the functional protein S result, sometimes dramatically. Factor VIII elevations also occur during acute phase reactions and thus factor VIII levels should be measured if the PTT-based functional protein S level is reduced. If factor VIII is elevated, repeat testing of protein S should be performed after the acute phase reaction has subsided. Some reports have found falsely decreased functional protein S levels as a result of the presence of FV_{Leiden}.[115–117] Because antigen assays are not affected, such interference can give the incorrect appearance of a type II deficiency. The Staclot Protein S assay (Diagnostica Stago, Asnieres-Sur-Seine, France) supplies normal factor Va and consequently appears to be less impacted by FV_{Leiden} than some other assays. In our experience with the Staclot assay, FV_{Leiden} has not interfered significantly with protein S determinations. Nevertheless, before confirming a diagnosis of type II protein S deficiency in a patient with FV_{Leiden}, it is necessary to either confirm protein S deficiency in a relative without FV_{Leiden}, measure protein S on increasing dilutions of patient plasma (the suspected FV_{Leiden} interference usually disappears upon higher dilution), or isolate the patient's protein S from the patient's plasma before quantitating it.[115] It is important to note that with PTT-based assays, an artifactually low protein S owing to elevated factor VIII will normalize upon dilution of the patient plasma or upon isolation of protein S from patient plasma.

Total and free protein S antigen levels are measured by a variety of immunological methods, ranging from Laurell-type assays (Helena Laboratories, Beaumont, Texas) to enzyme-linked immunosorbent assays (ELISAs) to automated latex bead agglutination-based assays (Instrumentation Laboratories, Bedford, Massachusetts, and Chromogenix, Milano, Italy). They measure the quantity of protein S regardless of its function. Although earlier assays relied on precipitation of C4bBP-bound protein S with polyethylene glycol (PEG) to distinguish between free and total protein S, the advent of monoclonal antibodies specific for free protein S has eliminated the need for PEG-precipitation and significantly improved the accuracy of the test result.[109]

Several conditions are known to cause acquired protein S deficiency. Oral anticoagulants, vitamin K deficiency, liver disease, active thrombosis, surgical procedures, DIC, and L-asparaginase therapy can cause decreased protein S, for the same reasons as described for protein C. Occasionally, liver disease can exhibit normal levels of protein S but decreased levels of protein C and antithrombin, even though all three proteins are hepatically synthesized. This is speculated to be because of additional synthesis of protein S by endothelial cells (protein S is also synthesized in megakaryocytes). As with protein C, protein S measurements cannot be reliably inter-preted during warfarin therapy. Patients should not have received warfarin for at least 20 days before testing. Hormonal status can also decrease protein S levels, including pregnancy, oral contraceptive (OCP) use, and hormone replacement therapy.[105,106,118–120] In interesting contrast, one group reported that progestin-only contraceptives can *elevate* protein S.[120] Protein S may become decreased in nephrotic syndrome as well as some infectious and autoimmune conditions such as HIV infection,[121] recent varicella infection,[122,123] Crohn's disease,[124,125] and ulcerative colitis.[124,125] Protein S inhibitors have been reported infrequently, and can be assessed by mixing studies, where the mixed plasma is incubated for 1 hour before to measuring protein S in the mixture.[126]

Finally, apart from these acquired causes, protein S antigen levels are also affected by age and gender. In this regard, women have slightly lower protein S levels than men, and total protein S levels increase with age in women, although protein S func-tion was not measured in these studies.[96,106] The complexities of protein S regulation (functional versus total versus free antigen level) are matched by the difficulties in measuring them precisely. The ECAT study showed that protein S parameters ex-hibited the highest inter- and intralaboratory variability, compared with protein C and antithrombin. Protein S function and total antigen and free antigen levels showed an interlaboratory variability of 36.9%, 17.2%, and 17.7%, respectively, and an intra-laboratory variability of 17.2%, 13.4%, and 14.1%, respectively.[93] Taken together, this demonstrates the importance and complexity in measuring protein S parameters in patients and study groups alike.

Special Considerations for Protein S Testing in Pediatrics

At birth, protein S total antigen levels are decreased to 36% (range 12%–60%) of normal adult values.[97,99] Levels rise into the adult normal range by age 6 months. Protein S in newborns is largely or entirely in the free (active) form, because C4bBP is low or undetectable in newborns.[127,128] This is proposed to help compensate for the low amount of total protein S in the neonate.

Recommendations for Testing for Protein S Deficiency

A functional protein S assay should be used for initial screening, because it detects all three types of deficiency (but the limitations of the functional assays should be taken into consideration as described earlier in this article). If this result is decreased, free protein S antigen should be measured. If free protein S antigen is decreased, a total antigen assay can also be performed, although it is not necessary to routinely measure total protein S antigen.[114] Because factor VIII elevations can artifactually decrease protein S in PTT-based assays, factor VIII levels should be measured when protein S is low by this method. In addition, elevated factor VIII may indicate an acute phase response, which could result in increased C4bBP and thus decreased free protein S levels. Because the different acute phase reactants do not elevate and resolve at the same time, an additional acute phase reactant, such as fibrinogen, can be measured to further assess for an acute phase reaction. This testing is best performed by reflexive laboratory analysis on a single specimen. If a decreased protein S value is attributed to an acute phase reaction, the protein S assay(s) may be repeated after recovery from the presumed acute phase reaction, when factor VIII and C4bBP will likely have returned to normal. Patients should not have received estrogen and not have been pregnant within the preceding 3 months before testing. In addition, patients should not have received warfarin for 20 days before testing.

Acquired causes of protein S deficiency must be excluded before making a diagnosis of hereditary protein S deficiency. Laboratory tests to assess for acquired causes of decreased protein S are the same as described earlier in this article for protein C, with the addition of urine albumin for proteinuria. Because confirmatory DNA testing is not routinely available, confirmation of the diagnosis may require demonstrating decreased protein S in a relative with a history of thrombosis.

ANTITHROMBIN DEFICIENCY

Antithrombin is a serpin that inhibits not only thrombin and factor Xa, but also factors IXa, XIa, XIIa, kallikrein, and plasmin.[129] Like other serpins, antithrombin acts as a suicide substrate inhibitor, covalently binding to and inactivating thrombin.[129] Antithrombin's activity is greatly accelerated by interaction with the heparan sulfate family of glycosaminoglycans, which includes heparin.[130] In vivo, heparan sulfate is found on the endothelial cell surface, thus localizing antithrombin activity.[130] The interaction of antithrombin with heparan sulfate on the endothelial cell surface also appears to result in release of prostacyclin, a platelet inhibitor.[131]

Significant advances have been made in understanding the molecular mechanism of antithrombin activity. The gene that encodes antithrombin, SERPINC1, comprises seven exons spanning 13.5 kb on chromosome 1. The 1392-bp mRNA encodes a 432-amino acid, 58-kDa glycoprotein that contains three β-sheets and nine α-helices with an active site region and a heparin binding site (HBS).[132] Heparin binds to the D-helix of antithrombin, exposing antithrombin's reactive center and accelerating its inhibitory activity approximately 1000-fold. Although inhibition of thrombin requires the formation of a trimolecular complex between antithrombin, thrombin, and a heparin longer than 18 saccharides (including a specific pentasaccharide sequence), inhibition of factor Xa by antithrombin can be accelerated by just the pentasaccharide of heparin.[129,130] Antithrombin circulates in the plasma at a concentration of 112 to 140 mg/L and a half life of 2 to 3 days.[129]

Antithrombin deficiency is inherited in an autosomal dominant fashion with variable clinical penetrance, occurring in 0.02% to 0.17% of the general population and in 0.5% to 4.9% of patients with VTE.[84,132–135] Antithrombin deficiency is associated almost exclusively with venous thrombosis; the magnitude of this risk is estimated at 5- to 50-fold.[83,85,129,136] A recent study found that antithrombin deficiency is not associated with an increased risk of arterial thrombosis.[86] As in protein C and protein S deficiency, the first thrombotic event tends to present between the ages of 10 and 50 years (peak 15 to 35 years). There is also a high risk of developing VTE during the patient's lifetime (50%) or during pregnancy (50%).[137] In general, the risk of thrombosis appears to be higher for antithrombin deficiency than for protein C or protein S deficiency, activated protein C resistance, or prothrombin G20210A. Homozygous type I antithrombin deficiency has not been described in patients and is thought to be incompatible with life. Consistent with this notion, homozygous knockout of the antithrombin gene is lethal in mice.[130] However, patients homozygous for type II HBS mutations have been described; they have severe venous thrombosis as well as an increased incidence of arterial thrombosis.[129,130] As with other hereditary hypercoagulable conditions, the presence of a second risk factor further increases the risk for thrombosis.

Antithrombin deficiencies can be divided into two types: quantitative (type I) or qualitative (type II) (**Table 3**). Type I deficiencies are characterized by decreased antithrombin functional and antigen levels; typically both are below 70%,[132] although values up to 78% to 80% have also been observed (Van Cott EM, unpublished

Type	Functional Antithrombin	Antithrombin Antigen	Molecular Basis
Table 3 Classification and molecular basis of antithrombin deficiencies			
I	Low	Low	92 unique mutations described, mostly missense mutations; deletions and insertions have also been described
II (RS)	Low	Normal	12 known reactive site mutations, all missense. Because this prevents interaction with target proteases, these mutations do not exhibit progressive activity
II (HBS)	Low	Normal	12 known heparin binding site mutations, all missense. The reactive site is unaffected, and these mutations exhibit progressive activity
II (pleiotrophic)	Low	Slightly low to normal	11 known mutations, all missense, with multiple (pleiotrophic) effects

observations, 1996). Type II deficiencies are qualitative defects resulting in the production of a variant protein with decreased function. Because antigen levels are often normal in type II deficiencies, functional assays should be used instead for initial screening. If the result is decreased, an antigen assay can be used to distinguish between type I and type II defects.

Type II deficiencies can be further subdivided into three subtypes, namely reactive site (RS), heparin binding site (HBS), and pleiotropic defects (mutations clustered in a region called s1C-s4B).[132,138] Both type II HBS and RS mutations are associated with decreased functional and normal antigenic levels; however, only type II HBS mutations are associated with progressive activity (see later in this article).[132,139] Type II pleiotropic defects are associated with a moderate decrease in both antithrombin function and antigen levels (typically antithrombin function lower than antigen levels) with genetic mutation in the s1C-s4B region.[132,140] The decreased antigen level may be a result of a combination of factors, including reduced synthesis and secretion as well as increased catabolism.[129] Clinically, type II HBS mutations occur in the general population at about 0.03% to 0.04% and are associated with a low risk of thrombosis in heterozygous carriers.[139,141,142] This raises the possibility that it may be useful to distinguish HBS defects from other type II defects.

Commercially available assays of antithrombin function predominantly use chromogenic amidolytic methods. Heparin and excess thrombin are added to the patient's plasma and the patient's endogenous antithrombin inactivates the thrombin. The amount of thrombin remaining is spectrophotometrically measured by its cleavage of a chromogenic peptide substrate, and is inversely proportional to the patient's antithrombin level. Factor Xa can be used in place of thrombin, because antithrombin also inhibits factor Xa. This can reduce the contribution of other natural thrombin inhibitors like heparin cofactor II, which can cause overestimation of antithrombin levels by thrombin-based assays but not by factor Xa-based assays.[143] However, one study suggested that the factor Xa-based assay may be less sensitive to type II deficiencies than the thrombin-based assay.[144] To further reduce the contribution of nonspecific cleavage by other natural proteases, assays have used protease inhibitors such as aprotinin, as well as bovine thrombin, which is resistant to cleavage facilitated by heparin cofactor II.[129] Because this method measures the heparin cofactor activity of antithrombin, it depends on both the HBS and the RS of antithrombin, and thus identifies all types of antithrombin deficiency without distinguishing type II HBS from other defects.[139] A variant of this assay, performed in the absence of heparin with a prolonged incubation time (300 seconds), is much slower (progressive activity) and measures activity independent of the HBS. Thus, a type II HBS deficiency would exhibit progressive activity (ie, increased activity with prolonged incubation time), unlike a type II RS defect.[139,145,146] Because the progressive activity assay can be affected by other inhibitors such as trypsin inhibitor and a2-macroglobulin, it is not commonly used as a screening assay.[147] Overall, with antithrombin III activity assays the ECAT study shows an interlaboratory and intralaboratory variability of 7.4% and 5.8% to 10.3% respectively, lower than of assays for protein C and protein S activity.[93] This likely reflects the higher complexity in the performance of clotting-based assays, compared to chromogenic assays.

Antigen levels were first tested by radial immunodiffusion and Laurell rocket electrophoresis. Newer methods include ELISAs and immunoturbidimetric methods. The 2008 ECAT data show a similar coefficient of variation (CV) of 6.0% and 9.1% for measurements of antithrombin function and antigen respectively (ECAT 2008 data).[129]

Over 127 distinct mutations are known to confer antithrombin deficiency (see **Table 3**)[148,149] (http://www1.imperial.ac.uk/medicine/about/divisions/is/haemo/coag/antithrombin); therefore, DNA testing is generally not available outside of specialized research laboratories. Although most of these mutations are private mutations dispersed throughout the gene, a recent study identified one mutation (antithrombin Cambridge II, A384S) that is relatively common in British and Spanish populations and seems to confer a ninefold increased risk of venous thrombosis.[149] Notably, this mutation is not associated with decreased functional or antigenic levels and could be underdiagnosed. However, a review of the Paris PATHROS cohort showed a much lower prevalence of this mutation, and its significance remains unclear.[132]

Several conditions can give rise to acquired antithrombin deficiency. These include liver disease, active thrombosis, surgical procedures, DIC, and L-asparaginase therapy for the same reasons outlined with regard to protein C and protein S. In addition, low antithrombin levels can be seen with inflammatory bowel disease and significant proteinuria such as in nephrotic syndrome. Anticoagulants affect antithrombin levels differently from protein C and protein S levels. Full-dose heparin administration can cause up to a 30% reduction in antithrombin levels within several days; antithrombin levels return to normal when heparin is discontinued.[150] Antithrombin levels may *increase* during oral anticoagulation, in contrast with protein C and protein S. Antithrombin levels can be decreased by oral contraceptives and pregnancy, and are lower in premenopausal women but higher in postmenopausal women, compared with men.[151]

Interestingly, a growing body of work is describing other possible roles for antithrombin testing. Antithrombin levels appear to decrease significantly in septic patients (as expected if DIC is present), and a study of patients with systemic inflammatory response syndrome (SIRS) found antithrombin activity to be the most useful predictor of organ dysfunction.[152,153] Moreover, antithrombin appears to have thrombin-independent effects on the function of endothelial cells and leukocytes.[154,155] Recent work suggests this may be in part attributable to antithrombin interacting with cell-surface glycosaminoglycans, leading to blocking NF-κB activation and modulation of gene expression.[156] These studies raise the possibility that testing for distinct functions of antithrombin in various clinical contexts may become important in the future.

Special Considerations for Antithrombin Testing in Pediatrics

At birth, antithrombin levels are on average decreased to 63% (range 39% to 87%) of adult normal values. Antithrombin rises to adult normal values within 6 months.[97]

Alpha-2-macroglobulin, a natural thrombin inhibitor, is elevated in newborns and children relative to adult values. It has been proposed that the elevated alpha-2-macroglobulin helps compensate for the low antithrombin observed at birth.[157] Between the ages of 1 and 16 years, antithrombin levels tend to be higher than adult levels.[98,99]

Recommendations for Testing for Antithrombin Deficiency

A functional assay should be used for screening. If the result is decreased, an antigenic assay may be performed to distinguish type I and type II deficiencies. As with low protein C and low protein S, confirmatory testing on a repeat specimen should be performed. Acquired causes of antithrombin deficiency must be excluded before making a diagnosis of hereditary antithrombin deficiency. Laboratory tests used to assess for acquired causes of decreased antithrombin are the same as listed above for protein S. Because DNA testing is not routinely available, confirmation of a hereditary deficiency may require demonstrating decreased antithrombin in a relative with a history of thrombosis.

PROTHROMBIN G20210A

Prothrombin (factor II) is hepatically synthesized, and its activity is vitamin K dependent. Prothrombin is activated by factor Xa cleavage to generate the serine protease thrombin. The gene encoding prothrombin comprises 14 exons spread over 21 kb on chromosome 11.[158] A candidate gene approach revealed a mutation in the 3′ untranslated region of the prothrombin gene (G20210A) to be associated with slightly increased plasma levels of prothrombin and a 2.8-fold increased risk of venous thrombosis.[83,158] Similarly, a pooled case-control study showed a three- to fivefold lifetime increased risk of venous thrombosis.[25] In adults, there has not been a consistent association of prothrombin G20210A with either ischemic stroke[28] or myocardial infarction.[30]

Prothrombin G20210A is a gain-of-function mutation that affects plasma protein levels by increasing mRNA formation by affecting 3′ end processing and/or enhancing translation efficiency.[159,160] Increased prothrombin level is itself correlated with increased thrombotic risk (odds ratio 2.1 for levels >115%).[158] The mechanism of this hypercoagulability is unclear. Although data are consistent with hyperprothrombinemia leading to increased thrombin generation, a recent study suggests that other mechanisms, such as thrombin activatable fibrinolysis inhibitor (TAFI)-mediated inhibition of fibrinolysis, may also be important.[161,162]

Prothrombin G20210A is thought to arise from a founder mutation about 24,000 years ago and differs with geographic and ethnic factors.[11] This mutation is present in heterozygous form in 2% to 4% of Europeans, and is rare in Asians and Africans.[11,158] It is present in 6% to 8% of patients with venous thrombosis[83,130,158] and in 18% of patients with venous thrombosis from thrombophilic families.[158] Testing for the mutation relies on molecular methods including PCR-based assays paired with various detection methods, and methods that do not rely on template amplification as mentioned for FV$_{Leiden}$.[158,163]

ANTIPHOSPHOLIPID ANTIBODIES

Antiphospholipid antibody syndrome is an important cause of acquired thrombophilia associated with an increased risk of arterial thrombosis, venous thrombosis, and recurrent pregnancy loss.[164] Diagnosis of antiphospholipid antibody syndrome requires demonstrating persistently elevated levels of antiphospholipid antibodies

(APAs) in the setting of thrombosis or certain pregnancy complications.[165] APAs are acquired autoantibodies directed against phospholipid-protein complexes. They can be found in 3% to 5% of the general population, and even more frequently in patients with systemic lupus erythematosis (SLE) and other autoimmune conditions. Current diagnostic criteria require a lupus anticoagulant (LA), a medium- or high-titer anticardiolipin (aCL) antibody, or medium- or high-titer anti-β_2-glycoprotein I (anti-β_2GP1) antibodies (although the authors did not reach consensus on the inclusion of anti-β_2GP1).[165] Of these, a study suggests that LAs pose the highest risk for arterial and venous thrombosis.[166,167] In individuals with high-titer IgG aCL antibodies (>40 IgG phospholipid units [GPL]), a prospective study found a rate of thrombosis of 6.1% per year, compared with 0.95% per year in individuals with no history of thrombosis, 4.3% in patients with SLE, and 5.5% in patients with a history of thrombosis.[168] Pregnancy loss has been linked to APAs in several studies, including the Thrombosis: Risk and Economic Assessment of Thrombophilia Screening (TREATS) study, which reported an odds ratio (OR) of 3.40 with aCL antibodies and an OR of 2.97 with LAs.[169,170]

Assays for APAs can be complex, and they exhibit high levels of interlaboratory variability.[165] Assays for LA are clotting time–based, such as dilute RVV-, PT-, or PTT-based assays, where "dilute" indicates a low concentration of phospholipid. LAs are thought to prolong clotting times in vitro by interfering with phospholipid's ability to serve as a cofactor in the coagulation cascade. To improve sensitivity, LA assays are usually performed with low concentrations of phospholipid and two or more screening tests for LA are suggested. An abnormal (prolonged) screening result is typically repeated on a 1:1 mix of patient plasma and normal plasma. If the clotting time remains prolonged in this mixture, confirmatory testing is then performed to demonstrate that the clotting time shortens toward normal after adding excess phospholipid. Mixing studies are often falsely normal despite the presence of LA;[171] therefore, some laboratories perform confirmatory testing if the screen is prolonged, regardless of the mixing study result. Both samples and normal plasmas used for the mixing studies should be depleted of platelets before freezing to prevent platelet phospholipid from decreasing sensitivity.[172] Importantly, LAs may or may not prolong routine PTTs, depending on the amount of phospholipid in the PTT reagent. Because heparin can cause false positive mixing studies and also interfere in confirmatory testing, some (but not all) commercial LA assays incorporate heparin neutralizers. New anticoagulants, namely the thrombin inhibitors argatroban, hirudin, and bivalirudin, can also cause false positive mixing studies and interfere with LA assays.[173]

Commercially available assays for aCL and anti-β_2GP1 antibodies rely on ELISA techniques. In these assays, cardiolipin or β_2GP1 are bound to a solid phase and bind any aCL or anti-β_2GP1 antibody in the patient sample respectively. Bound antibody is subsequently detected using a secondary antibody labeled for colorimetric quantitation. ELISA assays are also available for other phospholipids. Interlaboratory agreement is marginal. False positive IgM aCL results can be associated with rheumatoid factor and cryoglobulins.[174,175] The Royal College of Pathologists of Australasia Immunology Quality Assurance Program (QAP) study among 20 laboratories found total consensus in 41% of specimens with interlaboratory quantitative results showing CV greater than 50%.[176] Similarly, a study of 10 centers offering testing for several different APA antibodies found a clear diagnostic consensus in only 55% of patients.[177]

Special considerations may apply in pediatric populations, including different cutoff values and increased prevalence of APAs induced by infections, but further studies are needed to delineate these clearly.[178] Pediatric populations may also exhibit clinically important distinctions, including increased incidence of sinus vein thrombosis and stroke.[179]

Recommendations for Testing

The diagnosis of antiphospholipid antibody syndrome requires a positive test in the antiphospholipid antibody test panel (lupus anticoagulant, aCL, and/or anti-β_2GP1 antibodies) on two separate occasions, at least 12 weeks apart, in the setting of thrombosis or pregnancy complications. The aCL and anti-β_2GP1 antibodies should be of moderate or high titer.

SUMMARY

Laboratory testing plays an important role in identifying a growing number of hypercoagulable states in the thrombophilic patient. The presence of multiple risk factors appears to synergistically increase the risk for thrombosis. Advances in our understanding of the molecular underpinnings of these hypercoagulable conditions have important implications not just in how the performance of existing assays can be improved, but also in pointing out relevant new diagnostic targets. It is likely that future laboratory evaluation will be enhanced not just by DNA-based assays that identify heritable defects in hemostatic proteins, but also by rapidly expanding discovery of their novel interacting partners and pathways.

REFERENCES

1. Griffin JH, Fernandez JA, Gale AJ, et al. Activated protein C. J Thromb Haemost 2007;1(Suppl 5):73–80.
2. Nesheim M, Wang W, Boffa M, et al. Thrombin, thrombomodulin and TAFI in the molecular link between coagulation and fibrinolysis. Thromb Haemost 1997;78: 386–91.
3. Dahlback B. Resistance to activate protein C, the Arg506 to Gln mutation in the factor V gene, and venous thrombosis. Functional tests and DNA-based assays, pros and cons. Thromb Haemost 1995;73:739–42.
4. Dahlback B, Carlsson M, Svensson PJ. Familial thrombophilia due to a previously unrecognized mechanism characterized by poor anticoagulant response to activated protein C: prediction of a cofactor to activated protein C. Proc Natl Acad Sci U S A 1993;90:1004–8.
5. Griffin JH, Evatt B, Wideman C, et al. Anticoagulant protein C pathway defective in majority of thrombophilic patients. Blood 1993;82:1989–93.
6. Koster T, Rosendaal FR, de Ronde H, et al. Venous thrombosis due to poor anticoagulant response to activated protein C: Leiden Thrombophilia Study. Lancet 1993;342:1503–6.
7. Svensson PJ, Dahlback B. Resistance to activated protein C as a basis for venous thrombosis. N Engl J Med 1994;330:517–22.
8. Bertina RM, Koeleman BP, Koster T, et al. Mutation in blood coagulation factor V associated with resistance to activated protein C. Nature 1994;369:64–7.
9. Greengard JS, Sun X, Xu X, et al. Activated protein C resistance caused by Arg506Gln mutation in factor Va. Lancet 1994;343:1361–2.
10. Zoller B, Dahlback B. Linkage between inherited resistance to activated protein C and factor V gene mutation in venous thrombosis. Lancet 1994;343:1536–8.

11. Zivelin A, Mor-Cohen R, Kovalsky V, et al. Prothrombin 20210G>A is an ancestral prothrombotic mutation that occurred in whites approximately 24,000 years ago. Blood 2006;107:4666–8.
12. Voorberg J, Roelse J, Koopman R, et al. Association of idiopathic venous thromboembolism with single point-mutation at Arg506 of factor V. Lancet 1994;343:1535–6.
13. Chan LC, Bourke C, Lam CK, et al. Lack of activated protein C resistance in healthy Hong Kong Chinese blood donors—correlation with absence of Arg506-Gln mutation of factor V gene. Thromb Haemost 1996;75:522–3.
14. Hooper WC, Dilley A, Ribeiro MJ, et al. A racial difference in the prevalence of the Arg506–>Gln mutation. Thromb Res 1996;81:577–81.
15. Kohler HP, Boothby M, McCormack L, et al. Incidence of Arg506–> Gln mutation (factor V Leiden) in Pima Indians. Thromb Haemost 1997;78:961–2.
16. Ozawa T, Niiya K, Sakuragawa N. Absence of factor V Leiden in the Japanese. Thromb Res 1996;81:595–6.
17. Rees DC, Cox M, Clegg JB. World distribution of factor V Leiden. Lancet 1995;346:1133–4.
18. Ridker PM, Miletich JP, Hennekens CH, et al. Ethnic distribution of factor V Leiden in 4047 men and women. Implications for venous thromboembolism screening. JAMA 1997;277:1305–7.
19. Ridker PM, Hennekens CH, Lindpaintner K, et al. Mutation in the gene coding for coagulation factor V and the risk of myocardial infarction, stroke, and venous thrombosis in apparently healthy men. N Engl J Med 1995;332:912–7.
20. Rosendaal FR, Koster T, Vandenbroucke JP, et al. High risk of thrombosis in patients homozygous for factor V Leiden (activated protein C resistance). Blood 1995;85:1504–8.
21. Bloemenkamp KW, Rosendaal FR, Helmerhorst FM, et al. Enhancement by factor V Leiden mutation of risk of deep-vein thrombosis associated with oral contraceptives containing a third-generation progestagen. Lancet 1995;346:1593–6.
22. Dizon-Townson DS, Nelson LM, Jang H, et al. The incidence of the factor V Leiden mutation in an obstetric population and its relationship to deep vein thrombosis. Am J Obstet Gynecol 1997;176:883–6.
23. Koeleman BP, van Rumpt D, Hamulyak K, et al. Factor V Leiden: an additional risk factor for thrombosis in protein S deficient families? Thromb Haemost 1995;74:580–3.
24. Ridker PM, Glynn RJ, Miletich JP, et al. Age-specific incidence rates of venous thromboembolism among heterozygous carriers of factor V Leiden mutation. Ann Intern Med 1997;126:528–31.
25. Emmerich J, Rosendaal FR, Cattaneo M, et al. Combined effect of factor V Leiden and prothrombin 20210A on the risk of venous thromboembolism—pooled analysis of 8 case-control studies including 2310 cases and 3204 controls. Study Group for Pooled-Analysis in Venous Thromboembolism. Thromb Haemost 2001;86:809–16.
26. de Paula Sabino A, Ribeiro DD, Carvalho MG, et al. Factor V Leiden and increased risk for arterial thrombotic disease in young Brazilian patients. Blood Coagul Fibrinolysis 2006;17:271–5.
27. Juul K, Tybjaerg-Hansen A, Steffensen R, et al. Factor V Leiden: The Copenhagen City Heart Study and 2 meta-analyses. Blood 2002;100:3–10.
28. Rahemtullah A, Van Cott EM. Hypercoagulation testing in ischemic stroke. Arch Pathol Lab Med 2007;131:890–901.
29. Segers K, Dahlback B, Nicolaes GA. Coagulation factor V and thrombophilia: background and mechanisms. Thromb Haemost 2007;98:530–42.

30. Van Cott EM, Laposata M, Prins MH. Laboratory evaluation of hypercoagulability with venous or arterial thrombosis. Arch Pathol Lab Med 2002;126:1281–95.

31. Castoldi E, Brugge JM, Nicolaes GA, et al. Impaired APC cofactor activity of factor V plays a major role in the APC resistance associated with the factor V Leiden (R506Q) and R2 (H1299R) mutations. Blood 2004;103:4173–9.

32. Bernardi F, Faioni EM, Castoldi E, et al. A factor V genetic component differing from factor V R506Q contributes to the activated protein C resistance phenotype. Blood 1997;90:1552–7.

33. Biswas A, Bajaj J, Ranjan R, et al. Factor V Leiden: is it the chief contributor to activated protein C resistance in Asian-Indian patients with deep vein thrombosis? Clin Chim Acta 2008;392:21–4.

34. de Visser MC, Guasch JF, Kamphuisen PW, et al. The HR2 haplotype of factor V: effects on factor V levels, normalized activated protein C sensitivity ratios and the risk of venous thrombosis. Thromb Haemost 2000;83:577–82.

35. Steen M, Norstrom EA, Tholander AL, et al. Functional characterization of factor V-Ile359Thr: a novel mutation associated with thrombosis. Blood 2004;103: 3381–7.

36. Franco RF, Elion J, Tavella MH, et al. The prevalence of factor V Arg306–>Thr (factor V Cambridge) and factor V Arg306–>Gly mutations in different human populations. Thromb Haemost 1999;81:312–3.

37. Norstrom E, Thorelli E, Dahlback B. Functional characterization of recombinant FV Hong Kong and FV Cambridge. Blood 2002;100:524–30.

38. Chan WP, Lee CK, Kwong YL, et al. A novel mutation of Arg306 of factor V gene in Hong Kong Chinese. Blood 1998;91:1135–9.

39. de Visser MC, Rosendaal FR, Bertina RM. A reduced sensitivity for activated protein C in the absence of factor V Leiden increases the risk of venous thrombosis. Blood 1999;93:1271–6.

40. Kamphuisen PW, Haan J, Rosekrans PC, et al. Deep-vein thrombosis and coumarin skin necrosis associated with a factor V inhibitor with lupus-like features. Am J Hematol 1998;57:176–8.

41. Ortel TL. Clinical and laboratory manifestations of anti-factor V antibodies. J Lab Clin Med 1999;133:326–34.

42. Ortel TL, Charles LA, Keller FG, et al. Topical thrombin and acquired coagulation factor inhibitors: clinical spectrum and laboratory diagnosis. Am J Hematol 1994;45:128–35.

43. Negaard HF, Iversen PO, Ostenstad B, et al. Increased acquired activated protein C resistance in unselected patients with hematological malignancies. J Thromb Haemost 2008;6:1482–7.

44. Andre E, Hacquard M, Alnot Y, et al. Activated protein C resistance test using factor VIII-deficient plasma: a new approach to the venous thrombotic risk? Thromb Haemost 2007;98:693–4.

45. Mosnier LO, Zlokovic BV, Griffin JH. The cytoprotective protein C pathway. Blood 2007;109:3161–72.

46. Domotor E, Benzakour O, Griffin JH, et al. Activated protein C alters cytosolic calcium flux in human brain endothelium via binding to endothelial protein C receptor and activation of protease activated receptor-1. Blood 2003;101:4797–801.

47. Riewald M, Petrovan RJ, Donner A, et al. Activation of endothelial cell protease activated receptor 1 by the protein C pathway. Science 2002;296:1880–2.

48. Riewald M, Ruf W. Protease-activated receptor-1 signaling by activated protein C in cytokine-perturbed endothelial cells is distinct from thrombin signaling. J Biol Chem 2005;280:19808–14.

49. Toltl LJ, Beaudin S, Liaw PC. Activated protein C up-regulates IL-10 and inhibits tissue factor in blood monocytes. J Immunol 2008;181:2165–73.

50. Xue M, March L, Sambrook PN, et al. Differential regulation of matrix metalloproteinase 2 and matrix metalloproteinase 9 by activated protein C: relevance to inflammation in rheumatoid arthritis. Arthritis Rheum 2007;56:2864–74.

51. Rosendorff A, Dorfman DM. Activated protein C resistance and factor V Leiden: a review. Arch Pathol Lab Med 2007;131:866–71.

52. Strobl FJ, Hoffman S, Huber S, et al. Activated protein C resistance assay performance: improvement by sample dilution with factor V-deficient plasma. Arch Pathol Lab Med 1998;122:430–3.

53. Sweeney JD, Blair AJ, King TC. Comparison of an activated partial thromboplastin time with a Russell viper venom time test in screening for factor V(Leiden) (FVR506Q). Am J Clin Pathol 1997;108:74–7.

54. Zehnder JL, Benson RC. Sensitivity and specificity of the APC resistance assay in detection of individuals with factor V Leiden. Am J Clin Pathol 1996;106:107–11.

55. de Ronde H, Bertina RM. Laboratory diagnosis of APC-resistance: a critical evaluation of the test and the development of diagnostic criteria. Thromb Haemost 1994;72:880–6.

56. Trossaert M, Conard J, Horellou MH, et al. Influence of storage conditions on activated protein C resistance assay. Thromb Haemost 1995;73:163–4.

57. Jorquera JI, Montoro JM, Fernandez MA, et al. Modified test for activated protein C resistance. Lancet 1994;344:1162–3.

58. Trossaert M, Conard J, Horellou MH, et al. The modified APC resistance test in the presence of factor V deficient plasma can be used in patients without oral anticoagulant. Thromb Haemost 1996;75:521–2.

59. Rosen S, Andersson N-E, Andersson M, et al. Modified COATEST(R) APCTM resistance assay including V-DEF plasma with a heparin antagonist: analysis of heparin and OAC plasmas and influence of preanalytical variables. Blood Coagul Fibrinolysis 1996;7:390.

60. Shaikh S, Van Cott EM. The effect of argatroban on activated protein C resistance. Am J Clin Pathol 2009;131:828–33.

61. Saenz AJ, Van Cott EM. Clinical significance of acquired activated protein C resistance caused by lupus anticoagulants. Mod Pathol 2008;21:273A.

62. Coatest APC Resistance V assay. Chromogenix/Instrumentation Laboratory. Milano, Italy; 2008 [package insert].

63. Ragland BD, Reed CE, Eiland BM, et al. The effect of lupus anticoagulant in the second-generation assay for activated protein C resistance. Am J Clin Pathol 2003;119:66–71.

64. Martorell JR, Munoz-Castillo A, Gil JL. False positive activated protein C resistance test due to anti-phospholipid antibodies is corrected by platelet extract. Thromb Haemost 1995;74:796–7.

65. Brandt G, Gruppo R, Glueck CJ, et al. Sensitivity, specificity and predictive value of modified assays for activated protein C resistance in children. Thromb Haemost 1998;79:567–70.

66. Tripodi A, Chantarangkul V, Negri B, et al. Standardization of the APC resistance test. Effects of normalization of results by means of pooled normal plasma. Thromb Haemost 1998;79:564–6.

67. Voelkerding KV, Wu L, Williams EC, et al. Factor V R506Q gene mutation analysis by PCR-RFLP: optimization, comparison with functional testing for resistance to activated protein C, and establishment of cell line controls. Am J Clin Pathol 1996;106:100–6.

68. Wilmer M, Stocker C, Buhler B, et al. Improved distinction of factor V wild-type and factor V Leiden using a novel prothrombin-based activated protein C resistance assay. Am J Clin Pathol 2004;122:836–42.

69. Le DT, Griffin JH, Greengard JS, et al. Use of a generally applicable tissue factor–dependent factor V assay to detect activated protein C-resistant factor Va in patients receiving warfarin and in patients with a lupus anticoagulant. Blood 1995;85:1704–11.

70. van Oerle R, van Pampus L, Tans G, et al. The clinical application of a new specific functional assay to detect the factor V(Leiden) mutation associated with activated protein C resistance. Am J Clin Pathol 1997;107:521–6.

71. Male C, Mitchell L, Julian J, et al. Acquired activated protein C resistance is associated with lupus anticoagulants and thrombotic events in pediatric patients with systemic lupus erythematosus. Blood 2001;97:844–9.

72. Schrijver I, Lay MJ, Zehnder JL. Diagnostic single nucleotide polymorphism analysis of factor V Leiden and prothrombin 20210G > A. A comparison of the Nanogen Eelectronic Microarray with restriction enzyme digestion and the Roche LightCycler. Am J Clin Pathol 2003;119:490–6.

73. Liebman HA, Sutherland D, Bacon R, et al. Evaluation of a tissue factor dependent factor V assay to detect factor V Leiden: demonstration of high sensitivity and specificity for a generally applicable assay for activated protein C resistance. Br J Haematol 1996;95:550–3.

74. Uttenreuther-Fischer MM, Ziemer S, Gaedicke G. Resistance to activated protein C (APCR): reference values of APC-ratios for children. Thromb Haemost 1996;76:813–4.

75. Nowak-Gottl U, Kohlhase B, Vielhaber H, et al. APC resistance in neonates and infants: adjustment of the APTT-based method. Thromb Res 1996;81:665–70.

76. Inbal A, Kenet G, Zivelin A, et al. Purpura fulminans induced by disseminated intravascular coagulation following infection in 2 unrelated children with double heterozygosity for factor V Leiden and protein S deficiency. Thromb Haemost 1997;77:1086–9.

77. Pipe SW, Schmaier AH, Nichols WC, et al. Neonatal purpura fulminans in association with factor V R506Q mutation. J Pediatr 1996;128:706–9.

78. Press RD, Bauer KA, Kujovich JL, et al. Clinical utility of factor V leiden (R506Q) testing for the diagnosis and management of thromboembolic disorders. Arch Pathol Lab Med 2002;126:1304–18.

79. Taylor LJ, Oster RA, Fritsma GA, et al. Screening with the activated protein C resistance assay yields significant savings in a patient population with low prevalence of factor V leiden. Am J Clin Pathol 2008;129:494–9.

80. Stenflo J. A new vitamin K-dependent protein. Purification from bovine plasma and preliminary characterization. J Biol Chem 1976;251:355–63.

81. Miletich J, Sherman L, Broze G Jr. Absence of thrombosis in subjects with heterozygous protein C deficiency. N Engl J Med 1987;317:991–6.

82. Tait RC, Walker ID, Reitsma PH, et al. Prevalence of protein C deficiency in the healthy population. Thromb Haemost 1995;73:87–93.

83. van der Meer FJ, Koster T, Vandenbroucke JP, et al. The Leiden Thrombophilia Study (LETS). Thromb Haemost 1997;78:631–5.

84. Melissari E, Monte G, Lindo VS, et al. Congenital thrombophilia among patients with venous thromboembolism. Blood Coagul Fibrinolysis 1992;3:749–58.

85. Vossen CY, Conard J, Fontcuberta J, et al. Familial thrombophilia and lifetime risk of venous thrombosis. J Thromb Haemost 2004;2:1526–32.

86. Mahmoodi BK, Brouwer JL, Veeger NJ, et al. Hereditary deficiency of protein C or protein S confers increased risk of arterial thromboembolic events at a young age: results from a large family cohort study. Circulation 2008;118:1659–67.
87. Finazzi G, Barbui T. Different incidence of venous thrombosis in patients with inherited deficiencies of antithrombin III, protein C and protein S. Thromb Haemost 1994;71:15–8.
88. Reitsma PH. Protein C deficiency: from gene defects to disease. Thromb Haemost 1997;78:344–50.
89. Reitsma PH, Bernardi F, Doig RG, et al. Protein C deficiency: a database of mutations, 1995 update. On behalf of the Subcommittee on Plasma Coagulation Inhibitors of the Scientific and Standardization Committee of the ISTH. Thromb Haemost 1995;73:876–89.
90. Ireland H, Bayston T, Thompson E, et al. Apparent heterozygous type II protein C deficiency caused by the factor V 506 Arg to Gln mutation. Thromb Haemost 1995;73:731–2.
91. Vasse M, Borg JY, Monconduit M. Protein C: Rouen, a new hereditary protein C abnormality with low anticoagulant but normal amidolytic activities. Thromb Res 1989;56:387–98.
92. Wojcik EG, Simioni P, d Berg M, et al. Mutations which introduce free cysteine residues in the Gla-domain of vitamin K dependent proteins result in the formation of complexes with alpha 1-microglobulin. Thromb Haemost 1996;75:70–5.
93. Meijer P, Kluft C, Haverkate F, et al. The long-term within- and between-laboratory variability for assay of antithrombin, and proteins C and S: results derived from the external quality assessment program for thrombophilia screening of the ECAT Foundation. J Thromb Haemost 2003;1:748–53.
94. Mitchell CA, Rowell JA, Hau L, et al. A fatal thrombotic disorder associated with an acquired inhibitor of protein C. N Engl J Med 1987;317:1638–42.
95. Malm J, Laurell M, Dahlback B. Changes in the plasma levels of vitamin K-dependent proteins C and S and of C4b-binding protein during pregnancy and oral contraception. Br J Haematol 1988;68:437–43.
96. Henkens CM, Bom VJ, Van der Schaaf W, et al. Plasma levels of protein S, protein C, and factor X: effects of sex, hormonal state and age. Thromb Haemost 1995;74:1271–5.
97. Andrew M, Paes B, Milner R, et al. Development of the human coagulation system in the full-term infant. Blood 1987;70:165–72.
98. Andrew M, Vegh P, Johnston M, et al. Maturation of the hemostatic system during childhood. Blood 1992;80:1998–2005.
99. Monagle P, Barnes C, Ignjatovic V, et al. Developmental haemostasis. Impact for clinical haemostasis laboratories. Thromb Haemost 2006;95:362–72.
100. Toh CH, Samis J, Downey C, et al. Biphasic transmittance waveform in the APTT coagulation assay is due to the formation of a Ca($++$)-dependent complex of C-reactive protein with very-low-density lipoprotein and is a novel marker of impending disseminated intravascular coagulation. Blood 2002;100:2522–9.
101. Maurissen LF, Thomassen MC, Nicolaes GA, et al. Re-evaluation of the role of the protein S-C4b binding protein complex in activated protein C-catalyzed factor Va-inactivation. Blood 2008;111:3034–41.
102. Yegneswaran S, Hackeng TM, Dawson PE, et al. The thrombin-sensitive region of protein S mediates phospholipid-dependent interaction with factor Xa. J Biol Chem 2008;283:33046–52.

103. Garcia de Frutos P, Fuentes-Prior P, Hurtado B, et al. Molecular basis of protein S deficiency. Thromb Haemost 2007;98:543–56.

104. Rosing J, Maurissen LF, Tchaikovski SN, et al. Protein S is a cofactor for tissue factor pathway inhibitor. Thromb Res 2008;1(Suppl 122):S60–3.

105. Castoldi E, Hackeng TM. Regulation of coagulation by protein S. Curr Opin Hematol 2008;15:529–36.

106. Dykes AC, Walker ID, McMahon AD, et al. A study of protein S antigen levels in 3788 healthy volunteers: influence of age, sex and hormone use, and estimate for prevalence of deficiency state. Br J Haematol 2001;113:636–41.

107. Ten Kate MK, Platteel M, Mulder R, et al. PROS1 analysis in 87 pedigrees with hereditary protein S deficiency demonstrates striking genotype-phenotype associations. Hum Mutat 2008;29:939–47.

108. Strater R, Becker S, von Eckardstein A, et al. Prospective assessment of risk factors for recurrent stroke during childhood—a 5-year follow-up study. Lancet 2002;360:1540–5.

109. Aillaud MF, Pouymayou K, Brunet D, et al. New direct assay of free protein S antigen applied to diagnosis of protein S deficiency. Thromb Haemost 1996;75:283–5.

110. Pegelow CH, Ledford M, Young JN, et al. Severe protein S deficiency in a newborn. Pediatrics 1992;89:674–6.

111. Carter IS, Hewitt J, Pu CH, et al. Severe protein S deficiency resulting from two novel mutations in PROS1 presenting with a relatively mild clinical phenotype. J Thromb Haemost 2008;6:1237–9.

112. Heeb MJ, Gandrille S, Fernandez JA, et al. Late onset thrombosis in a case of severe protein S deficiency due to compound heterozygosity for PROS1 mutations. J Thromb Haemost 2008;6:1235–7.

113. Simmonds RE, Zoller B, Ireland H, et al. Genetic and phenotypic analysis of a large (122-member) protein S-deficient kindred provides an explanation for the familial coexistence of type I and type III plasma phenotypes. Blood 1997; 89:4364–70.

114. Goodwin AJ, Rosendaal FR, Kottke-Marchant K, et al. A review of the technical, diagnostic, and epidemiologic considerations for protein S assays. Arch Pathol Lab Med 2002;126:1349–66.

115. D'Angelo SV, Mazzola G, Della Valle P, et al. Variable interference of activated protein C resistance in the measurement of protein S activity by commercial assays. Thromb Res 1995;77:375–8.

116. Faioni EM, Boyer-Neumann C, Franchi F, et al. Another protein S functional assay is sensitive to resistance to activated protein C. Thromb Haemost 1994; 72:648.

117. Jennings I, Kitchen S, Cooper P, et al. Sensitivity of functional protein S assays to protein S deficiency: a comparative study of three commercial kits. J Thromb Haemost 2003;1:1112–4.

118. Carr Jr. ME, Steingold KA, Zekert SL. Protein S levels during the normal menstrual cycle and during estrogen therapy for premature ovarian failure. Am J Med Sci 1993;306:212–7.

119. Gilabert J, Estelles A, Cano A, et al. The effect of estrogen replacement therapy with or without progestogen on the fibrinolytic system and coagulation inhibitors in postmenopausal status. Am J Obstet Gynecol 1995;173:1849–54.

120. Hughes Q, Watson M, Cole V, et al. Upregulation of protein S by progestins. J Thromb Haemost 2007;5:2243–9.

121. Stahl CP, Wideman CS, Spira TJ, et al. Protein S deficiency in men with long-term human immunodeficiency virus infection. Blood 1993;81:1801–7.

122. Nguyen P, Reynaud J, Pouzol P, et al. Varicella and thrombotic complications associated with transient protein C and protein S deficiencies in children. Eur J Pediatr 1994;153:646–9.
123. Peyvandi F, Faioni E, Alessandro Moroni G, et al. Autoimmune protein S deficiency and deep vein thrombosis after chickenpox. Thromb Haemost 1996; 75:212–3.
124. Aadland E, Odegaard OR, Roseth A, et al. Free protein S deficiency in patients with chronic inflammatory bowel disease. Scand J Gastroenterol 1992;27:957–60.
125. Koutroubakis IE, Sfiridaki A, Mouzas IA, et al. Resistance to activated protein C and low levels of free protein S in Greek patients with inflammatory bowel disease. Am J Gastroenterol 2000;95:190–4.
126. Sorice M, Arcieri P, Griggi T, et al. Inhibition of protein S by autoantibodies in patients with acquired protein S deficiency. Thromb Haemost 1996;75:555–9.
127. Fernandez JA, Estelles A, Gilabert J, et al. Functional and immunologic protein S in normal pregnant women and in full-term newborns. Thromb Haemost 1989; 61:474–8.
128. Melissari E, Nicolaides KH, Scully MF, et al. Protein S and C4b-binding protein in fetal and neonatal blood. Br J Haematol 1988;70:199–203.
129. Kottke-Marchant K, Duncan A. Antithrombin deficiency: issues in laboratory diagnosis. Arch Pathol Lab Med 2002;126:1326–36.
130. Dahlback B. Advances in understanding pathogenic mechanisms of thrombophilic disorders. Blood 2008;112:19–27.
131. Okajima K, Uchiba M. The anti-inflammatory properties of antithrombin III: new therapeutic implications. Semin Thromb Hemost 1998;24:27–32.
132. Picard V, Nowak-Gottl U, Biron-Andreani C, et al. Molecular bases of antithrombin deficiency: twenty-two novel mutations in the antithrombin gene. Hum Mutat 2006;27:600.
133. De Stefano V, Finazzi G, Mannucci PM. Inherited thrombophilia: pathogenesis, clinical syndromes, and management. Blood 1996;87:3531–44.
134. Rodeghiero F, Tosetto A. The epidemiology of inherited thrombophilia: the VITA Project. Vicenza Thrombophilia and Atherosclerosis Project. Thromb Haemost 1997;78:636–40.
135. Tait RC, Walker ID, Perry DJ, et al. Prevalence of antithrombin deficiency in the healthy population. Br J Haematol 1994;87:106–12.
136. Demers C, Ginsberg JS, Hirsh J, et al. Thrombosis in antithrombin-III-deficient persons. Report of a large kindred and literature review. Ann Intern Med 1992;116:754–61.
137. Duhl AJ, Paidas MJ, Ural SH, et al. Antithrombotic therapy and pregnancy: consensus report and recommendations for prevention and treatment of venous thromboembolism and adverse pregnancy outcomes. Am J Obstet Gynecol 2007;197:457, e451–421.
138. Lane DA, Bayston T, Olds RJ, et al. Antithrombin mutation database: 2nd (1997) update. For the Plasma Coagulation Inhibitors Subcommittee of the Scientific and Standardization Committee of the International Society on Thrombosis and Haemostasis. Thromb Haemost 1997;77:197–211.
139. Rossi E, Chiusolo P, Za T, et al. Report of a novel kindred with antithrombin heparin-binding site variant (47 Arg to His): demand for an automated progressive antithrombin assay to detect molecular variants with low thrombotic risk. Thromb Haemost 2007;98:695–7.
140. Lane DA, Olds RJ, Conard J, et al. Pleiotropic effects of antithrombin strand 1C substitution mutations. J Clin Invest 1992;90:2422–33.

141. Girolami A, Lazzaro AR, Simioni P. The relationship between defective heparin cofactor activities and thrombotic phenomena in AT III abnormalities. Thromb Haemost 1988;59:121.

142. Wells PS, Blajchman MA, Henderson P, et al. Prevalence of antithrombin deficiency in healthy blood donors: a cross-sectional study. Am J Hematol 1994;45:321–4.

143. Demers C, Henderson P, Blajchman MA, et al. An antithrombin III assay based on factor Xa inhibition provides a more reliable test to identify congenital antithrombin III deficiency than an assay based on thrombin inhibition. Thromb Haemost 1993;69:231–5.

144. Ungerstedt JS, Schulman S, Egberg N, et al. Discrepancy between antithrombin activity methods revealed in Antithrombin Stockholm: do factor Xa-based methods overestimate antithrombin activity in some patients? Blood 2002;99: 2271–2.

145. Odegard OR, Lie M, Abildgaard U. Antifactor Xa activity measured with amidolytic methods. Haemostasis 1976;5:265–75.

146. Sas G, Pepper DS, Cash JD. Further investigations on antithrombin III in the plasmas of patients with the abnormality of antithrombin III Budapest. Thromb Diath Haemorrh 1975;33:564–72.

147. Downing MR, Bloom JW, Mann KG. Comparison of the inhibition of thrombin by three plasma protease inhibitors. Biochemistry 1978;17:2649–53.

148. Bayston TA, Lane DA. Antithrombin: molecular basis of deficiency. Thromb Haemost 1997;78:339–43.

149. Corral J, Hernandez-Espinosa D, Soria JM, et al. Antithrombin Cambridge II (A384S): an underestimated genetic risk factor for venous thrombosis. Blood 2007;109:4258–63.

150. Rao AK, Niewiarowski S, Guzzo J, et al. Antithrombin III levels during heparin therapy. Thromb Res 1981;24:181–6.

151. Meade TW, Dyer S, Howarth DJ, et al. Antithrombin III and procoagulant activity: sex differences and effects of the menopause. Br J Haematol 1990;74:77–81.

152. Iba T, Gando S, Murata A, et al. Predicting the severity of systemic inflammatory response syndrome (SIRS)-associated coagulopathy with hemostatic molecular markers and vascular endothelial injury markers. J Trauma 2007;63:1093–8.

153. Opal SM, Kessler CM, Roemisch J, et al. Antithrombin, heparin, and heparan sulfate. Crit Care Med 2002;30:S325–31.

154. Dunzendorfer S, Kaneider N, Rabensteiner A, et al. Cell-surface heparan sulfate proteoglycan-mediated regulation of human neutrophil migration by the serpin antithrombin III. Blood 2001;97:1079–85.

155. Souter PJ, Thomas S, Hubbard AR, et al. Antithrombin inhibits lipopolysaccharide-induced tissue factor and interleukin-6 production by mononuclear cells, human umbilical vein endothelial cells, and whole blood. Crit Care Med 2001;29:134–9.

156. Oelschlager C, Romisch J, Staubitz A, et al. Antithrombin III inhibits nuclear factor kappaB activation in human monocytes and vascular endothelial cells. Blood 2002;99:4015–20.

157. Ling X, Delorme M, Berry L, et al. alpha 2-Macroglobulin remains as important as antithrombin III for thrombin regulation in cord plasma in the presence of endothelial cell surfaces. Pediatr Res 1995;37:373–8.

158. Poort SR, Rosendaal FR, Reitsma PH, et al. A common genetic variation in the 3'-untranslated region of the prothrombin gene is associated with elevated plasma prothrombin levels and an increase in venous thrombosis. Blood 1996;88:3698–703.

159. Gehring NH, Frede U, Neu-Yilik G, et al. Increased efficiency of mRNA 3' end formation: a new genetic mechanism contributing to hereditary thrombophilia. Nat Genet 2001;28:389–92.
160. Pollak ES, Lam HS, Russell JE. The G20210A mutation does not affect the stability of prothrombin mRNA in vivo. Blood 2002;100:359–62.
161. Colucci M, Binetti BM, Tripodi A, et al. Hyperprothrombinemia associated with prothrombin G20210A mutation inhibits plasma fibrinolysis through a TAFI-mediated mechanism. Blood 2004;103:2157–61.
162. Eikelboom JW, Ivey L, Ivey J, et al. Familial thrombophilia and the prothrombin 20210A mutation: association with increased thrombin generation and unusual thrombosis. Blood Coagul Fibrinolysis 1999;10:1–5.
163. Ripoll L, Paulin D, Thomas S, et al. Multiplex PCR-mediated site-directed mutagenesis for one-step determination of factor V Leiden and G20210A transition of the prothrombin gene. Thromb Haemost 1997;78:960–1.
164. McNeil HP, Chesterman CN, Krilis SA. Immunology and clinical importance of antiphospholipid antibodies. Adv Immunol 1991;49:193–280.
165. Miyakis S, Lockshin MD, Atsumi T, et al. International consensus statement on an update of the classification criteria for definite antiphospholipid syndrome (APS). J Thromb Haemost 2006;4:295–306.
166. Galli M, Luciani D, Bertolini G, et al. Anti-beta 2-glycoprotein I, antiprothrombin antibodies, and the risk of thrombosis in the antiphospholipid syndrome. Blood 2003;102:2717–23.
167. Galli M, Luciani D, Bertolini G, et al. Lupus anticoagulants are stronger risk factors for thrombosis than anticardiolipin antibodies in the antiphospholipid syndrome: a systematic review of the literature. Blood 2003;101:1827–32.
168. Finazzi G, Brancaccio V, Moia M, et al. Natural history and risk factors for thrombosis in 360 patients with antiphospholipid antibodies: a four-year prospective study from the Italian Registry. Am J Med 1996;100:530–6.
169. Bates SM, Greer IA, Pabinger I, et al. Venous thromboembolism, thrombophilia, antithrombotic therapy, and pregnancy: American College of Chest Physicians Evidence-Based Clinical Practice Guidelines. 8th edition. Chest 2008;133:844S–86S.
170. Robertson L, Wu O, Langhorne P, et al. Thrombophilia in pregnancy: a systematic review. Br J Haematol 2006;132:171–96.
171. Zhang L, Whitis JG, Embry MB, et al. A simplified algorithm for the laboratory detection of lupus anticoagulants: utilization of two automated integrated tests. Am J Clin Pathol 2005;124:894–901.
172. Brandt JT, Triplett DA, Alving B, et al. Criteria for the diagnosis of lupus anticoagulants: an update. On behalf of the Subcommittee on Lupus Anticoagulant/ Antiphospholipid Antibody of the Scientific and Standardisation Committee of the ISTH. Thromb Haemost 1995;74:1185–90.
173. Genzen JR, Miller JL. Presence of direct thrombin inhibitors can affect the results and interpretation of lupus anticoagulant testing. Am J Clin Pathol 2005;124:586–93.
174. Bahar AM, Kwak JY, Beer AE, et al. Antibodies to phospholipids and nuclear antigens in non-pregnant women with unexplained spontaneous recurrent abortions. J Reprod Immunol 1993;24:213–22.
175. Spadaro A, Riccieri V, Terracina S, et al. Class specific rheumatoid factors and antiphospholipid syndrome in systemic lupus erythematosus. Lupus 2000;9:56–60.

176. Favaloro EJ, Wong RC, Jovanovich S, et al. A review of beta2 -glycoprotein-I antibody testing results from a peer-driven multilaboratory quality assurance program. Am J Clin Pathol 2007;127:441–8.
177. Kutteh WH, Franklin RD. Assessing the variation in antiphospholipid antibody (APA) assays: comparison of results from 10 centers. Am J Obstet Gynecol 2004;191:440–8.
178. Avcin T, Silverman ED. Antiphospholipid antibodies in pediatric systemic lupus erythematosus and the antiphospholipid syndrome. Lupus 2007;16:627–33.
179. Avcin T, Cimaz R, Silverman ED, et al. Pediatric antiphospholipid syndrome: clinical and immunologic features of 121 patients in an international registry. Pediatrics 2008;122:e1100–1107.

Molecular Diagnostics in Hemostatic Disorders

Peter L. Perrotta, MD[a,b,*], Annika M. Svensson, MD, PhD[a,b,c,d]

KEYWORDS

- Hemostasis • Coagulation • Thrombophilia • Molecular
- Testing • Genetic

The underlying molecular defects for many human disorders that are associated with imbalances in blood procoagulant and anticoagulant activities have been determined.[1] Some of these have been described in this issue (see the article by Korh and Van Cott, elsewhere in this issue). Classic family- and population-based genetic studies led to the discovery of coagulation factors with anticoagulant activity, including antithrombin (AT), protein C (PC), and protein S (PS). Later, advances in molecular biology allowed the genes coding for these proteins to be cloned and sequenced.[2–4] DNA technologies, including polymerase chain reaction (PCR), were used to identify specific mutations that result in the production of abnormal clotting proteins. Molecular diagnostic assays were then developed to detect these genetic disruptions associated with hemostatic diseases in a highly sensitive and specific manner. These assays are becoming more amenable to high-throughput testing and have gained widespread clinical use. In fact, factor V Leiden (FVL) and prothrombin (PT) G20210A mutation assays are two of the most commonly performed genetic tests. Other molecular hemostatic tests remain mainly research tools. The issues that laboratorians face in using DNA-based testing for coagulation disorders encompass those encountered in coagulation and molecular laboratories.

MOLECULAR TESTING FOR INHERITED THROMBOPHILIA

A predisposition to thrombosis, or thrombophilia, may be genetically predetermined based on overexpression of procoagulant proteins or underexpression of anticoagulant proteins. Thrombophilia is termed *acquired* when it is associated with external risk factors for thrombosis, including oral contraceptive or estrogen therapy, pregnancy or

[a] Department of Pathology, West Virginia University Health Sciences Center, Morgantown, WV 26506–9203, USA
[b] Clinical Laboratories, West Virginia University Hospital, Morgantown, WV, USA
[c] Department of Pathology, University of Utah, Salt Lake City, UT, USA
[d] ARUP Laboratories, Salt Lake City, UT, USA
* Corresponding author.
E-mail address: pperrotta@hsc.wvu.edu (P.L. Perrotta).

Clin Lab Med 29 (2009) 367–390
doi:10.1016/j.cll.2009.04.001
0272-2712/09/$ – see front matter © 2009 Elsevier Inc. All rights reserved.

labmed.theclinics.com

postpartum state, antiphospholipid syndrome, cancer, chemotherapy, and so forth. Major anticoagulant proteins include PC, AT, and PS. The serine protease inhibitor AT inhibits thrombin, F9a, F10, F11a, and F12 by irreversibly binding to active sites on these clotting factors. Activated protein C (APC) inactivates F5 and F8 in the presence of PS. With the exception of specific mutations that lead to reduced affinity for heparin, homozygosity for AT mutations seems to be incompatible with life. Homozygosity for PC and PS mutations may lead to neonatal purpura fulminans. Mutations that result in AT, PC, or PS deficiency are found in a few patients who have thrombotic disease, and these mutations are spread throughout the corresponding genes. Furthermore, correlations between genotype and phenotype are not yet fully understood. In cases with strong suspicion for a quantitative or qualitative defect of a specific factor, full gene sequencing may be attempted to confirm the diagnosis and to help direct specific therapy. In the United States, however, such analyses are available only in research laboratories. One US laboratory performs targeted mutation analysis for a PS mutation (PS Herleen, S460P) that results in poor APC cofactor activity when FVL is used as an APC substrate.[5,6]

The PT G20210A mutation is a gain-of-function mutation that affects the 3′ untranslated region of the gene. The mutation enhances the efficiency of the 3′ end cleavage signal, which results in increased mRNA accumulation and protein synthesis, ultimately leading to increased levels of PT in plasma.[7] The mutation seems to have originated in white populations approximately 20,000 years ago and is rarely seen in other ethnic groups. The carrier frequency is approximately 2% in the US population. The PT G20210A mutation increases the risk for venous thrombosis by a factor 2 to 3. Because the reference range for plasma PT activity is relatively wide, PT levels cannot be used to detect carriers of the PT gene mutations; molecular analysis is required. Genetic analysis must be able to differentiate the PT G20210A mutation from an unusual variant of uncertain significance, C20209T, that can interfere with these assays.[8,9] The two PT mutations can be discerned through melt analysis (**Fig. 1**). The variant can be detected by restriction enzyme treatment. The C20209T mutation can also be confirmed using bidirectional sequencing.

The FVL mutation (c.G1691A, p. R506Q) abolishes a recognition site for the Mnl I endonuclease, which renders the mutation detectable by restriction fragment length polymorphism (RFLP) methodology.[10,11] After PCR amplification of a DNA fragment containing the mutation, the amplicon is treated with Mnl I endonuclease. Genotyping is then performed by sizing the ensuing fragments by gel electrophoresis. This method is still used in some laboratories; however, it is not well-suited for high-throughput testing and is being replaced by other technologies. Allele-specific probe hybridization is based on the principle that probes specific to a mutated site bind efficiently to the target sequence only when the target is a perfect match (ie, in the presence or absence of the mutation, depending on the probe design). This methodology has been incorporated into various molecular platforms. One commercial assay (Invader; Third Wave Technology, Madison, Wisconsin) uses a non-PCR allele-specific hybridization method. Because the target DNA is not amplified, the platform can be placed in laboratories that are not specifically designed for molecular testing (ie, with separate areas for pre-PCR, PCR, and post-PCR procedures to minimize contamination by amplicon). Furthermore, the royalty fees that are associated with PCR amplification are avoided. The plate format makes this technology well suited to high-throughput settings. The assay is somewhat sensitive to sample quality or DNA concentration variation; however, it is generally regarded as a robust platform.

Several FVL and PT 20210G>A mutation assays have been approved by the US Food and Drug Administration (FDA) for clinical testing; a list of these is maintained

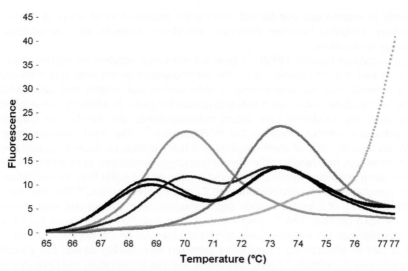

Fig. 1. Melt assay for PT G20210A mutation reveals a peak with a lower melting temperature (T_m) than would be expected for the PT G20210A mutation in a sample tested in triplicate (*black curves*). This peak corresponds to the PT G20209A mutation. Color code: red, wild type; green, PT G20210A homozygous; blue, PT G20210A heterozygous; yellow, nontemplate control; black, PT C20209T mutation tested in triplicate. (*Courtesy of* ARUP Laboratories, Salt Lake City, UT; with permission.)

by the Association for Molecular Pathology.[12] Per FDA requirements, all steps in the assay procedure, including sample preparation, must be performed exactly as described in the manufacturer's instructions. Validating FDA-approved assays is considerably less complicated than validating laboratory-developed tests ("homebrews"). In the case of an FDA-approved test, the laboratory is only required to show that the assay is applicable to the test population of that laboratory. If any changes are made to the protocol, however, the laboratory must perform extensive test validation, essentially to the extent required to validate a laboratory-developed test.

Currently, one real-time PCR assay has been approved by the FDA for FVL and PT G20210A mutation testing (Factor V Leiden Kit, Factor II G20210A Kit; Roche Diagnostics, Laval, Quebec, Canada). This assay uses two fluorescently labeled probes to detect the amplified product. The probes bind adjacent to the amplified fragment during the annealing phase of the PCR reaction. The proximity of the donor fluorophore (fluorescein) at the 3'end of one probe to the acceptor fluorophore (LightCycler Red 640) on the 5'end of the other probe enables fluorescence resonance energy transfer between the two fluorophores after excitation of the donor fluorophore. The intensity of fluorescence emitted from the acceptor fluorophore is then measured by the real-time PCR instrument. After amplification, a melting curve analysis is performed to confirm the presence of a specific mutation. The temperature is gradually increased beyond the point at which the shorter fluorescein-labeled probe, which spans the mutation site, dissociates (melts) from the template. The melting temperature (T_m) of the probe corresponds to the temperature at which 50% of the probes have dissociated from the templates. It varies based on the presence or absence of a mutation. When there is a discrepancy between the probe sequence and the target sequence, the binding between the probe and the template is less stable and melting occurs at a lower temperature. Real-time PCR with melt analysis methodology is currently in widespread use for detecting point mutations in all areas of molecular pathology, including inherited disorders, infectious diseases, and hematology or oncology applications.

High-resolution melting (HRM) analysis is a rapid and sensitive method for mutation scanning and targeted single-nucleotide polymorphism genotyping. This technology is made feasible by the engineering of plate-format instruments that can maintain stable temperatures within each well and across the plate. In addition, newer intercalating dyes (eg, LCGreen) can detect heteroduplexes and function at saturating concentrations without inhibiting the PCR reaction.[13] The least complex form of HRM monitors the melt of short amplicons. It is not always possible to design amplicon melt assays that reliably differentiate homozygous mutants from wild type. HRM assays using sequence-specific unlabeled probes do not suffer from this limitation. In HRM, genotypes can be distinguished by T_m and by curve shape.[14] The main factors affecting the T_m of a probe include oligonucleotide length (size) and total guanine-cytosine (GC) content. The T_m shift induced by a mutation depends on the binding strength between the mutated base and its counterpart on the opposite strand. The shift is further affected by interactions between neighboring bases, the so-called "nearest-neighbor effects." Assay conditions, such as temperature and ionic strength, can be modified to optimize detection of specific mutations. A clever technique devised to discriminate sequence variants better incorporates locked nucleic acids (LNAs) into the probe. LNAs are modified RNA nucleotides that significantly increase the T_m of oligonucleotide probes.[15] Alleles with a similar probe T_m can be better resolved using "masking" probes that neutralize the effects of polymorphisms near the mutation of interest.[16] Several high-throughput instruments have recently been developed that perform real-time PCR combined with HRM analysis in an automated fashion in one closed tube.[17] FVL and PT assays that use a single short unlabeled probe together with a saturating heteroduplex-detecting double-strand DNA dye can be performed on an integrated real-time PCR/HRM closed-tube platform (Light-Cycler 480 System; Roche Diagnostics, Indianapolis, Indiana). DNA is extracted using a robotic system to reduce hands-on time and to decrease overall turnaround time. Analysis software uses a proprietary algorithm that identifies samples as wild type, heterozygous, or homozygous by clustering groups based on T_m and curve shape. Samples that do not cluster into any of these groups are flagged as outliers (**Fig. 2**). These and other high-resolution assays are relatively sensitive to sample quality issues, including low template concentration or variation in ionic strength (ie, salt concentration) in the reaction mixture. Such problems can alter temperature transition rates, and hence T_ms, within a cluster, confounding the separation of wild-type and mutated sample groups.[18,19] In cases in which genotyping is suboptimal, samples may be re-extracted using a manual extraction method.

The automated and multiplexed INFINITI platform has been approved by the FDA for FVL and PT gene mutation testing (INFINITI; AutoGenomics, Carlsbad, California). This system is designed to operate in random access mode, such that FVL and PT testing can be performed separately or as a panel. A test for variants of the MTHFR gene is also available on this platform; however, it is not approved by the FDA for diagnostic testing. The INFINITI Analyzer (AutoGenomics) measures fluorescence signals emitted by labeled DNA targets hybridized to a microarray (BioFilmChip, Auto-Genomics). The three-dimensional film matrix consists of multiple layers, including (1) a polyester film base, (2) an optical blocking layer of proprietary composition that reduces intrinsic fluorescence, and (3) a hydrogel linker layer in which capture oligonucleotides are bound to streptavidin. DNA is first extracted and amplified by PCR off-line to generate amplicon that is loaded onto the INFINITI analyzer. The

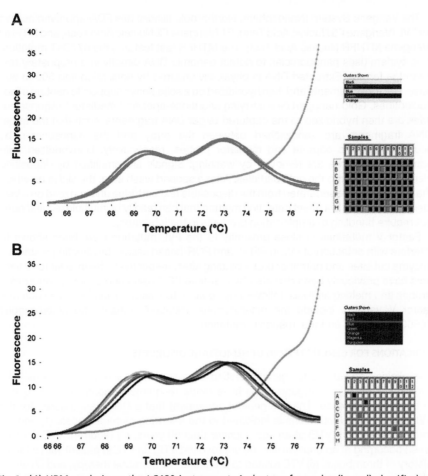

Fig. 2. (*A*) HRM analysis on the LC480 instrument. A cluster of samples (in red) classified as heterozygous based on T$_m$ and curve shape. (*B*) HRM analysis on the LC480 instrument. The figure shows several samples that were not included in a cluster (various colors). These samples are tentatively classified as heterozygous but are flagged for confirmatory review. (*Courtesy of* ARUP Laboratories, Salt Lake City, UT; with permission.)

amplicon is then detected using "detection primer extension," wherein complementary primers are first allowed to hybridize to their targets in the reaction mixture. The primers are then extended at their 3′ end by DNA polymerase. During this process, fluorescently labeled cytosine bases are incorporated into the extended product. After denaturation, the reaction mixture is transferred to the microarray. The extended primers contain a "flap" sequence at their 5′ end that is complementary to specific oligonucleotides trapped in discrete "spots" in the matrix that correspond to different genotypes. After hybridization of the flaps to the corresponding microarray oligonucleotides, laser scanning confocal microscopy detects fluorescence emanating from the cytosine bases incorporated into the extended primers. Each spot is assigned a fluorescence intensity value. All processes downstream of amplification are contained within the INFINITI Analyzer. Using this platform for genotyping requires handling of amplicon in the laboratory.

The Verigene System (Nanosphere, Northbrook, Illinois) has FDA-approved assays for FVL (Verigene F5 Nucleic Acid Test), PT (Verigene F2 Nucleic Acid Test), and MTFHR (Verigene MTHFR Nucleic Acid Test). The MTHFR test features the 677C>T mutation. This system uses nanoparticles to detect genomic DNA directly in a proprietary test cartridge format. Extracted DNA is physically sheared by sonication into 300 to 500 base-pair (bp) fragments and then hybridized on a solid phase support to capture oligonucleotides. Gold nanoparticles carrying sequence-specific "mediator" oligonucleotides are then hybridized to the captured target DNA fragments, such that the target DNA fragments are sandwiched between the array and the nanospheres by sequence-specific capture and mediator probes, respectively. Unhybridized gold nanoparticle probes are removed by washing. Signals are amplified by depositing elemental silver onto the gold particles. After a second wash step, the slides on which the matrix rests are separated from the disposable text cartridge unit and read on a Verigene reader. This is a direct detection method that can readily be multiplexed and does not require handling of amplification products in the laboratory.

Factor V mutations in close proximity to the FVL mutation have been shown to interfere with detection of FVL in RFLP- and PCR-based assays by affecting restriction enzyme cut sites and primer or probe binding sites, respectively. Several factor V variants have previously been detected by real-time PCR using fluorescent hybridization probes and melting analysis, followed by confirmatory sequencing.[20] Three such rare factor V variants include the heterozygous 1689G>A variant, the heterozygous 1690C>T variant, and the 1690delC mutation.

INDICATIONS FOR GENETIC TESTING OF HEMOSTATIC DISORDERS

The clinical indications for genetic testing in coagulation disorders are constantly evolving. Professional organizations have made recommendations for such testing in thrombotic disease. There is general agreement that a DNA-based assay for the FVL and PT gene mutations is indicated in the following circumstances: (1) venous thromboembolism (VTE) at an age younger than 50 years, (2) recurrent VTE, (3) VTE when occurring at an unusual site, (4) unprovoked VTE, (5) VTE in patient with a family history of thrombosis, (6) VTE related to pregnancy or hormone therapy, and (7) unexplained second- or third-trimester pregnancy loss.[21,22] In these scenarios, the FVL can be detected by an APC resistance assay using factor V-deficient plasma or a DNA-based test. These guidelines are not universally accepted, however, and laboratory testing for inherited thrombosis is widely variable.[23] Furthermore, the detection of a genetic abnormality in a patient who develops venous or arterial thrombosis does not necessarily change how that patient is managed.[24] There are no current recommendations for screening the general population for FVL during pregnancy or before surgery or oral contraceptive use. Several screening strategies have been proposed, but further studies are needed to determine their clinical effectiveness. The role of genetic testing for thrombotic risk in patients who have cancer is also unclear.[25]

STRENGTHS OF MOLECULAR TESTING FOR HEMOSTATIC DISEASE

Molecular testing is extremely useful for resolving patients as heterozygous or homozygous for a particular mutation associated with a coagulation disorder. Because clot-based assays have relatively wide analytic variability and carrier levels may overlap the "normal" ranges, this cannot be reliably done by assays based on factor levels. In addition, activity levels of homozygotes and heterozygotes may overlap. Other difficulties with factor assays, activity-based and antigenic, are that test results can be significantly influenced by many factors that do not affect molecular assays. These include external factors, such as exposure to hormones, drugs, and anticoagulation therapy. Increases in "acute-phase" proteins that occur during an inflammatory response can alter coagulation enzymes to levels outside reference ranges. Protein or activity assays are likely to continue to provide important phenotype information, however, and are not likely to be replaced by molecular assays for the foreseeable future.

PRACTICAL ISSUES IN MOLECULAR HEMOSTASIS TESTING

Pathology laboratories that perform molecular diagnostic testing for coagulation disorders are faced with the same practical and ethical issues that are encountered in other types of genetic testing.[26] Informed consent is typically required for all genetic testing. A recognized exception includes FVL testing; the American College of Medical Genetics (ACMG) recommends that formal informed consent not be required for FVL testing and that laboratories assume that informal consent was obtained.[21] Nevertheless, individuals who are tested for FVL should be informed that they are undergoing genetic testing and that the results may have implications for themselves and other family members. Confidentiality of test results is assured as for any diagnostic test becoming part of the patient's medical record.

In general, when genetic testing is performed, genetic counseling should be offered before and after the testing. Patients who undergo testing for inherited thrombophilia may be counseled by their physician or by a genetic counselor. In clinical practice, most patients undergoing thrombophilia evaluation receive this counseling from their physician. The ACMG has also developed recommendations for preparing informative laboratory reports. Key components of reports include comments regarding implications of the test result, the risk for the patient's relatives, and, if indicated, recommendations for further testing for other inherited hypercoagulabilities.[27]

Whereas hemophilia is usually diagnosed in childhood, the most common types of thrombophilia (those associated with FVL and PT mutations) manifest mainly in adults. Requests for testing minors for these mutations are uncommon. Generally, screening asymptomatic children and adolescents for adult-onset diseases is not recommended, unless the benefits of testing outweigh any possible harm.[28] It is difficult to justify testing a child for FVL or PT mutations unless the child has a clinical thrombotic disorder.[29]

Some individuals diagnosed with genetic disorders remain concerned over losing medical insurance or facing workplace discrimination. These concerns, which also exist for thrombophilia testing, are being addressed by the Genetic Information Nondiscrimination Act (GINA) enacted in 2008.[30] The GINA prohibits health insurers from requiring genetic information about individuals or family members, requesting genetic testing, or using genetic test information to make enrollment or coverage decisions. Genetic information cannot be used to establish a "preexisting condition." Likewise, employers may not request genetic information about an individual or family member or use such genetic information in making decisions regarding hiring, promotion, compensation, or termination. Only companies with 15 or more employees must adhere to these regulations, however, and the GINA does not apply to individuals in the US military.

PHARMACOGENOMICS IN TREATING THROMBOSIS: MOLECULAR TESTING FOR "PERSONALIZED" COUMADIN DOSING

One purpose of "personalized medicine" is to identify genetic differences that affect the metabolism or action of a drug. Ideally, these differences would be detected before prescribing a medication, allowing drug doses to be tailored to an individual's genetic composition. One such example is using cytochrome P450 (2C9) and vitamin K epoxide reductase (VKORC1) genotyping to select a warfarin dose. Warfarin has a narrow therapeutic range, and adverse drug reactions are common.[31] Drug requirements may differ by more than a factor of 10 among individuals, and the international normalized ratio (INR) of patients treated with warfarin is outside of target ranges approximately one third of the time.[32] Many other factors, including concurrent medications and dietary changes, may alter a patient's response to warfarin.

A major goal of genotyping patients before initiating warfarin treatment is to individualize dosing so that a therapeutic INR is rapidly achieved while minimizing bleeding risk from over-anticoagulation or thrombotic risk from undercoagulation. Two major genes that affect warfarin activity have been implicated in warfarin sensitivity: cytochrome P4502C9 (CYP2C9) and vitamin K epoxide reductase complex 1 (VKORC1).[33] The VKORC1 gene located on chromosome 16 produces an enzyme, VKOR, that reduces vitamin K 2,3-epoxide to an enzymatically activated form required for the posttranslational modification of vitamin K-dependent coagulation factors. Warfarin decreases VKOR activity. Polymorphisms of the VKORC1 gene result in warfarin sensitivity. These variations occur as a "haplotype block" (ie, a sequential set of genetic markers for which there is no evidence of historical recombination in the population).[34] The promoter polymorphism (−1639G>A), and the exonic polymorphism 1173C>T have been associated with reduced expression of the VKOR enzyme. Because these polymorphisms belong to the same haplotype, they can be targeted interchangeably during analysis. The contribution of the VKORC1 genotype to the variability of warfarin dose requirement has been estimated to be between 15% and 30%.[35] There is further variation among various ethnic groups. Although few African Americans are homozygous carriers of the VKORC1 mutant AA genotype, approximately 80% of Chinese are of the warfarin-sensitive AA genotype.

The CYP2C9 gene codes for an enzyme that metabolizes the more potent S-isomer of warfarin, in addition to several other drugs in the liver and kidney. Polymorphisms of the CYP2C9 gene are associated with reduced enzymatic activity, which leads to significant reductions in drug metabolism.[36,37] This decreased enzymatic activity leads to reduced warfarin clearance; thus, lower warfarin doses are required to reach a therapeutic INR. In this setting, standard warfarin doses may result in an increased risk for bleeding when therapy is initiated.[38] The highly polymorphic CYP2C9 gene is located on chromosome 10. The most common allelic variants in Caucasian are CYP2C9*2 (430C>T) and CYP2C9*3 (1075A>C). These polymorphisms confer approximately 70% and 20% of the wild-type enzyme activity, respectively.

The CYP2C9 and VKORC1 polymorphisms can be detected using various laboratory-developed tests based on real-time PCR with melt or HRM curve analysis.[39] Commercially available platforms are also available to identify these polymorphisms associated with warfarin sensitivity, several of which have obtained FDA approval for clinical diagnostic testing.[40] These systems are extremely accurate for detecting the three most common genetic variants discussed previously. One of these platforms simultaneously detects six allelic variants of CYP2C9 and eight variants of VKORC1 genes (INFINITI; AutoGenomics). Another specifically targets the *2 and *3 alleles of the CYP2C9 gene and a single-point polymorphism (C>T 1173) of the VKORC1 gene (Verigene). Proficiency testing for pharmacogenomics (PGx)-based warfarin dosing is available through the College of American Pathologists.

The differences in the platforms are related to their base technology, which affects the time and technical expertise required to perform the assays. One of the newest technologies to receive FDA clearance uses electrochemical detection technology to detect nucleic acids on a microarray (eSensor XT-8; Osmetech, Pasadena, California). Isolated genomic DNA is amplified and treated with exonuclease to produce single-stranded target DNA, which is hybridized to oligonucleotide capture probes attached to gold electrodes on a printed circuit board. Soluble allele-specific signal probes then bind to the target sequence adjacent to the base of the capture probe, creating a complex between the capture probe, target, and signal probe. This process brings the ferrocene (an organometallic compound) labels associated with the 5′ end of the signal probe in close proximity to the electrode surface, where they are detected by alternating current voltammetry. The signal probes that are complimentary to the mutant and wild-type sequences carry ferrocene labels with different electrochemical potentials, allowing them to be distinguished from each other. Genotyping is determined by calculating the ratio of wild-type to mutant signals.

Several studies suggest that warfarin can be dosed more precisely when genotypic information is available. This includes a small number of prospective trials that associate genotype-specific dosing with decreased duration to achieve a target INR with fewer dose changes. A large randomized controlled trial did not observe a reduction in INRs outside the therapeutic range ("out-of-range INRs") when comparing standard and PGx-guided warfarin dosing.[41] PGx-guided dosing did provide smaller and fewer dosing changes.

Currently, clear guidelines for how warfarin dosing should be altered based on a patient's genotype are lacking. Pharmacogenetic "algorithms" have recently been developed and validated to help guide dosing based on major independent predictors of warfarin metabolism. These include the *VKORC1*, *CYP2C9*2*, and *CYP2C9*3* polymorphisms, in addition to patient age, body surface area, race, target INR, smoker status, and current thrombosis.[41–45] An algorithm supported by the Barnes-Jewish Hospital at Washington University Medical Center and the National Institutes of Health (NIH) is freely available.[46] Adding genetic data seems to help explain variation in warfarin response not predicted based on clinical parameters alone, even across racially diverse groups.[47,48] A recent international trial used mathematic models that were based on clinical factors alone or a combination of clinical and genetic factors to dose warfarin.[49] Although it was a retrospective study, stable warfarin doses were better predicted by the pharmacogenetic algorithm, which included clinical and genetic factors, as compared with clinical factors alone.

One obstacle for the widespread adoption of PGx testing for dosing warfarin is the difficulty in proving improvements in health outcomes or cost. Compared with the targeted therapies used in oncology, warfarin is a relatively inexpensive drug. Many clinicians who prescribe warfarin are not convinced that PGx testing can improve their ability to achieve warfarin therapeutic levels. This is despite the FDA requiring manufacturers of warfarin to explain that genetics can influence response to warfarin and that genetic testing may help to optimize warfarin dosing. These recent labeling requirements are based on the drug's narrow therapeutic concentration and high incidence of adverse bleeding events; however, PGx testing is not required or suggested by the FDA.[50] Furthermore, several professional societies, including the ACMG and Americal College of Chest Physicians (ACCP), do not currently recommend routine screening of patients before warfarin treatment.[51,52]

Variability in warfarin dose-response is not entirely explained, and other as yet unidentified factors play a role.[53] Most pharmacogenetic trials exclude individuals with coexisting morbidity or who are receiving other medications, factors that clearly affect drug metabolism. Algorithms used to dose warfarin may become more complex when patients are further stratified based on comorbid conditions and other genetic predisposition for clotting, such as FVL and PT gene mutations.[54] Large multicenter trials that are currently underway, including studies sponsored by the FDA, may better help to define the role of PGx in warfarin dosing.

HEMOPHILIA A

Hemophilia A (HA) is a well-characterized X-linked recessive bleeding disorder resulting from deficient or defective factor VIII (F8) protein. Clinical disease severity correlates with residual F8 activity, ranging from less than 1% for severe, 1% to 5% for moderate, and 5% to 40% (IU/dL) for mild HA. Most carriers of an HA mutation have F8 levels of greater than 35%; thus, they may not be detected by F8 activity assays that have wide reference ranges (~50%–150%). Only approximately 10% of female carriers have less than 30% F8 clotting activity and may bleed abnormally. These individuals may have Turner syndrome (45X) or, alternatively, skewed X-inactivation, in which the normal allele has been inactivated through random events to a higher extent than the mutated allele. Other rare causes of low F8 activity in women include (1) the presence of two mutated alleles resulting from mating of an affected man and a female carrier, (2) translocation between the X chromosome and an autosome involving a breakpoint within the F8 gene, and (3) uniparental disomy with both X chromosomes emanating from the parent who carries the mutated X chromosome.

The factor 8 gene encompasses approximately 186 kilobases (kb), is located on chromosome Xq28, and has 26 exons. More than 1200 mutations (missense, nonsense, splicing, and small or large deletions and insertions) have been documented in the F8 gene (see the article by Wagenman and colleagues, elsewhere in this issue). Polymorphisms of the F8 gene are also defined for use in linkage analysis as described elsewhere in this article.[55] Mutations are spread across the F8 gene, with some concentration to exon 14. The intron 22 inversion (int22) is the most prevalent factor 8 gene defect seen in severe HA, accounting for 40% to 45% of all mutations. This intron contains two genes: the 2-kb F8-associated gene A, which is transcribed in the opposite direction of F8, and the 2.5-kb F8-associated gene B, which is transcribed in the same direction as F8. The function, if any, of these genes remains unclear. Furthermore, the F8-associated gene A is replicated in two other locations on the X-chromosome external to the F8 gene (INT22H2 and INT22H3). The F8-associated gene A sequences have the potential to interact through homologous recombination to create a gene rearrangement, the int22 inversion mutation, which places exons 1 to 22 of the F8 gene approximately 500 kb upstream of exons 23 to 26 and oriented in the opposite direction.[56,57] Because of gene disruption, patients with int22 inversions demonstrate severe HA. The recombinatory events leading to int22 inversions occur mostly during male meiosis (spermatogenesis). A female conceptus that receives the mutated X chromosome carries the trait to her offspring, meaning the mother of a male child with an int22 inversion is almost invariably a carrier of the mutation.[58]

An inversion involving exon 1 is present in approximately 5% of patients who have severe HA.[59] Almost 200 smaller deletions have been characterized, most of which produce reading frame shifts, and thus nonfunctional gene products. Large deletions constitute approximately 15% of HA.[55] The resulting phenotype ranges from moderate to severe depending on whether the deletions are located in the distal or proximal part of the gene and whether or not they cause in-frame splicing of remaining exons. Larger deletions result in truncated transcripts that are nonfunctional, poorly expressed, or rapidly inactivated. Patients who have severe HA caused by large deletions or nonsense mutations of the F8 gene also have a considerable risk (40%–60%) for developing F8 inhibitory antibodies.[60,61] Moreover, immune tolerance therapy used to eliminate these inhibitors is less successful in patients with large deletions.[62]

The diagnosis of HA is established by measuring plasma F8 clotting activity. Suboptimal handling of samples may result in some loss of F8 activity, such that repeat testing may be required to confirm mildly reduced factor activity. Furthermore, von Willebrand disease (vWD) type 2N must be excluded. A rare mutation in the *ERGIC-53* gene, which encodes a transport protein used by F5 and F8, may lead to a combined deficiency of these two factors, with F8 in the mildly deficient range.[63,64]

Occasionally, individuals with bleeding symptoms may have seemingly normal or near-normal F8 activity levels when measured by conventional one-stage clotting assays, whereas two-stage (chromogenic) clotting assays show deficient F8 activity. The mutation responsible for these "discrepant F8" results has been detailed in a family.[65] Other conditions, including pregnancy, oral contraceptive use, exercise, and inflammatory processes, may transiently elevate F8 activity. In such cases, molecular testing can be used to confirm the diagnosis of mild HA. Because F8 activity assays cannot determine HA carrier status, molecular testing is crucial for carrier testing. It is also used to identify family members with yet undiagnosed disease. To perform prenatal diagnostics, the family-specific mutation must have been previously identified. HA is not an absolute indication for cesarean section if the delivery is otherwise uncomplicated. Testing helps to avoid such procedures as circumcision and intramuscular injections and to initiate preventive treatment as soon as possible. Establishing mutation type (eg, inversion, deletion, nonsense) may also alter disease prognosis; for example, the risk for developing F8 inhibitors in response to factor replacement therapy correlates with mutation type, as previously discussed. Prepartum knowledge of a severe HA genotype in the fetus may also theoretically be used to allow for prophylaxis to decrease more intensive factor therapy, possibly decreasing the risk for inhibitor development. Preimplantation genetic diagnosis of HA may be performed at the cytogenetic level (selection of female embryos for transfer) or by molecular genetic testing for the family-specific mutation.

At least two laboratories in the United States perform full sequencing of the F8 gene. Two other laboratories perform targeted mutation analysis for int22 inversions, and one laboratory performs linkage analysis.[66] These laboratories also offer prenatal testing. An assay for the common intron 22 inversion is the most logical test to perform for patients with a severe HA phenotype. This mutation is usually tested for using restriction digestion followed by Southern blotting. Alternative methods to characterize mutations in HA include long-range PCR.[67] Using a blend of Taq polymerase and a proof-reading enzyme with 3' to 5' exonuclease activity, long DNA fragments (up to 10–20 kb), can be amplified with high efficiency and maximum fidelity. Other more esoteric methods, such as emulsion PCR, have been suggested for identifying int22 HA inversions.[68] In cases in which the results of int22 testing are negative, assays for the recurrent inversion in intron 1 and vWD type 2N (Normandy variant) should be considered. If the proband is not available for testing, an obligate carrier, such as the mother of a proband with int22 inversion, the mother of two sons who have HA, or a woman with one son and one other close relative with HA, may be tested.

The molecular diagnosis of HA in cases not caused by the common inversions is difficult because of the size of the F8 gene and the heterogeneity of the mutations spread across the gene. Full gene sequencing remains a labor-intensive and expensive technique. A database listing previously characterized mutations and polymorphisms in the F8 gene is available to use in conjunction with sequence data to diagnose HA.[55] In general, mutation databases should be used cautiously to classify gene variants, and the accuracy of references should be confirmed. Evaluating "novel" genetic variants that have not been previously reported in data repositories or the literature is challenging. In these cases, the bleeding propensity of the proband

and other affected family members must be weighed against the possible structural and functional changes in the F8 protein molecule.

In general, deletions, insertions, frameshift mutations, and mutations leading to premature stop codons alter protein expression, although mutations located close to the end of an expressed sequence may be less severe. Variants located in exons can be evaluated to determine if they result in an amino acid change. Mutations within exons that "conserve" amino acid sequences may still affect protein expression by causing base changes that affect putative regulatory regions within that exon. If the mutation results in an amino acid substitution, the significance of this change can be estimated to some extent based on the properties of the altered amino acid, whether it is localized in a region of the protein that is considered functional, and whether the amino acid is conserved among species.

Intronic mutations can be investigated using various algorithms or software tools that evaluate sequence changes with respect to assumed effects on splicing. Sequences beyond 20 to 50 bases from each exon are generally not evaluated unless a specific deep intronic variant is targeted. To determine the effects of a base change conclusively, expression studies must be performed; however, such studies are only undertaken in research laboratories.

To decrease assay costs, various screening techniques can be applied to determine which exons should be targeted for sequencing in a second step. Screening techniques for unknown variants include single-strand conformation polymorphism (SSCP) and denaturing high-pressure liquid chromatography (dHPLC). SSCP screening is based on the principle that under fixed assay conditions, a single-stranded DNA molecule assumes a specific secondary structure based on its sequence.[69] Under conditions of constant pH, ionic strength, and temperature, the mobility of a certain fragment in a gel depends on fragment length and conformation. This allows detection of mutations in amplicons based on deviations in migration speed during gel separation. Amplicons that migrate abnormally are then subjected to traditional Sanger sequencing to determine the exact location of the mutation. SSCP sensitivity decreases for amplicons larger than approximately 200 bp. To minimize the number of amplification reactions, larger amplicons can be subjected to restriction enzyme digestion. dHPLC separates DNA heteroduplexes (mutated DNA) from homoduplexes (wild type) on a liquid chromatography column in a partially denaturing environment. In the case of a male patient being tested for HA (ie, only one allele is present), the patient sample must be mixed with an equal amount of wild-type sample to produce heteroduplexes. Optimal fragment length is up to 500 bp for this technique.[70]

Large heterozygous deletions on the X chromosome cannot be detected in female patients through gene sequencing. This is because in the presence of a second wild-type allele, this normal allele is amplified and sequenced, and the sample seems to be homozygous wild type. In hemizygous male patients, a large deletion results in the absence of amplification of certain gene segments. If a deletion has already been characterized in the family, a molecular assay can be specifically designed to amplify across the breakpoints of the deletion. A newly developed method for dosage analysis, multiplex ligation-dependent probe amplification (MLPA, MRC-Holland),[71] may be used to detect larger deletions in male and female patients without any need for specific assay design.

In MLPA analysis, two hybridization probes are allowed to anneal side-by-side to the target sequence. The annealed probes are then ligated by a thermostable ligase and amplified. If the target sequence is not present, the corresponding probes will not anneal, and no ligation or amplification will take place. Because the probes contain consensus primer sites, as many as 45 ligated probe targets can be simultaneously amplified using the same primer pair. The probes also contain a stuffer sequence (DNA sequence of predefined length) that facilitates separation of the ligated amplified probe products by fragment analysis. The amount of probe amplification product from the patient sample is then compared with that from a reference sample group to determine the relative copy number, which indicates the presence of a duplication or deletion of the target sequence in the patient sample (**Fig. 3**). The MLPA technique for detection of copy number aberrations is presently available for several hundred different gene variants.

In rare cases, when extensive molecular testing cannot identify a mutation, linkage analysis may be used to trace the mutation through the pedigree. This method is also used in developing countries with limited access to advanced molecular testing.[62] In linkage analysis, several polymorphisms close to and within the F8 gene are analyzed in the affected individual and in both parents. "Informative" polymorphisms that differ between the maternally and paternally inherited chromosomes can then be used as indirect markers for the unknown mutation. The error rate of this method is minimal for cases in which intragenic polymorphisms are informative. When extragenic polymorphisms are used, however, error rates are higher because of the possibility of recombination events that lead to a separation between the polymorphic marker and the unknown mutation. Linkage analysis is considered a cumbersome technique that relies on access to accurate pedigree data and to samples from the proband and both parents. Furthermore, linkage analysis confers the risk for revealing nonpaternity, and genetic counseling should be offered before the analysis is undertaken. Currently, at least one laboratory in the United States performs linkage analysis for HA.[66]

Approximately one third of individuals who have HA are "simplex" cases, meaning that there is no known family history of hemophilia. These cases presumably result from de novo mutations in the proband or in the patient's mother. Alternatively, the mutation may have been carried through several generations of asymptomatic female carriers. Mutations may be somatic (occurs in any cell of the body except the germ cells) or germline (mutation in cell destined to become a germ cell or at the one-cell zygote stage), or they may represent so-called "germline mosaicism," in which some of the mother's germ cells harbor the mutation and some do not. Somatic mutations are not passed on to offspring and may or may not be detected in an individual's blood cells. Conversely, germline mutations are passed on to the offspring and should be detectable in the offspring's blood cells. In the case of germline mutation or germline mosaicism in the mother, the mutation would not be detectable in the mother's blood cells; this may complicate the assessment of pedigrees.

The first step in assessing the risk for HA in siblings of a proband is to determine whether the mother is a carrier. In most cases, this requires molecular methodology because F8 activity is likely to be within the reference range, as noted previously. If a mutation can be found in the mother's blood cells, one can conclude that she has a germline mutation that may be passed on to the offspring. Because the offspring can receive a mutated or nonmutated X-chromosome, the risk for her sons to manifest HA is 50% and the risk for her daughters to become carriers is likewise 50%. If a mutation cannot be found in the mother's blood cells, however, the risk is more difficult to determine. There is also a possibility that the mother is a germline mosaic for the mutation; in such a case, the mutation is present only in a subpopulation of her germ cells and is not detectable in blood samples. In this scenario, the risk for her offspring cannot be precisely quantified; however, it is much lower than 50%.[72] If a family-specific mutation is detected, all at-risk relatives should be tested

1. Denaturation and Hybridization

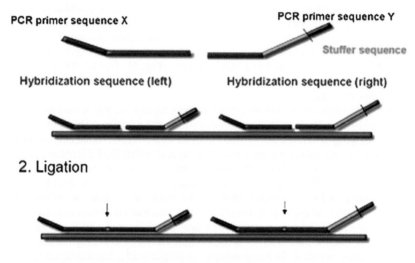

2. Ligation

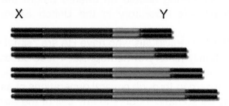

3. PCR with universal primers X and Y
exponential amplification of ligated probes only

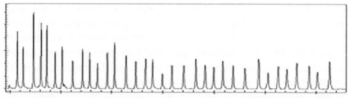

4. Fragment analysis

Fig. 3. Illustration of the principle for the MLPA technique. (1) The test sample is denatured, and two hybridization probes, one of which is a perfect match to the interrogated site, anneal side by side to the target sequence. (2) The annealed probes are then ligated by a thermostable ligase. If a mutation is present, the corresponding probe does not anneal and no ligation takes place. (3) Ligated probes (exclusively) amplify. A stuffer sequence confers different lengths to different probes, which facilitates separation of the ligated amplified probe products by fragment analysis (see text). (*Courtesy of* MRC Holland, Amsterdam, The Netherlands; with permission.)

for F8 activity (male relatives) or for the family-specific mutation (male and female relatives).

HEMOPHILIA B

Hemophilia B (HB) is an X-linked recessive bleeding disorder caused by a deficiency of coagulation factor IX (F9). The F9 gene is located on Xq27.1 to Xq27.2 and contains eight exons. The HB bleeding disorder is clinically indistinguishable from HA. A database encompassing known mutations in the F9 gene is also available.[73] Notable entries include several promoter mutations (HB Leyden 1, 2, 3) that are associated with a phenotype characterized by severe disease at birth and significant improvement or even normalization after puberty.[74,75] Several mutations that affect the alanine-10 locus confer an acquired hemophilia phenotype, specifically increased sensitivity to warfarin treatment as manifested by excessive bleeding despite a therapeutic INR, and are also associated with a disproportionately prolonged activated partial thromboplastin time.[76]

The diagnosis of HB is established by measuring plasma F9 activity. Vitamin K deficiency should be excluded in all mild or moderate cases of F9 deficiency. Similar to HA, molecular testing is required to identify carriers of F9 mutations who have normal F9 activity. Knowledge of mutation status does not directly affect clinical management but may help to predict risk for the development of inhibitors and anaphylactic reactions in response to F9 therapy.[77] A comprehensive listing of currently offered molecular laboratory testing for HB is available.[66] Approximately 25% of all patients diagnosed with HB carry one of three founder mutations (Gly60Ser, Ile397Thr, or Thr296Met), whereas the remainder of the mutations are distributed across the entire F9 gene. Therefore, an algorithm for F9 mutation testing may incorporate an initial test for these prevalent mutations. If a mutation is not identified, or if the patient has severe disease, the next step involves screening functional regions of the F9 gene. An MLPA assay is available to screen for large deletions.[71] At least two laboratories in the United States perform full gene sequencing analysis for the F9 gene.[66] One of these laboratories also performs prenatal diagnostics in cases in which the targeted mutation is known.

VON WILLEBRAND DISEASE

The most commonly diagnosed inherited bleeding disorder, vWD, is caused by a qualitative or quantitative abnormality of the von Willebrand factor (vWF), a multimeric glycoprotein that plays a critical role in primary hemostasis and serves as a protective carrier protein for F8. After binding to the platelet glycoprotein Ib receptor, vWF forms a bridge between the platelet surface and subendothelial collagen exposed by vascular injury. vWF consists of low, intermediate, and high molecular weight multimers; the higher weight multimers confer more efficient adhesion, whereas the lower weight multimers act as carriers for F8. Diagnosing inherited vWD and determining disease subtypes can be a complex process as described elsewhere (see the article by Torres and Fedoriw, elsewhere in this issue).[78] Molecular testing is not yet part of the standard investigation of this disorder but may help to establish a diagnosis of vWD in unusual cases. This information might help to optimize treatment and genetic counseling strategies and enable prenatal diagnosis.

The large vWF gene is located on the short arm of chromosome 12 (12p13.3). It spans approximately 180 kb and consists of 52 exons. A partial nonexpressed pseudogene corresponding to exons 23 to 34 present on Chr22q11.2 must be considered when designing assays for the vWF gene. Sequencing of the entire coding region is currently performed in only one US laboratory, whereas sequencing of select exons representing regions in which mutations are clustered is performed by several specialized laboratories. One molecular approach is to sequence exon 28 to target a diagnosis of type 2A, type 2B, or type 2M vWD specifically. Prenatal diagnosis is offered by at least one US laboratory, but as previously noted, such testing requires that a family-specific mutation has already been identified.

Type I vWD is the most prevalent form of vWD and is generally associated with a quantitative defect in structurally normal vWF. The disorder is inherited in an autosomal dominant manner and displays markedly variable penetrance and clinical heterogeneity that may complicate tracing the trait through affected pedigrees. The symptoms are usually mild, and patients may go unrecognized until they bleed excessively after trauma or surgery. Laboratory testing for type I vWD is complicated by the fact that numerous external factors, such as stress, infection, inflammation, exercise, pregnancy, estrogen therapy, surgical procedure, and liver disease, can increase vWF levels. Thus, low but still normal levels of ristocetin cofactor activity or vWF antigen may not exclude mild vWD.

Although type 1 vWD is mild and often straightforward to diagnose, molecular diagnostic approaches could be used to resolve difficult cases when plasma and platelet aggregation studies are inconclusive. Such testing, which requires freshly drawn blood, is performed in only a few reference laboratories. A database covering mutations and polymorphisms in the human vWF gene is maintained by researchers at the University of Sheffield.[79] In this database, approximately 120 different mutations are listed as associated with type 1 vWD. Most of these are missense mutations, but several splice site mutations, frameshift mutations, small deletions, and duplications are represented. No large deletions have been reported in type 1 vWD to date. The mutations are found in all parts of the gene, including the promoter region. One mutation (Y1584C, tyrosine to cysteine at amino acid 1584) has been seen in a somewhat larger proportion of type 1 vWD cases.[80,81] The mutations leading to type 1 vWD are not well characterized in terms of genotype-phenotype correlation. In addition, locus heterogeneity for type 1 vWD (involvement of genes other than the vWF gene) further complicates the interpretation of genetic testing. In summary, genetic testing for type 1 vWD would be desirable in borderline cases but is generally not yet feasible.

The five subtypes of type 2 vWD (2A, 2B, 2C, 2M, and 2N) all result from a primary qualitative abnormality of vWF. The two most prevalent subtypes, 2A and 2B, are inherited in an autosomal dominant fashion. Type 2A shows normal or slightly reduced plasma levels of vWF antigen and F8 but has a discordant decrease in ristocetin cofactor activity, together with a marked reduction in high and intermediate weight multimer complexes. More than 60 mutations have been described in type 2A vWD. Most of these are missense mutations, and approximately 80% of the identified mutations are found in exon 28. Frequently reported mutations in exon 28 include 4517C>T, 4789C>T, and 4790G>A.[79] At the protein level, these mutations affect the A2 domain of vWF. No large deletions have yet been reported in association with type 2A vWD.

Type 2B patients have qualitatively abnormal vWF with an increased affinity for the platelet glycoprotein Ib, which leads to rapid clearance of platelet or multimer complexes and thrombocytopenia. During routine vWD testing, a mild quantitative defect in vWF, with a discordant reduction in ristocetin cofactor activity, and loss of high and intermediate multimers is seen along with an exaggerated response to ristocetin in platelet aggregation studies. Because platelet counts may vary over time in individuals who have type 2B vWD, platelet aggregation studies are required to distinguish these patients from those who have type 2A vWD. All the approximately 25 mutations currently associated with type 2B are located in exon 28. Frequently reported mutations include 3916C>T, 3922C>T, 3946G>A, and 4022G>A. These dominant gain-of-function mutations are located in the Gp1b-binding site in the A1 domain of the protein. It has been suggested that these mutations inactivate specific ligand binding sites or disrupt regulation of vWF binding to platelets.[82] It is important to distinguish type 2B from 2A vWD because their clinical management differs. In fact, administration of DDAVP (desmopressin acetate) may lead to severe thrombocytopenia in type 2B, and is therefore relatively contraindicated. Because most mutations in types 2A and 2B are clustered in exon 28 of the vWD gene, sequencing studies may be specifically targeted to this exon. Genotype-phenotype correlation is not always possible, however, because many loci have not yet been characterized at a functional level.

Type 2M vWD shows decreased ristocetin cofactor activity, whereas the vWF antigen and level of F8 activity are normal. Multimeric studies are typically normal except for the occasional case of ultrahigh molecular weight multimers occurring in a rare subtype of 2M.[83] More than 20 mutations are associated with type 2M, and more than 80% of these are located in exon 28. At the protein level, these mutations are found in the A domain and lead to decreased affinity for GP1b.

Type 2N vWD (Normandy variant) is inherited in an autosomal recessive manner. It is characterized by a shortened half-life of F8. Approximately 30 different mutations have been associated with type 2N, and 40% of these are located in exon 18. Mutations reported multiple times in the data repository include 2372C>T in exon 18, 2446C>T in exon 19, and 2561G>A in exon 20. Other mutations have been demonstrated in exons 24 to 25. At the protein level, this corresponds to deficiencies in the D'-D3 region of vWF, which represents the F8 binding domain. The second mutation seen in type 2N vWD is either another F8 binding region mutation or a null mutation.[62] Although patients may show reduced ristocetin cofactor activity, some individuals show only isolated and markedly reduced F8 activity. In the past, some patients who had type 2N vWD may have been misdiagnosed as having mild HA. It is important to distinguish type 2N vWD from HA because the former does not respond optimally to treatment with pure (ie, recombinant or highly purified plasma-derived) F8 concentrates. Type 2N vWD responds to concentrates with significant amounts of normal vWF (eg, Humate-P). The distinction is also essential for genetic counseling because, as opposed to HA, type 2N vWD is inherited as an autosomal recessive trait. The diagnosis should be considered in patients who have apparent mild HA and a pedigree inconsistent with X-linked recessive inheritance and when mutations cannot be found in the F8 gene. Initial sequencing analysis should focus on exons 18 to 20, followed by studies on exons 23 to 24.

The rare type 3 vWD variant is inherited in an autosomal recessive fashion. Most affected individuals are compound heterozygotes, but homozygous individuals have been identified in consanguineous pedigrees. Patients who have type 3 vWD show a virtual absence of vWF and severely reduced F8 levels. More than 90 different mutations associated with type 3 vWD have been reported, with most of these representing null (nonexpressed) alleles. The mutations are spread over the vWF gene with some concentration to exon 28. Currently, 11 entries in the vWD database represent large deletions.[79] The diagnosis of type 3 vWD does not, per se, require analysis at the molecular level. Because this variant can lead to potentially life-threatening bleeding, however, it is important to identify other at-risk family members. If a mutation can be identified, this locus can be targeted specifically in testing of at-risk family members, potential carriers, or a fetus. In patients who have type 3 vWD, several large deletions that are associated with an increased potential for developing vWF autoantibodies, the presence of which complicates treatment using vWF concentrates, have been identi-fied. Southern blotting can be used to detect large deletions; however, such analyses are currently only performed on a research basis. Linkage analysis may be indicated in type 3 vWD, but these studies are currently offered by only one US laboratory.[66]

GENOMICS AND PROTEOMICS IN HEMOSTASIS

The information gleaned from the Human Genome Project has not yet translated into a better understanding of the hemostatic system at the molecular level. Presumably, a detailed human genetic map would facilitate discovery of new genetic markers of bleeding and thrombophilia. Such knowledge could then be used more precisely to estimate hemostatic risk and to refine treatment of coagulation disorders.[84] Mutations in regions that are not routinely assessed, such as deep intronic portions of genes, or mutations currently considered "benign" because they do not result in amino acid substitution could, in fact, have phenotypic effects by enhancing or suppressing expression of other genes. DNA microarrays, used to determine gene expression profiles in many human diseases, have not been widely applied to blood hemostasis testing. One exception is the use of cDNA and oligonucleotide microarrays to study blood platelets. Platelets are well suited to certain genomic techniques because they lack nuclear DNA and contain fewer mRNA transcripts than other cells. These transcripts are presumably derived from precursor megakaryocytes. A challenging aspect of studying platelets with microarrays is removing white blood cells and retic-ulocytes that contain large amounts of RNA. Despite technical difficulties, the platelet "transcriptome" (all mRNAs in a platelet) has been cataloged using traditional micro-arrays, serial analysis of gene expression, and multiplexed PCR.[85–87] Interestingly, the gene expression patterns of normal platelets as determined by different groups agree reasonably well. Gene profiling experiments have been marginally successful in iden-tifying genes that are differentially expressed in platelet disorders, such as essential thrombocythemia.[88] Information obtained from microarray studies can provide clues that may help to clarify the pathogenesis of platelet disorders. Other common diseases in which hemostasis plays an important role, including myocardial infarction and stroke, are being studied more frequently by transcriptome profiling.[89,90]

The use of expression microarrays in clinical and experimental settings has been limited for several reasons. These include the requirements for relatively large amounts of high-quality RNA and the limitation that only genes that are prefabricated on the microarray are interrogated. More importantly, there are complex relations between genes and proteins that cannot be delineated through genomic information alone. For these reasons, investigators are turning toward "proteomic" techniques to study the ultimate products of DNA and mRNA, namely, proteins. As described previously for platelet genomics, the platelet proteome (all proteins comprising a platelet) has been cataloged using a variety of techniques, including two-dimensional electropho-resis, multidimensional protein identification technology, and other forms of mass spectrometry.[91,92] Other groups have studied proteins that are released from acti-vated platelets and the composition of platelet microparticles, which retain their hemostatic ability and participate in coagulation reactions.[93,94] Even with comprehen-sive genomic and proteomic data, it may be difficult to relate mRNA and protein levels to a phenotype associated with hemostatic disruption.

FUTURE OF GENETIC TESTING IN HEMOSTASIS

As knowledge of the human genome expands, layers of complexity beyond DNA and RNA sequences may be defined to the point at which analysis is useful in a clinical context. Epigenetic factors (changes in the genome that do not involve alterations in the DNA sequence, per se [eg, methylation of bases, modifications of proteins associated with the DNA]) and expression of microRNAs (short single-stranded regulatory RNA molecules) may prove useful in thrombophilia diagnostics. Furthermore, mutations in DNA regions presently not routinely assessed, such as deep intronic parts of genes or "silent" exonic mutations (mutations that do not result in amino acid substitution), may be shown to affect gene regulation and play a role maintaining balance in the hemostatic system.

As rapidly evolving molecular technology is applied to hemostatic diseases and the results of larger epidemiologic studies and meta-analysis become available, the effect of currently recognized risk factors may be better defined, suspected risk factors for thrombosis may be confirmed, and novel candidate risk factors for bleeding or thrombotic disorders may be identified. For example, mutations within genes that increase the expression of proteins that can enhance clot formation, such as tissue factor pathway inhibitor, may be clinically relevant in certain patient groups.[95] A better understanding of the genotype and phenotype correlations could also help to guide personalized recommendations for anticoagulant therapy dosing as previously discussed for Coumadin. One emerging example is identifying functional variants of genes coding for cytochrome P450 isoenzymes involved in clopidogrel metabolism. These polymorphisms (eg, CYP2C19*2, CYP2B6*5, CYP1A2*1F, CYP3A5*3) seem to influence platelet responsiveness to clopidogrel and may partially explain individual differences in response to this widely used drug.[96,97]

A primary goal of molecular hemostatic testing is to establish the total "current" risk for thrombosis for an individual. Thrombophilia is a multifactorial disease, however, and overall risk for clotting is influenced by genetic makeup and external risk factors, such as age and immobilization. Therefore, as in most other diseases, the presence of a molecular marker does not by itself predict future disease. This uncertainty is likely to drive the development not only toward the creation and application of refined molecular instruments, such as specifically designed microarrays or "next-generation sequencing," but of complex algorithms that include evaluation of extrinsic risk factors and molecular test results.

REFERENCES

1. Dahlback B. Advances in understanding pathogenic mechanisms of thrombophilic disorders. Blood 2008;112(1):19–27.
2. Bock SC, Wion KL, Vehar GA, et al. Cloning and expression of the cDNA for human antithrombin III. Nucleic Acids Res 1982;10(24):8113–25.
3. Beckmann RJ, Schmidt RJ, Santerre RF, et al. The structure and evolution of a 461 amino acid human protein C precursor and its messenger RNA, based upon the DNA sequence of cloned human liver cDNAs. Nucleic Acids Res 1985;13(14): 5233–47.
4. Lundwall A, Dackowski W, Cohen E, et al. Isolation and sequence of the cDNA for human protein S, a regulator of blood coagulation. Proc Natl Acad Sci U S A 1986; 83(18):6716–20.
5. Bertina RM, Ploos van Amstel HK, van Wijngaarden A, et al. Heerlen polymorphism of protein S, an immunologic polymorphism due to dimorphism of residue 460. Blood 1990;76(3):538–48.
6. Giri TK, Yamazaki T, Sala N, et al. Deficient APC-cofactor activity of protein S Heerlen in degradation of factor Va Leiden: a possible mechanism of synergism between thrombophilic risk factors. Blood 2000;96(2):523–31.

7. Gehring NH, Frede U, Neu-Yilik G, et al. Increased efficiency of mRNA 3' end formation: a new genetic mechanism contributing to hereditary thrombophilia. Nat Genet 2001;28(4):389–92.

8. Ozelo MC, Annichino-Bizzacchi JM, Pollak ES, et al. Rapid detection of the prothrombin C20209T variant by differential sensitivity to restriction endonuclease digestion. J Thromb Haemost 2003;1(12):2683–5.

9. Clench T, Standen GR, Ryan E, et al. Rapid detection of the prothrombin C20209T transition by Light Cycler analysis. Thromb Haemost 2005;94(5):1114–5.

10. Dahlback B, Carlsson M, Svensson PJ. Familial thrombophilia due to a previously unrecognized mechanism characterized by poor anticoagulant response to activated protein C: prediction of a cofactor to activated protein C. Proc Natl Acad Sci U S A 1993;90(3):1004–8.

11. Bertina RM, Koeleman BP, Koster T, et al. Mutation in blood coagulation factor V associated with resistance to activated protein C. Nature 1994;369(6475):64–7.

12. Association for Molecular Pathology. Available at: http://www.amp.org/. Accessed March 5, 2009.

13. Erali M, Voelkerding KV, Wittwer CT. High resolution melting applications for clinical laboratory medicine. Exp Mol Pathol 2008;85(1):50–8.

14. Margraf RL, Mao R, Highsmith WE, et al. Mutation scanning of the RET protooncogene using high-resolution melting analysis. Clin Chem 2006;52(1):138–41.

15. Chou LS, Meadows C, Wittwer CT, et al. Unlabeled oligonucleotide probes modified with locked nucleic acids for improved mismatch discrimination in genotyping by melting analysis. Biotechniques 2005;39(5):644, 646, 648 passim.

16. Margraf RL, Mao R, Wittwer CT. Masking selected sequence variation by incorporating mismatches into melting analysis probes. Hum Mutat 2006;27(3):269–78.

17. Herrmann MG, Durtschi JD, Wittwer CT, et al. Expanded instrument comparison of amplicon DNA melting analysis for mutation scanning and genotyping. Clin Chem 2007;53(8):1544–8.

18. Seipp MT, Durtschi JD, Liew MA, et al. Unlabeled oligonucleotides as internal temperature controls for genotyping by amplicon melting. J Mol Diagn 2007;9(3):284–9.

19. De Leeneer K, Coene I, Poppe B, et al. Rapid and sensitive detection of BRCA1/2 mutations in a diagnostic setting: comparison of two high-resolution melting platforms. Clin Chem 2008;54(6):982–9.

20. Lyon E. Discovering rare variants by use of melting temperature shifts seen in melting curve analysis. Clin Chem 2005;51(8):1331–2.

21. Grody WW, Griffin JH, Taylor AK, et al. American College of Medical Genetics consensus statement on factor V Leiden mutation testing. Genet Med 2001;3(2):139–48.

22. Van Cott EM, Laposata M, Prins MH. Laboratory evaluation of hypercoagulability with venous or arterial thrombosis. Arch Pathol Lab Med 2002;126(11):1281–95.

23. Jackson BR, Holmes K, Phansalkar A, et al. Testing for hereditary thrombophilia: a retrospective analysis of testing referred to a national laboratory. BMC Clin Pathol 2008;8:3.

24. Middeldorp S, van Hylckama Vlieg A. Does thrombophilia testing help in the clinical management of patients? Br J Haematol 2008;143(3):321–35.

25. Eroglu A, Ulu A, Cam R, et al. Prevalence of factor V 1691 G-A (Leiden) and prothrombin G20210A polymorphisms and the risk of venous thrombosis among cancer patients. J Thromb Thrombolysis 2007;23(1):31–4.

26. Bates BR, Templeton A, Achter PJ, et al. What does "a gene for heart disease" mean? A focus group study of public understandings of genetic risk factors. Am J Med Genet A 2003;119A(2):156–61.
27. American College of Medical Genetics. Available at: http://www.acmg.net/. Accessed March 6, 2009.
28. Points to consider: ethical, legal, and psychosocial implications of genetic testing in children and adolescents. American Society of Human Genetics Board of Directors, American College of Medical Genetics Board of Directors. Am J Hum Genet 1995;57(5):1233–41.
29. Albisetti M, Moeller A, Waldvogel K, et al. Congenital prothrombotic disorders in children with peripheral venous and arterial thromboses. Acta Haematol 2007; 117(3):149–55.
30. Asmonga D. Getting to know GINA. An overview of the genetic information nondiscrimination act. J AHIMA 2008;79(7):18, 20, 22.
31. Wadelius M, Pirmohamed M. Pharmacogenetics of warfarin: current status and future challenges. Pharmacogenomics J 2007;7(2):99–111.
32. Jones M, McEwan P, Morgan CL, et al. Evaluation of the pattern of treatment, level of anticoagulation control, and outcome of treatment with warfarin in patients with non-valvar atrial fibrillation: a record linkage study in a large British population. Heart 2005;91(4):472–7.
33. Wadelius M, Chen LY, Lindh JD, et al. The largest prospective warfarin-treated cohort supports genetic forecasting. Blood 2009;113(4):784–92.
34. Li T, Chang CY, Jin DY, et al. Identification of the gene for vitamin K epoxide reductase. Nature 2004;427(6974):541–4.
35. Hynicka LM, Cahoon WD Jr, Bukaveckas BL. Genetic testing for warfarin therapy initiation. Ann Pharmacother 2008;42(9):1298–303.
36. Geisen C, Watzka M, Sittinger K, et al. VKORC1 haplotypes and their impact on the inter-individual and inter-ethnical variability of oral anticoagulation. Thromb Haemost 2005;94(4):773–9.
37. Rieder MJ, Reiner AP, Gage BF, et al. Effect of VKORC1 haplotypes on transcriptional regulation and warfarin dose. N Engl J Med 2005;352(22):2285–93.
38. Aithal GP, Day CP, Kesteven PJ, et al. Association of polymorphisms in the cytochrome P450 CYP2C9 with warfarin dose requirement and risk of bleeding complications. Lancet 1999;353(9154):717–9.
39. Carlquist JF, McKinney JT, Nicholas ZP, et al. Rapid melting curve analysis for genetic variants that underlie inter-individual variability in stable warfarin dosing. J Thromb Thrombolysis 2008;26(1):1–7.
40. King CR, Porche-Sorbet RM, Gage BF, et al. Performance of commercial platforms for rapid genotyping of polymorphisms affecting warfarin dose. Am J Clin Pathol 2008;129(6):876–83.
41. Anderson JL, Horne BD, Stevens SM, et al. Randomized trial of genotype-guided versus standard warfarin dosing in patients initiating oral anticoagulation. Circulation 2007;116(22):2563–70.
42. Sconce EA, Khan TI, Wynne HA, et al. The impact of CYP2C9 and VKORC1 genetic polymorphism and patient characteristics upon warfarin dose requirements: proposal for a new dosing regimen. Blood 2005;106(7):2329–33.
43. Voora D, Eby C, Linder MW, et al. Prospective dosing of warfarin based on cytochrome P-450 2C9 genotype. Thromb Haemost 2005;93(4):700–5.
44. Hillman MA, Wilke RA, Yale SH, et al. A prospective, randomized pilot trial of model-based warfarin dose initiation using CYP2C9 genotype and clinical data. Clin Med Res 2005;3(3):137–45.

45. Gage BF, Eby C, Johnson JA, et al. Use of pharmacogenetic and clinical factors to predict the therapeutic dose of warfarin. Clin Pharmacol Ther 2008;84(3): 326–31.

46. Warfarindosing. Available at: http://www.warfarindosing.org/. Accessed March 5, 2009.

47. Wu AH, Wang P, Smith A, et al. Dosing algorithm for warfarin using CYP2C9 and VKORC1 genotyping from a multi-ethnic population: comparison with other equations. Pharmacogenomics 2008;9(2):169–78.

48. Limdi NA, Beasley TM, Crowley MR, et al. VKORC1 polymorphisms, haplotypes and haplotype groups on warfarin dose among African-Americans and European-Americans. Pharmacogenomics 2008;9(10):1445–58.

49. Klein TE, Altman RB, Eriksson N, et al. Estimation of the warfarin dose with clinical and pharmacogenetic data. N Engl J Med 2009;360(8):753–64.

50. FDA CDER. Available at: http://www.fda.gov/cder/. Accessed March 5, 2009.

51. Flockhart DA, O'Kane D, Williams MS, et al. Pharmacogenetic testing of CYP2C9 and VKORC1 alleles for warfarin. Genet Med 2008;10(2):139–50.

52. Hirsh J, Guyatt G, Albers GW, et al. Executive summary: American College of Chest Physicians evidence-based clinical practice guidelines (8th edition). Chest 2008;133(Suppl 6):71S–109S.

53. Sconce EA, Daly AK, Khan TI, et al. APOE genotype makes a small contribution to warfarin dose requirements. Pharmacogenet Genomics 2006;16(8):609–11.

54. Leung A, Huang CK, Muto R, et al. CYP2C9 and VKORC1 genetic polymorphism analysis might be necessary in patients with Factor V Leiden and prothrombin gene G2021A mutation(s). Diagn Mol Pathol 2007;16(3):184–6.

55. Haemophilia A mutation structure, test and resource site. Available at: http://europium.csc.mrc.ac.uk/. Accessed February 23, 2009.

56. Lakich D, Kazazian HH Jr, Antonarakis SE, et al. Inversions disrupting the factor VIII gene are a common cause of severe haemophilia A. Nat Genet 1993;5(3): 236–41.

57. Naylor J, Brinke A, Hassock S, et al. Characteristic mRNA abnormality found in half the patients with severe haemophilia A is due to large DNA inversions. Hum Mol Genet 1993;2(11):1773–8.

58. Rossiter JP, Young M, Kimberland ML, et al. Factor VIII gene inversions causing severe hemophilia A originate almost exclusively in male germ cells. Hum Mol Genet 1994;3(7):1035–9.

59. Bagnall RD, Waseem N, Green PM, et al. Recurrent inversion breaking intron 1 of the factor VIII gene is a frequent cause of severe hemophilia A. Blood 2002;99(1): 168–74.

60. Schwaab R, Brackmann HH, Meyer C, et al. Haemophilia A: mutation type determines risk of inhibitor formation. Thromb Haemost 1995;74(6):1402–6.

61. Gilles JG, Peerlinck K, Arnout J, et al. Restricted epitope specificity of anti-FVIII antibodies that appeared during a recent outbreak of inhibitors. Thromb Haemost 1997;77(5):938–43.

62. Peyvandi F, Jayandharan G, Chandy M, et al. Genetic diagnosis of haemophilia and other inherited bleeding disorders. Haemophilia 2006;12(Suppl 3):82–9.

63. Nichols WC, Seligsohn U, Zivelin A, et al. Mutations in the ER-Golgi intermediate compartment protein ERGIC-53 cause combined deficiency of coagulation factors V and VIII. Cell 1998;93(1):61–70.

64. Neerman-Arbez M, Johnson KM, Morris MA, et al. Molecular analysis of the ERGIC-53 gene in 35 families with combined factor V-factor VIII deficiency. Blood 1999;93(7):2253–60.

65. Lucia JF, Aguilar C, Dobon M, et al. Discrepant factor VIII activity in a family with mild haemophilia A and 531 mutation using various FVIII assays and APTT reagents. Haemophilia 2005;11(5):561–4.

66. GeneTests. Available at: http://www.genetests.org/. Accessed February 23, 2009.

67. Salviato R, Belvini D, Radossi P, et al. F8 gene mutation profile and ITT response in a cohort of Italian haemophilia A patients with inhibitors. Haemophilia 2007; 13(4):361–72.

68. Turner DJ, Shendure J, Porreca G, et al. Assaying chromosomal inversions by single-molecule haplotyping. Nat Methods 2006;3(6):439–45.

69. Orita M, Iwahana H, Kanazawa H, et al. Detection of polymorphisms of human DNA by gel electrophoresis as single-strand conformation polymorphisms. Proc Natl Acad Sci U S A 1989;86(8):2766–70.

70. Oldenburg J, Ivaskevicius V, Rost S, et al. Evaluation of DHPLC in the analysis of hemophilia A. J Biochem Biophys Methods 2001;47(1–2):39–51.

71. MRC Holland. Available at: http://www.mlpa.com/. Accessed February 23, 2009.

72. Leuer M, Oldenburg J, Lavergne JM, et al. Somatic mosaicism in hemophilia A: a fairly common event. Am J Hum Genet 2001;69(1):75–87.

73. Haemophilia B mutation. Available at: http://www.kcl.ac.uk/ip/petergreen/haem Bdatabase.html. Accessed February 23, 2009.

74. Veltkamp JJ, Meilof J, Remmelts HG, et al. Another genetic variant of haemophilia B: haemophilia B Leyden. Scand J Haematol 1970;7(2):82–90.

75. Reitsma PH, Mandalaki T, Kasper CK, et al. Two novel point mutations correlate with an altered developmental expression of blood coagulation factor IX (hemo-philia B Leyden phenotype). Blood 1989;73(3):743–6.

76. Oldenburg J, Quenzel EM, Harbrecht U, et al. Missense mutations at ALA-10 in the factor IX propeptide: an insignificant variant in normal life but a decisive cause of bleeding during oral anticoagulant therapy. Br J Haematol 1997;98(1): 240–4.

77. Thorland EC, Drost JB, Lusher JM, et al. Anaphylactic response to factor IX replacement therapy in haemophilia B patients: complete gene deletions confer the highest risk. Haemophilia 1999;5(2):101–5.

78. Sadler JE, Budde U, Eikenboom JC, et al. Update on the pathophysiology and classification of von Willebrand disease: a report of the Subcommittee on von Wil-lebrand Factor. J Thromb Haemost 2006;4(10):2103–14.

79. ISTH SSC VWF database. Available at: http://www.vwf.group.shef.ac.uk/. Accessed February 23, 2009.

80. James PD, Paterson AD, Notley C, et al. Genetic linkage and association analysis in type 1 von Willebrand disease: results from the Canadian type 1 VWD study. J Thromb Haemost 2006;4(4):783–92.

81. Eikenboom J, Van Marion V, Putter H, et al. Linkage analysis in families diagnosed with type 1 von Willebrand disease in the European study, molecular and clinical markers for the diagnosis and management of type 1 VWD. J Thromb Haemost 2006;4(4):774–82.

82. Sadler JE. Biochemistry and genetics of von Willebrand factor. Annu Rev Bio-chem 1998;67:395–424.

83. Rayes J, Hommais A, Legendre P, et al. Effect of von Willebrand disease type 2B and type 2M mutations on the susceptibility of von Willebrand factor to ADAMTS-13. J Thromb Haemost 2007;5(2):321–8.

84. Collins FS, McKusick VA. Implications of the Human Genome Project for medical science. JAMA 2001;285(5):540–4.

85. Gnatenko DV, Dunn JJ, McCorkle SR, et al. Transcript profiling of human platelets using microarray and serial analysis of gene expression. Blood 2003;101(6): 2285–93.
86. McRedmond JP, Park SD, Reilly DF, et al. Integration of proteomics and genomics in platelets: a profile of platelet proteins and platelet-specific genes. Mol Cell Proteomics 2004;3(2):133–44.
87. Rox JM, Bugert P, Muller J, et al. Gene expression analysis in platelets from a single donor: evaluation of a PCR-based amplification technique. Clin Chem 2004;50(12):2271–8.
88. Gnatenko DV, Cupit LD, Huang EC, et al. Platelets express steroidogenic 17beta-hydroxysteroid dehydrogenases. Distinct profiles predict the essential thrombocythemic phenotype. Thromb Haemost 2005;94(2):412–21.
89. Ma J, Liew CC. Gene profiling identifies secreted protein transcripts from peripheral blood cells in coronary artery disease. J Mol Cell Cardiol 2003;35(8):993–8.
90. Tang Y, Xu H, Du X, et al. Gene expression in blood changes rapidly in neutrophils and monocytes after ischemic stroke in humans: a microarray study. J Cereb Blood Flow Metab 2006;26(8):1089–102.
91. Maguire PB, Foy M, Fitzgerald DJ. Using proteomics to identify potential therapeutic targets in platelets. Biochem Soc Trans 2005;33(Pt 2):409–12.
92. Delahunty CM, Yates JR III. MudPIT: multidimensional protein identification technology. Biotechniques 2007;43(5):563, 565, 567 passim.
93. Coppinger JA, Cagney G, Toomey S, et al. Characterization of the proteins released from activated platelets leads to localization of novel platelet proteins in human atherosclerotic lesions. Blood 2004;103(6):2096–104.
94. Garcia A, Watson SP, Dwek RA, et al. Applying proteomics technology to platelet research. Mass Spectrom Rev 2005;24(6):918–30.
95. Lincz LF, Adams MJ, Scorgie FE, et al. Polymorphisms of the tissue factor pathway inhibitor gene are associated with venous thromboembolism in the antiphospholipid syndrome and carriers of factor V Leiden. Blood Coagul Fibrinolysis 2007;18(6):559–64.
96. Hulot JS, Bura A, Villard E, et al. Cytochrome P450 2C19 loss-of-function polymorphism is a major determinant of clopidogrel responsiveness in healthy subjects. Blood 2006;108(7):2244–7.
97. Geisler T, Schaeffeler E, Dippon J, et al. CYP2C19 and nongenetic factors predict poor responsiveness to clopidogrel loading dose after coronary stent implantation. Pharmacogenomics 2008;9(9):1251–9.

Global Hemostasis Testing Thromboelastography: Old Technology, New Applications

Alice Chen, MD, PhD[a,b], Jun Teruya, MD, DSc[c,d],*

KEYWORDS

- Thromboelastography • Review • Central laboratory
- Hemostasis • Whole blood assay

Thromboelastography (TEG) has been used for more than 60 years to assess primary and secondary hemostasis.[1,2] After the development of modern coagulation testing using plasma, such as prothrombin time (PT) and activated partial thromboplastin time (PTT), the utility of TEG became limited in clinical settings. With the increased frequency of complex surgeries such as liver transplants and cardiac bypass in the 1980s to early 1990s,[3–6] where a rapid assessment of global hemostatic function was needed, TEG, however, was revisited. Since then, numerous data have shown the utility of TEG in these settings for better management of bleeding, mainly by transfusion support. Although TEG tracing originally was plotted by ink and suffered from inconvenience, over the years there have been several technical improvements in the way TEG is performed that have improved its reliability, including computerized equipment, real-time view from remote computers, and automatic calculation of all TEG parameters. Currently, TEG is marketed by Haemonetics (Braintree, Massachusetts) in the United States. By contrast, thromboelastometry (ROTEM, Sysmex, Mioton Keynes, United Kingdom) is not widely used for clinical purposes in the United

[a] Molecular Laboratory, Blood Donor Center, Department of Pathology, St. Luke's Episcopal Hospital, 6720 Bertner Avenue, MC 4-265, Houston, TX 77030, USA
[b] Department of Pathology, Baylor College of Medicine, Houston, TX, USA
[c] Blood Bank and Coagulation, Texas Children's Hospital, 6620, Fannin Street, MC 1-2261, Houston, TX 77030, Texas, USA
[d] Division of Transfusion Medicine, Departments of Pathology, Pediatrics, and Medicine, Baylor College of Medicine, Houston, TX, USA
* Corresponding author. Blood Bank and Coagulation, Texas Children's Hospital, 6620 Fannin Street, MC 1-2261, Houston, TX 77030.
E-mail address: jteruya@bcm.edu (J. Teruya).

Clin Lab Med 29 (2009) 391–407
doi:10.1016/j.cll.2009.04.003
0272-2712/09/$ – see front matter labmed.theclinics.com

States as US Food and Drug Administration approval has not been granted. The difference between TEG and ROTEM has been reviewed elsewhere in detail.[7,8]

The TEG has been used primarily to manage transfusion therapy during surgery, with well-documented success.[9,10] This article focuses on the underdescribed utility of TEG when performed in central laboratories as part of nonurgent patient care. Because of the paucity of actual TEG patterns of various conditions in published literature, the authors' own experience was included in this article.

METHODOLOGY

The specimen type can be noncitrated or citrated whole blood. Citrated whole blood should be allowed to equilibrate at room temperature for 30 minutes, whereas the assay using noncitrated whole blood should be started within 4 to 6 minutes from draw, to avoid clot formation before testing. Calcium is added to TEG cup, and then the citrated specimen is added to initiate the coagulation process. The cup is raised, submerging a transducer pin. The cup moves 4.45° every 10 seconds, and as the specimen forms a clot, the pin moves with the cup. The movement of the pin is monitored electronically and translated into TEG tracing (**Fig. 1**). According to the manufacturer's guidelines, many parameters can be measured or calculated from the tracing. The normal ranges for each parameter may differ between arterial blood and venous blood samples.[11]

Measurements include:

Reaction time—the time in minutes from the start of a sample run until the first detectable levels of fibrin clot formation. Reaction time generally reflects coagulation factor levels, but does not always correlate with PT and PTT.

Angle—the size in degrees of the angle formed by the tangent line to TEG tracing measure at the reaction time. Angle reflects fibrinogen activity, but may not always correlate with direct measurements.

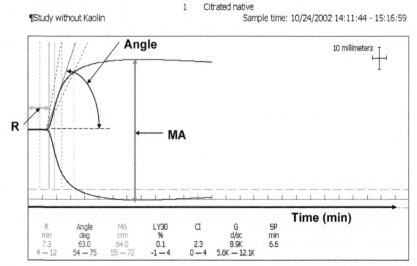

Fig. 1. Thromboelastography (TEG) profile parameters in normal TEG. *Abbreviations*: MA, maximum amplitude; R, reaction time.

Maximum amplitude (MA)—the width in millimeters of the widest gap in TEG tracing, reflecting the maximum strength of the final hemostatic plug. MA assesses the combination of platelet count and function plus fibrinogen activity, although it cannot be used to monitor antiplatelet therapy unless TEG platelet-mapping (Haemonetics) is employed. The clot firmness (G) is calculated by 5000 × MA/(100 − MA) and expressed in dyne per second.

When TEG assay is performed, kaolin or celite, as factor XII (FXII) activators, or tissue factor may be used in order to facilitate the clot formation. Tissue factor is used more widely for performing ROTEM in the European Union. If the specimen contains heparin, TEG assay is performed using a heparinase cup or with added prot-amine sulfate in the cup to remove the heparin effect, so that underlying coagulable states are assessed.

A major advantage of TEG is that it can be performed rapidly at the bedside as point-of-care-testing. A specimen is collected without citrate, and TEG assay is per-formed with or without an FXII activator. Because of the nonstandardized technique, TEG initially was limited to point-of-care-testing in environments such as emergency rooms or operating rooms for the urgent management of patients needing blood component therapy. Recently, however, TEG has been offered in central clinical labo-ratories in order to assess other contributors to hemostasis such as hyperfibrinolysis, factor XIII (FXIII) deficiency, and hypercoagulable states. Platelet function during anti-platelet therapy also may be monitored by TEG platelet mapping in central laborato-ries. If specimens may be potentially delivered by a pneumatic tube system to the central laboratory, the methods of specimen transportation should be validated by each institution, as vibration and shock may affect TEG results, especially platelet function.

THROMBOELASTOGRAPHY USING A FACTOR XII ACTIVATOR

When an FXII activator is used for TEG, the reaction time is shortened. When kaolin is used on a normal specimen, the only difference between the two tracings is the reac-tion time, with the shorter reaction time seen in TEG tracing with kaolin (**Fig. 2**). When the patient has a severe coagulation factor deficiency, however, there are substantial differences in TEG with and without kaolin. Without kaolin, TEG pattern is almost a flat

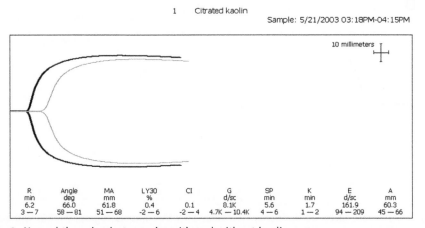

R min	Angle deg	MA mm	LY30 %	CI	G d/sc	SP min	K min	E d/sc	A mm
6.2	66.0	61.8	0.4	0.1	8.1K	5.6	1.7	161.9	60.3
3 — 7	58 — 81	51 — 68	-2 — 6	-2 — 4	4.7K — 10.4K	4 — 6	1 — 2	94 — 209	45 — 66

Fig. 2. Normal thromboelastography with and without kaolin.

line, with little clot formation recorded. When kaolin is used, however, TEG shows clot formation with a long reaction time and hyperfibrinolysis of some degree (**Fig. 3**). Drug effects on coagulation, such as with an antifibrinolytic or recombinant activated factor VII (Novoseven; Novo Nordisk, Princeton, New Jersey), were shown clearly by ROTEM with an added contact activator in a patient who had factor XI deficiency.[12] To predict bleeding after cardiac surgery, kaolin-activated TEG is more useful than nonkaolin-activated TEG.[13] The value of kaolin in other hemostatic settings is controversial, however. One study indicated poor correlation between nonkaolin-activated and kaolin-activated TEG,[14] whereas another report indicated better reproducibility with either kaolin-activated or tissue factor-activated TEG.[15]

UTILITY OF THROMBOELASTOGRAPHY FOR NEWBORNS

Because of the small specimen volume requirement, TEG often is utilized to assess hemostatic function for newborns. The reported normal range of reaction time in newborns is significantly shorter than adults and older children despite the fact that the PT and PTT are prolonged substantially for newborns compared with the adult reference range.[16–18] The reason for this difference has not been demonstrated

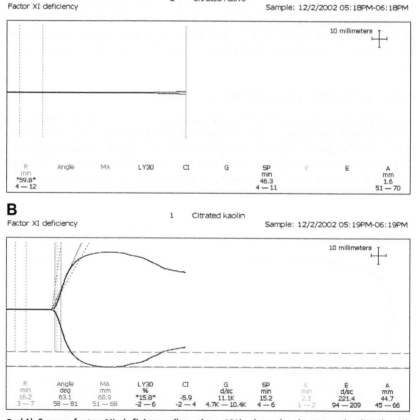

Fig. 3. (*A*) Severe factor XI deficiency (less than 1%); thromboelastography (TEG) without kaolin. (*B*) Severe factor XI deficiency (less than 1%); TEG with kaolin.

clearly. Because the specimen for TEG is whole blood, however, one reasonable hypothesis is that the cellular portion of red cells and platelets may be contributing to the shorter reaction time in newborns. **Fig. 4** depicts TEG of a normal newborn born at 39 weeks of gestation on the day of birth showing a low-normal reaction time. With its requirement for a small specimen volume and rapid testing, TEG may be useful for the early diagnosis and management of neonatal sepsis.[19] It also has been used to monitor the anticoagulant effect in neonates treated with extracorporeal membrane oxygenation (ECMO). Bleeding complications in patients on ECMO are especially common among newborns because of the prematurity of the coagulation system coupled with the use of unfractionated heparin as an anticoagulant. Because the individual PT, PTT, activated clotting time, and platelet count results either are overwhelmed by heparin effect or do not provide a global overview of the coagulation system, TEG showed significant value for managing bleeding complications.[20]

FACTOR XIII DEFICIENCY

Most laboratories use the 5 M urea solubility test or 1% monochloroacetic acid as a screening test for FXIII deficiency.[21,22] The sensitivity of the screening test is relatively low, however, detecting abnormalities only when FXIII activity is less than 5%, and the test is time-consuming, taking at least 24 hours.

The TEG pattern of FXIII deficiency, by contrast, shows a normal reaction time, low to low-normal maximal amplitude, and some degree of fibrinolysis (**Fig. 5**). Because results are available in 1 hour, TEG is more immediately useful than any screening tests. The TEG also can be used to monitor the therapeutic effect of FXIII replacement therapy.[23,24]

HYPERFIBRINOLYSIS

Tissue plasminogen activator, plasminogen activator inhibitor-1, alpha-2 antiplasmin, and thrombin-activatable fibrinolysis inhibitor may be measured individually to assess their particular contribution to fibrinolytic function. These tests are not routinely available in most hospitals, however, and there are no useful tests to detect overall hyperfibrinolysis. Euglobulin lysis time was used commonly in the past to detect hyperfibrinolysis, but fewer laboratories continue to perform this test, in part because of the nonautomated and time-consuming nature of the test. The TEG may be a good

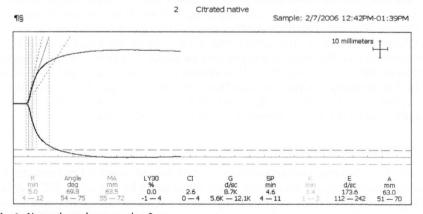

R min	Angle deg	MA mm	LY30 %	CI	G d/sc	SP min	K min	E d/sc	A mm
5.0	69.8	63.5	0.0	2.6	8.7K	4.6	1.4	173.6	63.0
4 — 12	54 — 75	55 — 72	-1 — 4	0 — 4	5.6K — 12.1K	4 — 11	1 — 3	112 — 242	51 — 70

Fig. 4. Normal newborn on day 0.

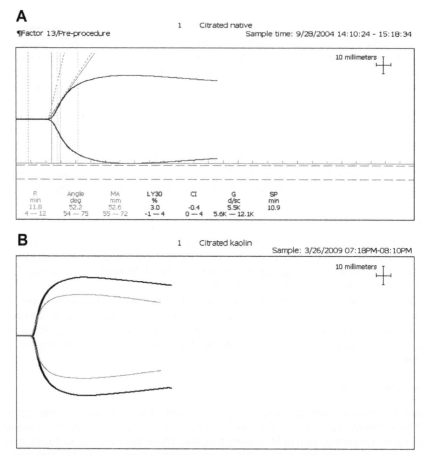

Fig. 5. (*A*) Mild factor XIII deficiency (13%). (*B*) Severe factor XIII deficiency (less than 3%) before and after transfusion of cryoprecipitate.

substitute laboratory test to detect hyperfibrinolysis. During liver transplant surgery, for example, patients have marked hyperfibrinolysis, seen on TEG as the combination of a normal reaction time, low to low-normal maximal amplitude, and some degree of fibrinolysis (**Fig. 6**A). **Fig. 6**B is another example of hyperfibrinolysis with a normal reaction time and angle in a patient who is on a ventricular assist device. When demonstrated by TEG, hyperfibrinolysis may be managed appropriately by administration of antifibrinolytic agents such as epsilon aminocaproic acid and tranexamic acid. The sensitivity for detecting hyperfibrinolysis and the degree of hyperfibrinolysis in relation to other markers for fibrinolysis are not known, however. In addition, TEG cannot detect a decrease in fibrinolytic activity, or hypofibrinolysis.

GLANZMANN'S THROMBASTHENIA

Glanzmann's thrombasthenia is characterized by either deficiency or functional abnormality of platelet glycoprotein IIb/IIIa, which is a receptor for fibrinogen. TEG may be utilized when a diagnosis of platelet dysfunction is suspected, and would show a normal reaction time, normal angle, and decreased maximum amplitude (**Fig. 7**).[25]

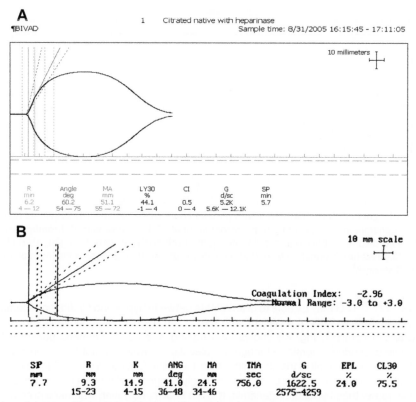

A

¶BIVAD

1   Citrated native with heparinase

Sample time: 8/31/2005 16:15:45 - 17:11:05

10 millimeters

R min	Angle deg	MA mm	LY30 %	CI	G d/sc	SP min
6.2	60.2	51.1	44.1	0.5	5.2K	5.7
4 — 12	54 — 75	55 — 72	-1 — 4	0 — 4	5.6K — 12.1K	

B

10 mm scale

Coagulation Index: -2.96
Normal Range: -3.0 to +3.0

SP mm	R mm	K mm	ANG deg	MA mm	TMA sec	G d/sc	EPL %	CL30 %
7.7	9.3	14.9	41.0	24.5	756.0	1622.5	24.0	75.5
	15-23	4-15	36-48	34-46		2575-4259		

Fig. 6. (*A*) Hyperfibrinolysis. (*B*) Hyperfibrinolysis during liver transplant surgery. Hemoglobin 7.6 g/dL, platelets 40,000/uL, prothrombin time 20.4 seconds, activated partial thromboplastin time 65.6 seconds, and fibrinogen activity 79 mg/dL.

In a Glanzmann's patient who presented with generalized purpura caused by platelet dysfunction, the PT, PTT, fibrinogen, thrombin time, and platelet count were all normal. The abnormal TEG pattern, however, suggested platelet function defects, and deficiency of glycoprotein IIb/IIIa was shown later, confirming Glanzmann's thrombasthenia. The TEG also has been used to monitor the therapeutic effect of recombinant activated factor VII (FVII) or platelet transfusion for patients who have Glanzmann's thrombasthenia, with a shortening of the reaction time or an increase in maximum amplitude, respectively, after treatment.[26,27]

HYPOFIBRINOGENEMIA AND DYSFIBRINOGENEMIA

The fibrinogen level is measured by the von Clauss method in an automated coagulation analyzer very easily. When the value is low, the diagnosis may be hypofibrinogenemia, but on occasion, the diagnosis may be dysfibrinogenemia. Although the reported incidence of congenital dysfibrinogenemia is low,[28] it may be under-recognized because of the lack of easy confirmatory tests. The recommended screening tests include a combination of fibrinogen activity and antigen or a combination of thrombin time and reptilase time.[29] Symptoms of dysfibrinogenemia are bleeding (20%), thrombosis (17%), bleeding plus thrombosis (20%), or poor wound healing. Approximately 50% of patients who have dysfibrinogenemia are asymptomatic,

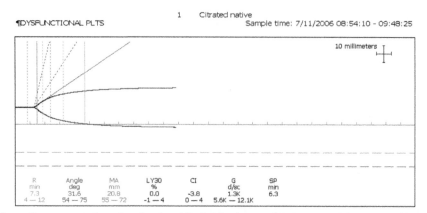

¶DYSFUNCTIONAL PLTS   Sample time: 7/11/2006 08:54:10 - 09:48:25

R min	Angle deg	MA mm	LY30 %	CI	G d/sc	SP min
7.3	31.6	20.8	0.0	-3.8	1.3K	6.3
4 — 12	54 — 75	55 — 72	-1 — 4	0 — 4	5.6K — 12.1K	

Fig. 7. Glanzmann's thrombasthenia with platelet count of 342,000/uL. (*A*) Suspected hypofibrinogenemia in a 3-year-old girl; prothrombin time 17.5 seconds, partial thromboplastin time 33.0 seconds, fibrinogen activity 96 mg/dL, fibrinogen antigen 77 mg/dL, thrombin time 28.3 seconds (normal 15.0 to 19.0 seconds), reptilase time 26.9 seconds (normal 13.5 to 19.5 seconds).

however.[30,31] TEG may be able to discriminate between hypo- and dysfibrinogenemia. As an illustration, TEG of a patient with suspected hypofibrinogenemia is shown in **Fig. 8A.** In contrast, **Fig. 8B** shows TEG tracing of an asymptomatic patient with possible dysfibrinogenemia. Although a molecular analysis has not been completed for this latter patient, all of the screening tests, including functional and antigenic fibrinogen, thrombin time, and reptilase time, strongly suggest a diagnosis of dysfibrinogenemia, rather than hypofibrinogenemia. It is not known, however, whether a normal or near-normal TEG in a patient who has dysfibrinogenemia predicts an absence of clinical bleeding.

HYPERCOAGULABLE STATES

If TEG parameters show an increased clot firmness, intuitively this may suggest a increase in thrombotic risk (**Fig. 9**). Although there are not a large number of prospective studies in the literature, some evidence suggests that TEG may yield information relevant to thrombotic risk. Increased maximum amplitude is considered to predict postoperative thrombotic complications.[32] Patients who had a history of venous or arterial thrombosis showed significantly shorter clotting times and an accelerated maximum velocity of clot propagation in ROTEM.[33]

DISSEMINATED INTRAVASCULAR COAGULATION

Disseminated intravascular coagulation (DIC) is characterized by continuous thrombin activation accompanied by a consumptive coagulopathy associated with predisposing conditions such as sepsis, malignancy, or obstetric complications.[34] The scoring system for the likelihood of the diagnosis of DIC published by the International Society on Thrombosis and Hemostasis includes the PT, fibrinogen, D-dimer, platelet count, and the presence of a predisposing condition.[35] To this scoring system, TEG may not add any additional utility in order to confirm the laboratory diagnosis of DIC. However, the effect of fibrin fragments on general hemostasis, and on the inhibition of thrombin and platelets may be monitored by TEG for appropriate management

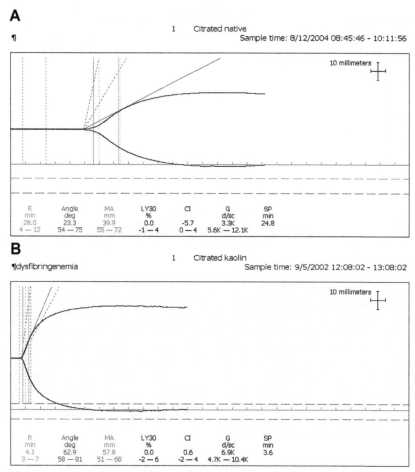

Fig. 8. (*A*) Suspected hypofibrinogenemia in a 3-year-old girl; prothrombin time 17.5 seconds, partial thromboplastin time 33.0 seconds, fibrinogen activity 96 mg/dL, fibrinogen antigen 77 mg/dL, thrombin time 28.3 seconds (normal 15.0 to 19.0 seconds), reptilase time 26.9 seconds (normal 13.5 to 19.5 seconds). (*B*) Suspected dysfibrinogenemia in a 6-year-old boy; fibrinogen activity 52 mg/dL, fibrinogen antigen 240 mg/dL, thrombin time 30.6 seconds (normal 15.0 to 19.0 seconds), reptilase time greater than 120.0 seconds (normal 14.8 to 20.4 seconds).

with blood component therapy. The case of **Fig. 10** shows how TEG can be used for transfusion support with plasma, cryoprecipitate, and platelets before invasive procedures in a patient who has DIC.

VON WILLEBRAND DISEASE

von Willebrand disease (vWD) is the most common hereditary bleeding disorder in the United States. It is postulated that as many as 1% to 2% of the population may have one form or another of vWD.[36] Type 1 vWD is characterized by a mild deficiency of von Willebrand factor; type 2 vWD is a qualitative deficiency of vWF, and type 3 vWD is complete absence of vWF. Interestingly, TEG does not show an abnormal pattern in

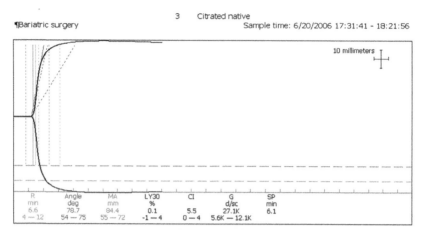

Fig. 9. Hypercoagulable state in a patient with morbid obesity before gastric bypass surgery.

vWD unless the factor VIII (FVIII) level is decreased substantially, mostly because vWF needs relatively high shear force to bind to the platelet glycoprotein Ib/V/IX complex, and TEG is a static assay. Thus, for most type 1 and type 2 vWD, TEG would not be diagnostic, because FVIII levels are relatively well-preserved. By contrast, **Fig. 11** shows TEG pattern of type 3 (severe) vWD. Because FVIII is severely decreased at 1% in this patient, TEG reaction time is prolonged. vWF antigen was 4%, and vWF activity was undetectable in this particular case. The angle and the maximum amplitude, however, were within normal limits. Therefore, TEG is not useful as a screening test for vWD, nor is it efficacious for monitoring the effect of replacement therapy with vWF or 1-Deamino-8-D-Arginine Vasopressin (DDAVP), unless FVIII levels are decreased significantly in severe vWD.

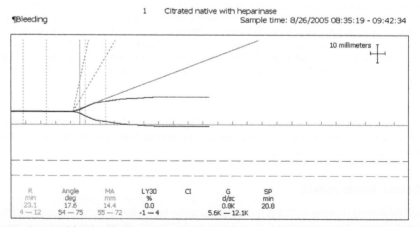

Fig. 10. 4-year-old girl with disseminated intravascular coagulation DIC associated with blue rubber bleb nevus syndrome. prothrombin time 19.0 seconds, activated partial thromboplastin time 47.2 seconds, fibrinogen activity 67 mg/dL, D-dimer greater than 4.00 µg/mL, platelet count 111,000/uL.

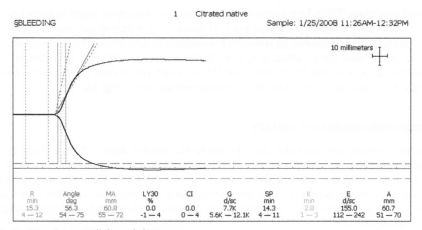

§BLEEDING

1   Citrated native

Sample: 1/25/2008 11:26AM-12:32PM

10 millimeters

R min 15.3 4 — 12	Angle deg 56.3 54 — 75	MA mm 60.8 55 — 72	LY30 % 0.0 -1 — 4	CI 0.0 0 — 4	G d/sc 7.7K 5.6K — 12.1K	SP min 14.3 4 — 11	K min 2.8 1 — 3	E d/sc 155.0 112 — 242	A mm 60.7 51 — 70

Fig. 11. Type 3 von Willebrand disease.

MONITORING RECOMBINANT ACTIVATED FVII

Recombinant activated FVII (rFVIIa) is indicated primarily for treating of hemophilia patients with inhibitors and for patients who have FVII deficiency. In addition, off-label use of FVIIa is common for treatment of patients with uncontrollable bleeding in the settings of trauma or severe liver disease (**Fig. 12**). There are no good laboratory methods for monitoring the efficacy of FVIIa or predicting effectiveness; certainly measuring the FVII level is not useful. The TEG, however, is considered to be a good test to predict the efficacy and risk of thrombotic complications of rFVIIa, because TEG tracing demonstrates not only the speed of clot formation, but also clot strength.[37,38] High clot strength may be predictive of restoration of hemostasis in bleeding patients.

POLYCYTHEMIA

In transgenic mice with an increased hematocrit level of 0.85 (85%), the angle and the maximum amplitude of TEG were decreased significantly using a noncitrated whole

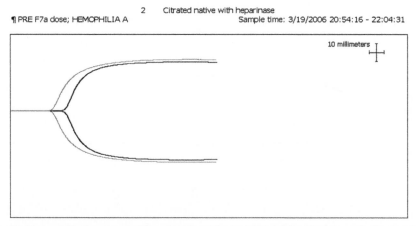

¶ PRE F7a dose; HEMOPHILIA A

2   Citrated native with heparinase

Sample time: 3/19/2006 20:54:16 - 22:04:31

10 millimeters

Fig. 12. Hemophilia A patient with a significant factor VIII inhibitor; before and after administration of recombinant activated factor VII.

blood specimen.[39] The high concentration of red cells was speculated to have interfered with the interactions of platelets and fibrin, thus affecting clot formation. The clot strength was recovered by reducing the hematocrit with reconstitution by plasma. Although citrated whole blood was used in the following instance, TEG pattern of a cardiac patient whose hematocrit was 73% showed similar findings of a decreased angle and maximum amplitude with a normal reaction time (**Fig. 13**).

MONITORING ANTIPLATELET THERAPY

Several methods are commercially available to monitor antiplatelet therapy. Each test has advantages and disadvantages. Although TEG can measure platelet function by maximum amplitude, it is not sensitive enough for dose adjustment of antiplatelet therapy. Recently, however, TEG platelet mapping has become available and has been used to monitor antiplatelet therapy in patients receiving aspirin, dipyridamole, or clopidogrel.

TEG platelet mapping uses four channels of TEG tracings: (1) kaolin-induced TEG, (2) activator F-induced TEG, (3) arachidonic acid (AA) plus activator F-induced TEG, and (4) adenosine diphosphate (ADP) plus activator F-induced TEG. Although the specimen for kaolin-induced TEG requires citrated whole blood, the other specimens require heparinized whole blood in order to suppress thrombin formation. Activator F consists of reptilase and activated FXIII (FXIIIa). Therefore, the maximum amplitude induced by activator F results from cross-linked fibrin only. Cup AA and cup ADP do not induce thrombin activation. The percentage of MA reduction is calculated using the following formula:

$$100 - [\text{MA of AA or ADP} - \text{MA of activator}]/$$
$$[\text{MA of kaolin} - \text{MA of activator}] \times 100$$

Representative tracings are shown in **Fig. 14**. TEG platelet mapping may prove to be a good laboratory candidate to monitor antiplatelet therapy because of its rapid results.[40] There remain questions to be answered regarding TEG platelet mapping for this indication, however. First, as with other tests to monitor antiplatelet therapy, the results are not always in agreement between assays.[41] Although a comparison of the

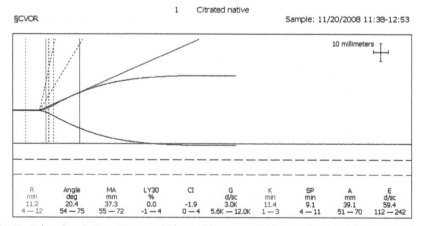

	R min	Angle deg	MA mm	LY30 %	CI	G d/sc	K min	SP min	A mm	E d/sc
	11.2	20.4	37.3	0.0	-1.9	3.0K	11.4	9.1	39.1	59.4
	4 — 12	54 — 75	55 — 72	-1 — 4	0 — 4	5.6K — 12.0K	1 — 3	4 — 11	51 — 70	112 — 242

Fig. 13. Polycythemia in a 17-year-old boy with congenital heart disease with hematocrit of 73%.

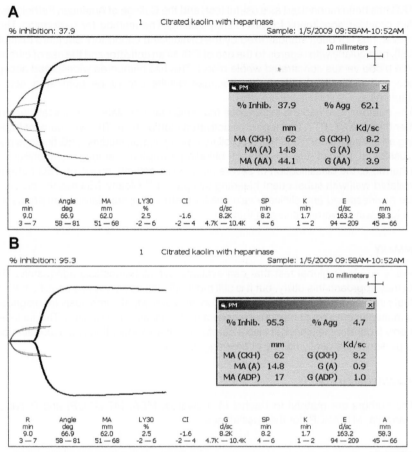

Fig. 14. (*A*) Thromboelastography (TEG) platelet mapping with arachidonic acid. (*B*) TEG platelet mapping with adenosine diphosphate.

results of each particular method is beyond the scope of this article (see the article by Tormey in this issue), platelet aggregometry using platelet-rich plasma has been used for many years and is considered the gold standard. Second, according to the company's instructions for TEG platelet mapping, the MA of the activator should be less than 20 mm. If the MA is greater than 20 mm, this is likely to be caused by increased thrombin formation due to either a low antithrombin level, high fibrinogen level, or an increase in circulating activated platelets. If antithrombin deficiency is present, p-pack, a thrombin inhibitor, should be used to suppress thrombin in the specimen. A comparable solution, however, is not yet evident when the MA is greater than 20 mm because of elevated fibrinogen or activated platelets. Whether this issue can be overcome to allow for routine platelet monitoring by TEG needs to be investigated.

OTHER ISSUES SURROUNDING THROMBOELASTOGRAPHY

One major issue that needs concerted investigation is whether TEG is more useful simply because it can be performed rapidly as a point-of-care test. In that situation, does TEG provide more or different information on hemostasis than the combination of the PT, PTT, fibrinogen, and platelets?

TEG has been recognized as a useful test, and the College of American Pathologists (CAP) provides specimens for proficiency testing. The method for performing TEG, however, has not been standardized by the Clinical and Laboratory Standard Institute (CLSI), particularly with regards to the use of FXII as an activator and the use of citrated whole blood versus noncitrated whole blood. This has hampered widespread acceptance and methods development, because results cannot be compared across institutions.

The authors have had the experience that TEG may correlate with clinical bleeding better than the PT, PTT, fibrinogen, or activated clotting time. This was demonstrated using an animal model[42] and has a corollary among human studies. TEG findings may be useful to predict the severity of bleeding symptoms among hemophiliacs.[43] Furthermore, the classification of severe hemophilia patients based on TEG patterns correlated well with subsequent bleeding symptoms.[44] Clearly TEG has the potential to be a widespread and clinically valuable laboratory tool; standardized methods will go a long way towards achieving that aim.

SUMMARY

There is no single global test that can evaluate overall hemostasis adequately. The TEG may approach this utility, but it is still most efficacious as one of a specific battery of tests in coagulation. The overall laboratory assessment of hemostasis for diagnosis and management should be done by collecting all pieces of information. This includes not only laboratory testing, but also a careful physical examination and ascertainment of a personal and family history of bleeding or thrombosis.

ACKNOWLEDGEMENTS

The authors are grateful to Rachel M. Edwards, MBA, MT (ASCP) and Purviben D. Jariwala, MT (ASCP) for their assistance.

REFERENCES

1. Hartert H. Blutgerninnungstudien mit der thromboelastographic, einen neven untersuchingsver fahren. Klin Wochenschr 1948;16:257–60 [German].
2. Howland WS, Castro EB, Fortner JB, et al. Hypercoagulability—thromboelastographic monitoring during extensive hepatic surgery. Arch Surg 1974;108:605–8.
3. Kang YC, Martin DJ, Marquez J, et al. Intraoperative changes in blood coagulation and thromboelastographic monitoring in liver transplantation. Anesth Analg 1985;64:888–96.
4. Spiess BD, Tuman KJ, McCarthy RJ, et al. Thromboelastography as an indicator of postcardiopuomonary bypass coagulopathies. J Clin Monit 1987;3(1):25–30.
5. Mallett SV, Cox DJ. Thromboelastography. Br J Anaesth 1992;69:307–13.
6. Tuman KJ, McCarthy RJ, Djuric M, et al. Evaluation of coagulation during cardiopuomonary bypass with a heparinase-modified thromboelastographic assay. J Cardiothorac Vasc Anesth 1994;8:144–9.
7. Luddington RJ. Thromboeastography/thromboelastometry. Clin Lab Haematol 2005;27:81–90.
8. Jackson GNB, Ashpole KJ, Yentis SM. The TEG vs the ROTEM thromboelastography/thromboelastometry systems. Anaesthesia 2009;64:212–5.

9. Depotis GJ, Joist JH, Goodnough LT. Monitoring of hemostasis in cardiac surgical patients: impact of point-of-care testing on blood loss and transfusion outcomes. Clin Chem 1997;43(9):1684–96.
10. Shore-Lesserson L, Manspeizer HE, DePerio M, et al. Thromboelastography-guided transfusion algorithm reduces transfusion in complex cardiac surgery. Anesth Analg 1999;88(2):312–9.
11. Frumento RJ, Hirsh AL, Parides MK, et al. Difference in arterial and venous thromboelastography paramteters: potential roles of shear stress and oxygen content. J Cardiothorac Vasc Anesth 2002;16(5):551–4.
12. Dirkmann D, Hanke AA, Gorlinger K, et al. Perioperative use of modified thromboelastography in factor XI deficiency: a helpful method to assess drug effects. Acta Anaesthesiol Scand 2007;51:640–3.
13. Welsby IJ, Jiao K, Orgel TL, et al. The kaolin-activated thromboelastograph predicts bleeding after cardiac surgery. J Cardiothorac Vasc Anesth 2006; 20(4):531–5.
14. Thalheimer U, Triantos CK, Samonakis DN, et al. A comparison of kaolin-activated versus nonkaolin-activated thromboelastography in native and citrated blood. Blood Coagul Fibrinolysis 2008;19(6):495–501.
15. Johansson PI, Bochsen L, Andersen S, et al. Investigation of the effect of kaolin and tissue factor-activated citrated whole blood, on clot-forming variables, as evaluated by thromboelastography. Transfusion 2008;48: 2377–83.
16. Kettner SC, Pollack A, Zimpfer M, et al. Heparinase-modified thromboelastography in term and preterm neonates. Anesth Analg 2004;98:1650–2.
17. Edwards RM, Naik-Mathuria B, Gay N, et al. Parameters of thromboelastography in the normal newborns. Am J Clin Pathol 2008;130:99–102.
18. Miller BE, Bailey JM, Mancuso TJ, et al. Functional maturity of the coagulation system in children: an evaluation using thromboelastography. Anesth Analg 1997;84(4):745–8.
19. Grant HW, Hadley GP. Prediction of neonatal sepsis by thromboelastography. Pediatr Surg Int 1997;12:289–92.
20. Zavadil DP, Stammers AH, Willett LD, et al. Hematological abnormalities in neonatal patients treated with extracorporeal membrane oxygenation (ECMO). J Extra Corpor Technol 1998;30(2):83–90.
21. Ikemori R, Gruhl M, Shrivastava S, et al. Solubility of fibrin clots in monochloroacetic acid. A reflection of serum pepsinogen levels. Am J Clin Pathol 1975;63(1): 49–56.
22. Miller J. Hemostasis and thrombosis. In: McPherson RA, Pincus MR, editors. Henry's clinical diagnosis and management by laboratory methods. 21st edition. Philadelphia: Saunders Elsevier; 2007. p. 742.
23. Nielse VG, Gurley WQ Jr, Burch TM. The impact of factor XIII on coagulation kinetics and clot strength determined by thromboelastography. Anesth Analg 2004;99:120–3.
24. Lovejoy AE, Reynolds TC, Visich JE, et al. Safety and pharmacokinetics of recombinant factor XIII-A2 administration in patients with congenital factor XIII deficiency. Blood 2006;108:57–62.
25. Macieira S, Rivard GE, Champagne J, et al. Glanzmann thrombasthenia in an Oldenbourg filly. Vet Clin Pathol 2007;36(2):204–8.
26. Male C, Koren D, Eichelberger B, et al. Monitoring survival and function of transfused platelets in Glanzmann thrombasthenia by flow cytometry and thrombelastography. Vox Sang 2006;91:174–7.

27. Lak M, Scharling B, Blemings A, et al. Evaluation of rFVIIa (NovoSeven) in Glanzmann patients with thromboelastogram. Haemophilia 2008;14: 103–10.

28. McDonagh J. Dysfibrinogenemia and other disorders of fibrinogen structure of function. In: Colman RW, Hirsh J, Marder VJ, et al. editors. hemostasis and thrombosis—basic principles and clinical practice. 4th edition. Philadelphia: Lippincott Williams & Wilkins; 2001. p. 855.

29. Cunningham MT, Brandt JT, Laposata M, et al. Laboratory diagnosis of dysfibrinogenemia. Arch Pathol Lab Med 2002;126(4):499–505.

30. Roberts HR, Escobar MA. Disorders of fibrinogen. In: Kitchens CS, Alving BM, Kessler CM, editors. Consultative hemostasis and thrombosis. 2nd edition. Saunders/Elsevier; 2007. p. 64–5.

31. Forman WB, Ratnoff OD, Boyer MH. An inheritied qualitative abnormality in plasma fibrinogen: fibrinogen Cleveland. J Lab Clin Med 1968;72: 455–72.

32. McCrath DJ, Cerboni E, Frumento, et al. Thromboelastography maximum amplitude predicts postoperative thrombotic complications including myocardial infarction. Anesth Analg 2005;100(6):1576–83.

33. Hvitfeldt Poulsen L, Christiansen K, Sorensen B, et al. Whole blood thromboelastographic coagulation profiles using minimal tissue factor activation can display hypercoagulation in thrombosis-prone patients. Scand J Clin Lab Invest 2006; 66(4):329–36.

34. LaBelle C, Kitchens CS. Disseminated intravascular coagulation. In: Kitchens CS, Alving BM, Kessler CM, editors. Consultative hemostasis and thrombosis. 2nd edition. Philadelphia: Saunders/Elsevier; 2007. p. 183–96.

35. Toh CH, Hoots WK. The scoring system of the Scientific and Standardization Committee on disseminated intravascular coagulation of the international society on thrombosis and haemostasis: a 5-year overview. J Thromb Haemost 2007;5: 604–6.

36. Nichols WL, Nultin MB, James AH, et al. von Willebrand disease (VWD): evidence-based diagnosis and management guidelines, the National Heart, Lung, and Blood Institute (NHLBI) expert panel report (USA). Haemophilia 2008;14:171–232.

37. Kawaguchi C, Takahashi Y, Hanesaka Y, et al. The in vitro analysis of the coagulation mechanism of activated factor VII using thromboelastogram. Thromb Haemost 2002;88:768–72.

38. Hendriks HG, Meijer K, de Wolf JT, et al. Effects of recombinant activated factor VII on coagulation measured by thromboelastography in liver transplantation. Blood Coagul Fibrinolysis 2002;13:309–13.

39. Shibata J, Hasegawa J, Siemens HJ, et al. Hemostasis and coagulation at a hematocrit level of 0.85: functional consequences of erythrocytosis. Blood 2003;101(11):4416–22.

40. Swallow RA, Agarwala RA, Dawkins KD, et al. Thromboelastography: potential bedside tool to assess the effects of antiplatelet therapy? Platelets 2006;17(6): 385–92.

41. Agarwal S, Coakely M, Reddy K, et al. Quantifying the effect of antiplatelet therapy. Anesthesiology 2006;105(4):676–83.

42. Martini WZ, Cortez DS, Dubick MA, et al. Thromboelastography is better than PT, aPTT, and activated clotting time in detecting clinically relevant clotteing abnormalities after hypothermia, hemorrhagic shock and resuscitation in pigs. J Trauma 2008;65(3):535–43.

43. Chitlur M, Warrier I, Rajpurkar M, et al. Thromboelastography in children with coagulation factor deficiencies. Br J Haematol 2008;142:250–6.
44. Ghosh K, Shetty S, Kulkarni B. Correlation of thromboelastographic patterns with clinical presentation and rationale for use of antifibrinolytics in severe haemophilia patients. Haemophilia 2007;13(6):734–9.

Index

Note: Page numbers of article titles are in **boldface** type.

A

Clin Lab Med 29 (2009) 409–420
doi:10.1016/S0272-2712(09)00079-1
0272-2712/09/$ – see front matter © 2009 Elsevier Inc. All rights reserved.

Moving?

Make sure your subscription moves with you!

To notify us of your new address, find your **Clinics Account Number** (located on your mailing label above your name), and contact customer service at:

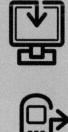

Email: journalscustomerservice-usa@elsevier.com

800-654-2452 (subscribers in the U.S. & Canada)
314-447-8871 (subscribers outside of the U.S. & Canada)

Fax number: 314-447-8029

Elsevier Health Sciences Division
Subscription Customer Service
3251 Riverport Lane
Maryland Heights, MO 63043